DISEASES of the ESOPHAGUS

CONTEMPORARY ISSUES in GASTROENTEROLOGY VOL. 1

SERIES EDITORS

Sidney Cohen, M.D.

Roger D. Soloway, M.D.

Forthcoming Volumes in the Series

DISEASES of the ESOPHAGUS

Edited by

Sidney Cohen, M.D.

Chief, Gastrointestinal Section
Department of Medicine
University of Pennsylvania School of Medicine
Philadelphia, Pennsylvania

and

Roger D. Soloway, M.D.

Associate Chief, Gastrointestinal Section
Department of Medicine
University of Pennsylvania School of Medicine
Philadelphia, Pennsylvania

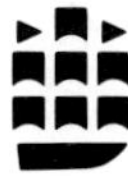

Churchill Livingstone
New York, Edinburgh, London, and Melbourne
1982

© Churchill Livingstone Inc. 1982

Distributed in the United Kingdom by Churchill Livingstone,
Robert Stevenson House, 1–3 Baxter's Place, Leith Walk,
Edinburgh EH1 3AF and associated companies, branches
and representatives throughout the world.

First published in 1982

Printed in U.S.A.

ISBN   0-443-08202-2

9 8 7 6 5 4 3 2 1

Library of Congress Cataloging in Publication Data

Main entry under title:

Diseases of the esophagus.

    (Contemporary issues in gastroenterology ; v. 1.)
    Includes bibliographies and index.
    1. Esophagus—Diseases. I. Cohen, Sidney, 1939–
II. Soloway, Roger D. III. Series: Contemporary issues
in gastroenterology ; 1. [DNLM: 1. Esophageal
diseases. W1 CO769MQR v.1./W1 250 D61103]
RC815.7.D57 1982   616.3′2   82-17681
ISBN 0-443-08202-2

Manufactured in the United States of America

Contributors

Jose Behar, M.D.
Associate Professor
Division of Gastroenterology
Brown University and Rhode Island Hospital
Providence, Rhode Island

John T. Boyle, M.D.
Assistant Professor
Department of Pediatrics
University of Pennsylvania School of Medicine
Assistant Physician
Department of Pediatric Gastroenterology and Nutrition
Children's Hospital of Philadelphia
Philadelphia, Pennsylvania

Douglas L. Brand, M.D.
Assistant Professor of Medicine
Head, Division of Gastroenterology-Hepatology
State University of New York
Stony Brook, New York
Chief, Gastroenterology Medical Service
Veterans Administration Medical Center
Northport, New York

Nicholas E. Diamant, M.D.
Associate Professor of Physiology and Associate Professor of Medicine
University of Toronto
Chief of Gastroenterology
Toronto Western Hospital
Toronto, Ontario, Canada

Harvey M. Friedman, M.D.
Associate Professor of Medicine
University of Pennsylvania School of Medicine
Philadelphia, Pennsylvania

Donald Gerhardt, M.D.
Assistant Professor of Medicine, Clinical Appointment
Gastroenterology Division
Department of Medicine
University of Missouri School of Medicine, and
Boone Clinic
Columbia, Missouri

Stephen J. Gluckman, M.D.
Assistant Clinical Professor of Medicine
University of Pennsylvania School of Medicine
Philadelphia, Pennsylvania

J. Hellemans, M.D., Agg. H.O.
Professor of Medicine
Head, Section of Geriatrics
Department of Medicine
University Hospitals of Leuven
Head, Remy Institute of Geriatrics
Leuven, Belgium

Richard H. Holloway, M.B., B.S., F.R.A.C.P.
Department of Medicine
Section of Gastroenterology
Yale University School of Medicine
New Haven, Connecticut, and
Veterans Administration Medical Center
West Haven, Connecticut

Igor Laufer, M.D.
Professor of Radiology
University of Pennsylvania School of Medicine
Chief, Gastrointestinal Radiology Section
Department of Radiology
Hospital of the University of Pennsylvania
Philadelphia, Pennsylvania

Marc S. Levine, M.D.
Assistant Professor of Radiology
University of Pennsylvania School of Medicine
Department of Radiology
Hospital of the University of Pennsylvania
Philadelphia, Pennsylvania

Alex G. Little, M.D.
Assistant Professor of Surgery
University of Chicago
Pritzker School of Medicine
Chicago, Illinois

Richard W. McCallum, M.D.
Associate Professor of Medicine
Department of Medicine
Section of Gastroenterology
Yale University School of Medicine
New Haven, Connecticut, and
Veterans Administration Medical Center
West Haven, Connecticut

Mark Mellow, M.D.
Assistant Professor of Medicine
Georgetown University School of Medicine
Chief, Intestinal Motility Unit
Veterans Administration Medical Center
Washington, D.C.

Ann Ouyang, M.D.
Assistant Professor of Medicine
University of Pennsylvania School of Medicine
Department of Medicine
Hospital of the University of Pennsylvania
Philadelphia, Pennsylvania

Konrad Schulze-Delrieu, F.R.C.P.(C)
Assistant Professor of Medicine
Division of Gastroenterology-Hepatology
University of Iowa
Iowa City, Iowa

David B. Skinner, M.D.
Dallas B. Phemister Professor, and
Chairman, Department of Surgery
University of Chicago, Pritzker School of Medicine
Chicago, Illinois

John Jones Thompson, M.D.
Assistant Professor of Pathology and Laboratory Medicine
University of Pennsylvania
Philadelphia, Pennsylvania

G. Vantrappen, M.D., Agg. H.O.
Professor of Medicine
Head, Department of Medicine and Division of Gastroenterology
University Hospitals of Leuven
Head, Laboratory of Gastrointestinal Pathophysiology
University of Leuven
Leuven, Belgium

Daniel Winship, M.D.
Professor of Medicine
University of Missouri School of Medicine
Gastroenterology Division
Department of Medicine
University of Missouri Medical Center, and
Harry S. Truman Memorial Veterans Hospital
Columbia, Missouri

Preface

The introduction of a new series of publications in a selected clinical sphere always raises the critical issue of whether further publication is needed. The broad area of gastroenterology and hepatology has shown rapid advancement during the past decade. From a field of clinical anecdotes and empiric therapy has emerged a highly complex science of diagnostic technology and therapy. It is our purpose to direct this series toward specific areas of this rapidly changing arena of activity. We will focus upon important topics of clinical interest to the specialist. Topics will be reviewed in depth. Controversial issues will be addressed.

Each volume will be oriented toward diseases in a specific organ or in a specific family of diseases. A multiauthor approach will encompass varied insights into a specific area. We expect to present timely issues, and to cover each topic thoroughly. At a time of rapid growth in knowledge, a series of this type can provide material that is not available in textbooks or in journals. The series will provide material in greater depth than is possible in a general text, and will synthesize data to a greater degree than can be done in a scientific journal. The series should thus interface with both of these already-available sources of medical information.

In a new publication, the editors always proceed with some caution and doubt. We hope that our readers feel free to offer their suggestions for future issues—contents or possible changes. The series can only be of value if it meets the ever-changing needs of its readers.

Sidney Cohen, M.D.
Roger D. Soloway, M.D.

Contents

1 | Normal Esophageal Physiology

Nicholas E. Diamant

INTRODUCTION

Normal esophageal motor activity consists of an orderly peristaltic contraction that passes through the esophageal body and terminates in closure of the lower esophageal sphincter (LES). The striated muscle upper esophageal sphincter (UES) and the smooth muscle LES are tonically closed, and they open in a precise coordinated fashion in concert with the body motor activity. This remarkable orchestration occurs in the face of marked in-species and between-species differences in the proportions of esophageal striated and smooth muscle.[1] Although in most species normal activity is programmed to proceed only in the aboral direction, in other species, such as the ruminants, there is coordinated peristalsis in both aboral and oral directions.[2] In those species where aboral progression is the rule, there is provision for those necessary retrograde activities—a belch and vomiting.

Radiological, manometric, and electrical recording techniques have provided accurate description of these motor phenomena in man. However, in man, detailed understanding of the control mechanisms responsible for the coordinated esophageal motor activity is limited, and little information is available for closely related species, such as the nonhuman primates. The bulk of data has been collected in species such as the cat, dog, sheep, and opossum. As a result, differences in species anatomy, physiology, and pharmacology, combined with differences in experimental technique have made it difficult to apply the animal observations to normal human esophageal physiology with confidence. This has been less of a problem for the striated muscle portion of the esophagus, where despite anatomical differences, the mechanisms of control are relatively limited and consistent. Control of the smooth muscle esophagus, including the LES, is, however, less well defined.

Several broad principles govern the control of motor function across species and at all levels of the gut including the esophagus:

(1)   The basic machinery consists of two components: (a) the muscle and (b) the innervation. Other factors act on either the muscle or nerve function.

(2)   For coordinated motor activity to occur, two fundamental functional mechanisms must operate: (a) an excitation mechanism and (b) a coordinating mechanism. These may be separate mechanisms, or one mechanism can serve both functions in part or in total.

(3)   There is frequently more than one control mechanism for initiation and/or production of a coordinated contraction pattern. As a result, a number of functional situations exist: (a) under normal circumstances, one control mechanism dominates. This activity in some way exerts its influence over, and integrates with, other levels and mechanisms of control, (b) there is a potential for control at different locations along the gut ("horizontal" integration) and/or at different levels extending from the gut to the central nervous system including the brain ("vertical" integration), and (c) if the usual dominant control mechanism fails or is removed (e.g., by disease, surgery, or experimental conditions), other mechanisms or levels of control will become evident and can take over to produce a functional coordinated motor pattern. These could be called "reserve" or "secondary" mechanisms of control, and if they are absent or fail to function, significant motor abnormality is likely to occur.

A number of recent reviews deal with the anatomy, innervation, and physiology of the esophagus and mechanisms for control of its motor activity.[3-13] The present review will concentrate on those areas with potential relevance to the situation in the human esophagus. The pharynx and its function will not be discussed in detail.[3,5,9,11,12]

THE NATURE OF ESOPHAGEAL MUSCLE

The nature of esophageal contraction can be affected by two interrelated characteristics of the muscle: its gross and microscopic anatomy on one hand and its physiological properties on the other. The pharynx, UES, and a variable length of esophageal body below the UES are composed of striated muscle in all species including the human. In the human, 2–4 cm of the upper esophagus is composed of striated muscle only, but rarely the entire esophageal body can be striated muscle. Normally, the LES and a variable length of the esophageal body above it (7–10 cm in man) are composed of smooth muscle. The two muscle types intermingle intimately over a variable length of the mid esophagus.[12,14-17]

The amount of striated and smooth muscle in the esophagus of other species is quite variable. In some animals, such as the rat, guinea pig, rabbit, dog, sheep, and cow, the esophageal body is composed almost entirely of striated muscle. In the amphibians and avian species the esophagus is smooth muscle. Yet other animals, such as the opossum, cat, monkey, pig, and horse, have a variable mixture of striated and smooth muscle. Unfortunately, the orientation of fiber bundles, the electron microscopic features, and the physiological characteristics vary considerably among these different animals and species. Therefore, and except for some broad generalization, drawing conclusions about human esophageal muscle from data in other species is fraught with potential problems.

Striated Muscle

Gross and Microscopic Anatomy. The upper esophageal sphincter (UES), a tonically closed high-pressure zone, has a length of 2–4.5 cm on manometry.[3,12] As pointed out by Goyal and Cobb, correlation between the anatomy and radiology in man indicates that the high-pressure zone is produced by the horizontal fibers of the cricopharyngeus muscle along with at least the caudad portion of the inferior pharyngeal constrictor muscle above it.[12] The inferior pharyngeal constrictor muscle consists of fibers that originate anteriorly on either side from both the thyroid cartilage and the upper lateral portions of the cricoid cartilage. These fibers sweep posteriorly and slightly superiorly to meet in the median raphe. The cricopharyngeus muscle fibers on either side arise anteriorly from the lower third of the cricoid cartilage and form a loop posteriorly with its upper border at approximately the C6 to C7 vertebral level. The lower border of this muscle is at the level of the lower border of the cricoid cartilage. The anterior wall of the UES is rigid and is composed of two major components, the curved back of the cricoid cartilage covered by the cricoarytenoid muscle, and more cranially a portion of the transverse and oblique arytenoid muscles forming part of the posterior wall of the larynx.[18,19] It is unclear whether circular muscle fibers of the upper esophageal body normally contribute actively to the sphincter zone. The high-pressure zone radiologically appears to end at the lower border of the cricopharyngeus muscle,[12] and this is also the level at which continuous electromyographic spiking activity ends in animals[8,4,20-22] and probably in humans.[14,24] There is usually a distinct separation between the cricopharyngeus muscle and the inner circular muscle fibers of the upper esophagus. However, occasionally this distinction is not present[19] and in this case the upper esophagus may also contribute actively to the high-pressure zone. Because of the anatomical features, the UES forms a transverse slit-like structure, when closed, which is convex posteriorly (Killian's "lip of the esophageal mouth").[1]

The striated muscle portion of the esophageal body begins at the inferior border of the cricopharyngeus muscle. Generally, in the human, there is a longitudinally oriented outer layer and a thicker circularly oriented inner layer. Muscle bundles of both layers have been described as taking a screw-type and/or oblique course. Vantrappen and Hellemans,[14] quoting from the study of Kaufmann et al.,[16] describe the two layers in humans as part of the same system of fiber bundles. These bundles begin on the exterior surface of the esophagus and penetrate toward the lumen as they travel either orally or caudally. The bundles also take a screw-like course either clockwise or counterclockwise. The outer bundles tend to be more longitudinally directed, while the deeper and end-parts of the bundles are more circularly wound to form an "inner circular" layer, with the ring fibers usually at 10 to 20° to the horizontal plane. This arrangement of fiber bundles can be described as an "apolar screw." Surprisingly, this description has generated little controversy, nor has it been fully confirmed, although other studies describe similar findings.[15,25] Separate from the above system, longitudinal fibers arising from the cricoid cartilage anterolaterally along with some bundles from the cricopharyngeus muscle posterolaterally, initially take an oblique course dorsally and caudally to join approximately 3 cm distal to the cricoid cartilage posteriorly. This forms the triangle of Laimer, a small area of the upper posterior esophageal body devoid of longitudinal muscle.[1,12,15,18,19] Obliquity of the longitudinally directed bundles is also dictated to some extent by a 45–90° twist of the esophagus to the left at its lower end.[14,16,26]

Human esophageal striated muscle has had only limited study by light mocroscopy and virtually no studies have been undertaken of its electronmicroscopic features. According to Rohen, fibers are larger in diameter (60–80μ) in the upper esophagus and become smaller distally (20μ) with some single fibers as tiny as 2–4μ.[25] There is an abundant and continuous fibro-elastic supporting stroma that appears to join with the sarcolemma of some muscle fibers while serving as a connecting link between other closely opposed muscle fibers.[25] Gruber describes striated muscle fibers of the rat esophagus connecting with each other through cholinesterase positive zones.[25] Similar junctions are described in sheep esophageal striated muscle[28] but this has not been confirmed in humans. Although the microstructure of rat esophageal striated muscle is similar to other rat skeletal muscle, similar information is unavailable in humans.[27] The length of fibers in humans is not reported. Rat fibers are greater than 10 mm in length[27] and sheep fibers are estimated to be about 50 mm in length.[28]

Physiological Characteristics. The physiological and biochemical nature of esophageal striated muscle in humans is unknown. One might have anticipated a "slow" striated muscle, perhaps more comparable to smooth muscle.[29] However, data from dogs,[30] sheep, and cats[31] indicate that the striated muscle is of the twitch type, but relatively slow mechanically, with a time to peak tension of approximately 75–80 msec, and a tetanic fusion frequency in the range of 28–40 stim/sec for all three species. The twitch contraction in the rat is much faster, with a time to peak tension of 30 msec and a tetanic fusion frequency of 75–100 stim/sec (unpublished observations). There are no studies attempting to distinguish between fibers in the longitudinal and circular orientations, or to demonstrate regional differences.

Smooth Muscle

Gross Anatomy. Smooth muscle in the human esophageal body also tends to have outer longitudinal and thicker inner circular layers. However, bundles of smooth muscle fibers are said to follow the same screw-type pathways as the striated muscle, both in the region of the body where the two types of muscle coexist and intermingle, and lower, where only smooth muscle is present.[14,16] That is, the two layers are not isolated from each other but are connected anatomically through the orientation of the bundles of fibers. The bundles of fibers are separated by prominent oblique connective tissue septa.[14] There are, in addition, so-called "bracket-fibers," bundles of longitudinally and obliquely oriented fibers internal to the circular layer in the lower esophagus.[15]

The presence of a high-pressure zone at the gastroesophageal junction and the functional and radiological characteristics of the zone have long been accepted as proof of the existence of a physiological sphincter at that site.[1,7,12,14] However, a convincing demonstration of a corresponding structural sphincter in humans has been absent until the recent elegant study of Lieberman-Meffert et al.[26] (Fig. 1-1). This study positions a thick gastroesophageal ring (GER) of muscle obliquely upward from lesser to greater curvature. The greatest thickness occurs at the greater

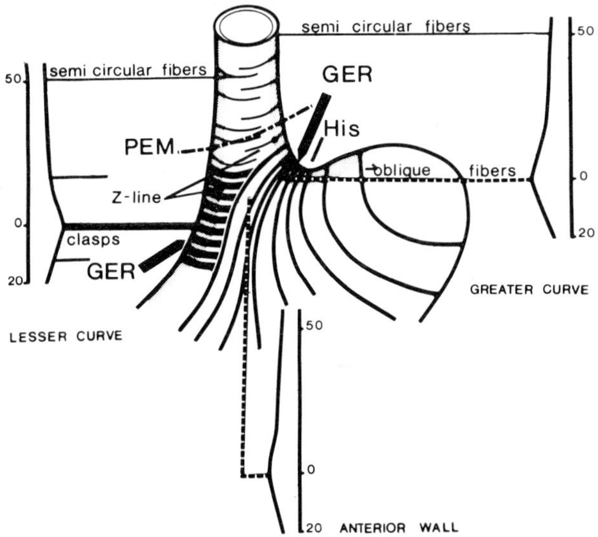

Fig. 1-1. The site of muscle thickness (GER), muscle fiber arrangement, phrenoesophageal membrane (PEM), and squamo columnar mucosal junction (Z-line). Scale is in mm. Reprinted by permission of the publisher from Muscular equivalent of the lower esophageal sphincter, by Liebermann-Meffert D, Allgower M, Schmid P, Blum AL, Gastroenterology 76:31–38. Copyright 1979 by the American Gastroenterological Association.

curvature, and the thickening occurs over approximately 2.3 to 3.1 cm, again greatest on the greater curvature side. The GER coincides with the transition from transverse gastric to longitudinally oriented esophageal mucosal folds. The squamo-columnar junction and attachment of the phreno-esophageal membrane are above the GER, and the angle of His is below it. Of interest is the orientation of the fibers in the muscular ring. On the lesser curve side, these are composed of short transverse semilunar clasps, rather than complete rings, while the bundles on the greater curve side form longer oblique gastric fiber loops.[26] A recent study by Jackson also supports the absence of a complete ring of circular muscle in this region.[32] The oblique gastric bundles appear to correspond to the gastric sling fibers described by numerous authors in the past[33] and Lieberman-Meffert's anatomical description would give these an important functional role. External to the muscular ring, the longitudinal fiber bundles are separate.[26,32] There is no indication that either the longitudinal or circular bundles in this region are an integral part of the apolar screw system of fiber bundles described for the esophageal body, although Jackson describes a more spiral course for the inner smooth muscle fibers.[32] This description of the LES anatomy bears some relationship to manometric and endoscopic findings. However, the relationship of anatomy to the radiologic landmarks is still uncertain.[12]

Microscopic Anatomy. The microscopic anatomy of the smooth muscle esophagus in humans and other species is even less clear. In humans, the cells are $4.5–8.0\mu$ in their widest diameter.[34] In the region of the LES, there are at least two cellular configurations. The first consists of cells with numerous branches, and the second of more oval or elliptical cells.[35] It is not known whether both types of cells are present in the smooth muscle body above the LES, where the unbranched cells appear to be the usual type.[34] Cell-to-cell contact is common in esophageal smooth muscle. However, a detailed study of these contacts is not available and descriptions of the types of contacts differ between authors.[34-36] Daniel et al. describe three types of contacts, nexuses or gap junctions, simple close apositions (100–250 Å), and intermediate contacts (500–750 Å), the latter with electron-dense beads in the adjacent basement membranes. In their study, both cell types in the circular layer have more cell-to-cell contacts than cells in the longitudinal layer. The branched cells are more abundantly supplied with cell-to-cell contacts than are the oval cells. The longitudinal layer has no gap junction.[35] Both Harman et al.[36] and Casella et al.[34] describe structures similar to the gap junctions and the intermediate contacts but failed to distinguish simple close appositions. They did not distinguish between longitudinal and circular muscle. In studies of cat and baboon esophageal smooth muscle, Gonella et al. feel that only the nexus or gap-junction type of contacts are present and these occur in both longitudinal and circular muscle.[37] In the cat, the nexuses are more common in the circular layer compared to the longitudinal layer. The opposite is true in the baboon. The role that different technique might play in dictating these differences within and among species has not been clarified. However, it is likely that true species differences do exist and further studies in humans are essential to establish the nature and function of cell-to-cell contacts.

Physiological Characteristics. There are virtually no studies of the physiological characteristics of human esophageal smooth muscle independent of the studies, usually pharmacological, dealing with the innervation and neuro-endocrine responsiveness of the muscle (see below). However, from studies in other species where some findings are relatively consistent, one can risk extrapolation of a few general characteristics to the human situation. The presence of cell-to-cell contacts in human muscle,[34-36] and circumstantial evidence for electrical coupling between cells in other species[37] provide a basis for esophageal smooth muscle to behave as a functional syncitium, as does gastric and intestinal muscle.[38] Although esophageal smooth muscle is not spontaneously active *in vivo* (except perhaps for LES tone in some species), and a peristaltic contraction is usually monophasic, the muscle from the chicken,[39] opossum,[40] cat,[41-45] and baboon[42] can exhibit oscillatory properties when excited. Slow membrane depolarizations[41-45] and/or associated repetitive contractions have been observed.[39-45] Esophageal smooth muscle therefore shares some of the characteristics of smooth muscle in the distal gut and can perhaps be considered as a relaxation oscillator—an excitable relaxation oscillator rather than the spontaneously active type used to describe gastric and small intestinal muscle.[46] If human esophageal muscle is like that of the opossum, cat, and monkey, it is likely that there are differences between the longitudinal and circular muscle layers.[4,41,42,47] Perhaps more important in these species, there appear to be significant regional differences not only between the esophageal body and the LES, but along the smooth muscle body itself.[40,47-51] Finally, in both the chicken and opossum smooth muscle esophagus, a peristaltic contraction can be induced that seems to be entirely myogenic.[39,52] It is not yet known whether myogenic peristalsis can occur in the human esophagus. However, in the human, it is reasonable to expect that muscle properties will influence and contribute to the nature of peristalsis, once induced by adequate excitation.

Regional differences in the physiological properties of esophageal smooth muscle fall into two broad inter-related areas—those differences that relate to the contractile properties and excitation contraction coupling of the muscle, and those that relate to the oscillatory properties of the muscle membrane. The only information available comes from animal studies, and in many of these studies it is difficult to distinguish between truly myogenic regional differences and those that result from differences in the innervation or neuroendocrine responsiveness of the muscle. *In vivo,* the LES in all species studied, including the human, is recognized by intraluminal manometry as a high-pressure zone which relaxes on swallowing. *In vitro,* LES muscle is usually identified by its ability to exhibit neurally mediated relaxation, as opposed to the neurally mediated contraction exhibited by more proximal esophageal body muscle under the same resting condition.[53-63] This latter method of definition has permitted studies of the potential myogenic differences between the LES and the esophageal body.

The presence of the LES high-pressure zone suggested that there was something different about LES muscle as compared to muscle from the esophageal body: the LES remained closed due to tonic contraction of the muscle localized to this region. The demonstration of many-branched cells and numerous cell-to-cell contacts in this region has provided a potential structural basis for this increased tone.[35] Debate has arisen as to the mechanism responsible for the tonic contraction. Is it myogenic or due to external influences such as innervation, hormones, etc., or a combination of these factors? Certainly in the opossum a significant portion of this resting tone is myogenic since it persists *in vivo* in the face of vagotomy and intravenous injection of tetrodotoxin,[58] and *in vitro* in the presence of atropine and/or tetrodotoxin.[64] However, in other species, such as the human, cat, dog and monkey, the resting LES tone *in vivo* is atropine sensitive or significantly reduced by vagal interruption implying that the neural component of tone is dominant.[65,66] The effect of neural blocking agents on *in vitro* LES tone in these latter species has not been adequately evaluated. It is proposed that differences in myogenic receptors, either in number or response to agonists, make LES muscle more sensitive to neural and endocrine stimulation. The dose response curves for agonists acting on the LES are shifted to the left[53,54] and the maximum tension developed by agonists can be higher for the LES than for the esophageal body.[54] One could argue that this also represents myogenic specialization in this region.

Independent of extrinsic innervation or hormones, studies with opossum and cat LES tissue show that active tension in the resting muscle as determined by length–tension measurements, is higher in LES than in body muscle.[54-56,63] Passive tension of the LES and body muscle is not different.[54,63] Since intramural nerves are still present in muscle strips, and studies of the length tension relationships have not been done in the presence of neural blocking agents, it is still not clear whether the difference at the LES is entirely a muscle property. It may also contain an element of neuroendocrine responsiveness. In the cat, the force of contraction induced by high potassium concentrations and measured at the length for maximum tension development (a length well beyond the *in vivo* length), is greater for LES muscle.[63] This appears to be due to a greater thickness of muscle at the LES.[63]

Regardless of the origin of the LES resting tone, it is calcium dependent in all species studied.[60,61,64,67,69] Daniel et al. proposed that this myogenic tension in the opossum is determined by a voltage-dependent leak of extracellular calcium, since they observed that the membrane potential of the LES muscle was 40 mV compared to the higher 50 mV of the esophageal body.[64] DeCarle et al. have argued that abolition of the tonic contraction by nitroprusside fits with the hypothesis that calcium acts through the T system of Golenhofen,[70] although Dent et al. were less convinced of this interpretation.[69] In a brief abstract, Mukhopadhyay and Kunneman did not confirm this effect of nitroprusside on KCL-induced contractions.[61] Although elevation of serum calcium in normal humans does not increase LES pressure,[71,72] the calcium blocking agents decrease it in nonhuman primates.[67] This knowledge has been used to treat patients with achalasia by reduction of the high LES pressure with nifedipine.[73]

In addition to dependency on calcium, the LES tonic contraction in the opossum is also oxygen dependent, and uses high-energy phosphate.[62] Contraction of the esophageal body muscle is less dependent on oxygen than the LES, although it is not clear whether this applies to both longitudinal and circular layers.[62] Similar studies have not been done with human LES muscle and the potential relationships of anoxia to LES dysfunction in humans has yet to be explored.

Except for a difference in resting membrane potential between the LES and the esophageal body, the membrane characteristics of the LES have not been compared with those of the body. There is some *in vivo* evidence in the dog and opossum that some type of periodic electrical activity (approximately 2/min in dogs, and 20–25/min in opossums) is associated with tone.[74,75] Similar activity has not been seen *in vitro* under resting conditions. *In vivo* this activity may be due to the addition of other influences, such as neural excitation.

There are differences between the circular and longitudinal muscle layers,[4,40-42] as well as differences along the body within each layer.[40,47-51] As in the LES, the muscle contractions in the body have in large part been defined by the responses to neural stimulation. This is true in all species studied, including the human. Longitudinal muscle responds with a contraction throughout most of the period of stimulation, the "duration response"; circular muscle responds with a contraction that follows with a variable delay after cessation of stimulation, the "off-response."[4,40-42,47,48,50,51,76-84] In addition, circular muscle can contract near the onset of stimulation in response to a neural mechanism[41,42,76,81,85] but also in response to direct electrical stimulation[78,79,84] or stimulation by stretch.[78-80] These latter circular muscle responses have been called the "on-response" or "on-contraction." Dodds et al. used the term "on-contraction" to define a neurally mediated event[81] as opossed to the earlier described "on-response," which was due to direct electrical or pharmacological stimulation.[79] In the present discussion, the terms are used interchangeably to indicate the timing of the event, not its mechanism of production. To date, there is a large fund of information exploring and establishing the neural basis for many of the different responses (see below). However, isolation of a myogenic contribution to the differences in the neurally mediated contractions has not been satisfactorily accomplished, or even attempted with any degree of sophistication. In particular, there are no such studies with human tissue.

As noted above, resting active tension in the circular muscle of the body is less than that in the LES muscle.[54-56,63] However, there is no consistent difference in active tension, and therefore no gradient in this parameter along the esophageal body of opossum,[55,56] cat,[63] or monkey.[55] Furthermore, no differences in force–velocity relationships are noted along the esophageal body or between the body and the LES of the opossum esophagus.[86] There are no reports of length–tension or force–velocity measurements with the esophageal smooth muscle in the longitudinal orientation.

There are reported regional differences in the response of the circular body muscle to stimulation with various agonists. In the cat, the amplitude of contractions in response to agonists is less proximally but this has been attributed to the increased proportion of striated muscle,[87] while differences in active stress (which decrease distally) have been accounted for on the basis of differences in thickness of the circular muscle layer.[63] In the opossum, the decreased responsiveness of the more proximal muscle to noradrenaline has been attributed to receptor differences,[53] similar to those proposed for differences between LES and body muscle.[54] This may also be true for the proximal increase in responsiveness to the inhibitory effect of isoproterenol.[88] Except possibly for the latter two findings, regional myogenic specialization is not evident from these types of studies. The effect of these particular regional differences on features such as the amplitude of the peristaltic contraction *in vivo* is not known. Amplitude of contraction in the opossum smooth muscle esophagus tends to decrease distally[82,89] while that in the cat[81] and human[90-92] tends to increase distally.

Both the "duration response" of longitudinal muscle and the "off-response" of circular muscle are calcium dependent.[70] Furthermore, the force–velocity characteristics of the "off-response" are sensitive to changes in extracellular calcium.[86,88,93] Also, calcium-blocking agents decrease the amplitude and duration of peristaltic contraction in the baboon esophagus, presumably through an action on the muscle.[67] To date, there are no studies establishing regional differences in the calcium dependence of the various muscle responses in the esophageal body. Using the nitroprusside effect, in this case failure of nitroprusside to abolish the contractions, DeCarle et al. have concluded that both the "duration" and "off-responses" result from calcium acting through the P system of Golenhofen.[70] The utilization of the P activation system in esophageal body and the T activation system in the LES would fit with the phasic and tonic activity, respectively, of the two muscle regions. DeCarle et al. also propose that a different kind of calcium activation is present for each of the two muscle responses but this requires confirmation. The role of calcium in the "on-response" contractions of the circular muscle has not been studied in detail. In the opossum, the acetylcholine-induced contraction is apparently independent of extracellular calcium,[70] as is contraction due to direct electrical stimulation of the muscle.[64] In the longitudinal muscle also, acetylcholine-induced contraction can occur in the absence of extracellular calcium.[70] Nevertheless, Cohen and Green have reported that acetylcholine, noradrenaline, and gastrin can alter the force–velocity characteristics of the "off-response" when extracellular calcium has been lowered. Although they were studying a neurally mediated response, the implication was that these agents affected mobilization of calcium by the muscle.[86,88,93] It is apparent, therefore, that in studies of neurally mediated responses, care must be taken to determine the role of calcium in nerve function as well as in muscle function, a difficult task.

Of particular interest are the oscillatory and membrane properties of esophageal body smooth muscle, which can show regional differences.[40,48,51] Interest in these properties began with the initial observation of Weisbrodt and Christensen that the time delay between the stimulus and the circular muscle "off-response" increased distally along the esophageal body of the opossum.[40] This observation, along with the fact that both the longitudinal and circular layers contract repetitively during prolonged continuous stimulation, raises the likely possibility that esophageal muscle has important relaxation oscillator properties. Although the method of stimulation is frequently neural, the repetitive activity may well have a major myogenic contribution.[40,43,51] If so, regional differences in these myogenic properties would also be of importance.

In the longitudinal muscle layer, the repetitive contractions are accompanied by bursts of electrical spiking activity.[41,42,77,94] With the usual extracellular recording techniques, a definite slow membrane depolarization or "slow-wave" with each contraction or burst of spiking has not been noted, although there is a strong suggestion these occur.[41,42,77] The repetitive contractions in this layer have been induced *in vitro* or *in vivo* in several species, including the chicken,[39] cat,[41,42,77] opossum,[79] and baboon.[42] *In vitro,* repetitive contractions occasionally occur spontaneously[77,79] or they occur in response to increased potassium concentration,[40] atropine at 10^{-4} g/ml or greater,[95] cholinergic and α adrenergic stimulation,[77] and stretch.[39] In the one instance where it was explored, with high concentration of potassium *in vitro,* a regional difference in contraction frequency was found in the longitudinal layer. The frequency was higher proximally and decreased distally.[40] *In vivo,* vagal stimulation and intraluminal distension readily produce repetitive activity in the longitudinal layer.[41,42]

In the circular muscle layer, repetitive mechanical and electrical activity is a feature of both the "on-response" or "on-contraction," and the "off-response."[40-42,44,45,52,85,95,96] Although the "off-response" has only a neural mode of initiation, the circular muscle *in vitro* can be stimulated to immediate repetitive contraction by increased KCL concentration,[40] high concentration of atropine,[95] field stimulation of an intramural cholinergic mechanism[44,85] cholinergic agonists,[44,45,52,85,96] α adrenergic agonists,[96] and stretch.[39] In a number of these instances, repetitive slow membrane depolarizations with or without superimposed spiking activity and repetitive contractions have been observed.[52,85,96] As with the longitudinal layer, prolonged continuous vagal stimulation or intraluminal balloon distension causes repetitive circular muscle contractions in a number of species,[41,42,44] including the human.[97-99]

In studies of circular muscular activity it is not clear whether various muscle properties relate equally to the "on-response" and "off-response," and to what extent neural mechanisms alone influence the nature of the responses. For example, the "off-response," a neurally mediated event shows a gradient in its delay along the esophagus, while in contrast to the longitudinal layer, KCL-induced contractions of the circular muscle show no gradient in contraction frequency along the esophagus.[40] This suggested that the main regional difference in the circular layer was in the innervation or the neuroendocrine responsiveness of the muscle. This hypothesis gains some support from more recent studies where the "off-response" characteristics are altered significantly and nonuniformly at each level by neural and neuropharmacological manipulations[48,50,51,81,82,89,100] (see below).

However, definite regional differences have been found in a number of membrane properties of the circular muscle. There is a resting membrane potential gradient along the opossum esophageal body from -52.8 ± 0.6 mV proximally to -43.5 ± 1.0 mV distally,[51] and approximately 40 mV at the LES.[64] If the membrane potential is in large part potassium dependent, the gradient in membrane potential of the circular layer would fit with the gradient in intracellular potassium concentration, which also decreases distally, although both muscle layers were included in the latter studies.[49] As opposed to the "on-response" contractions, where excitatory junction potentials (EJP) and slow membrane depolarizations are featured,[41,42,44] the "off-response" contraction is associated with a slow membrane depolarization (the electrical "off-response"), which is preceded by a membrane hyperpolarization, the latter composed of single or multiple inhibitory junction potentials (IJP).[43,51,94] Chan and Diamant proposed that the electrical "off-response" could represent a passive rebound oscillation of the membrane following its release from the active hyperpolarization.[43] Others have questioned whether the oscillation is entirely passive since in the opossum, transient passive hyperpolarization by electrical current injection is followed by little or no overshoot depolarization (Daniel EE, personal communication), and the "off-response" contraction is variably atropine sensitive or augmented by cholinesterase inhibitors in the cat[44,84] and opossum.[79] The "off-response" in opossum can also be selectively depressed by neurotropic veratum alkaloids.[47] Therefore, some degree of active excitation appears to be necessary for the "off-response." Whether this excitation alone causes the "off-response," or through its effect on the membrane facilitates or permits a passive oscillation, is yet to be determined. One would guess that the latter combination is most likely. In studies relating the "off-response" depolarization to the previous hyperpolarization, regional differences become apparent. The electrical "off-response" distally tends to be slower to peak, and for a given hyperpolarization of less amplitude.[48,51] From the oscillatory point of view, the distal muscle response appears more "damped."[43] If so, a functional frequency gradient, decreasing distally, could be present in this layer. Obviously, the innervation can affect the electrical "off-responses," but the effect is not uniform at each level[48,51] and some of the characteristics are likely myogenic. The functional role of these myogenic properties and differences is yet to be determined in all species, including the human.

INNERVATION AND PHARMACOLOGY

This review will not provide an exhaustive description of the esophageal innervation since several recent reviews deal with this subject in detail, both for the esophageal body and its sphincters.[4,6,11,12,101,102] The majority of detailed information has been derived from species other than the human. It is pertinent, however, to outline a number of features of the innervation with particular relevance to its role as a control mechanism for the peristaltic contraction of the esophagus, especially in the human. Newer information will be emphasized. Since pharmacological tools have served to define many of the characteristics of the innervation at the peripheral level, a discussion of the innervation is necessarily linked to the pharmacology of the esophagus. The local esophageal innervation must also be considered in light of recent views of the enteric nervous system elsewhere in the gut—a system with remarkable autonomy.[103] Finally, with the emerging concept of the "neuroendocrine" relationships, it is more appropriate to consider the role of the various peptide hormones within this broader context.[104]

Central

The "swallowing center," composed of two intimately connected half-centers, is located in the medulla and pons and has three functional components: an afferent reception system, an efferent system of motor neurons, and a complex organizing or internuncial system of neurons.[11,101,105,108] This center controls bucopharyngeal, as well as esophageal, motor activity on swallowing. Doty proposed that the central control mechanism should be viewed as containing three separable controls for the bucopharyngeal, esophageal, and gastroesophageal (LES) regions along the deglutition pathway.[101] Afferent information from the periphery ultimately funnels into the solitary tract, the afferent receptor center. The motor neurons lie mainly in the trigeminal, facial, and hypoglossal nuclei, nucleus ambiguous (for esophageal striated muscle), and dorsal motor nucleus of the vagus (esophageal smooth muscle). Some motor neurons for the smooth muscle esophagus may also originate in the nucleus ambiguous.[107] The internuncial system for organizing the entire motor sequence of deglutition is located in the solitary tract nucleus and neighboring reticular substance.

Afferent Connections. The swallowing center can be activated or influenced by afferent information from the periphery via the superior laryngeal branch of the vagus, the vagus itself, the glossopharyngeus, and the maxillary branch of the trigeminal nerve. Unilateral afferent stimulation can activate both halves of the swallowing center.[108] Sensory information can either reflexly initiate deglutition and a peristaltic sequence, or alternatively affect previously initiated activity in the swallowing center, and therefore ongoing motor activity. The reflexly elicited motor events may be limited to the bucopharyngeal phase only, or to all or part of the esophagus. The final effect depends on the species, the origin of the stimulus (site of stimulation in the intact animal, or nerve stimulated), intensity of stimulation, and the presence or absence of ongoing motor activity.[11,12,101] For initiation of reflex swallowing in man, the anterior and posterior tonsillar pillars and the posterior pharyngeal wall are the most sensitive areas.[12,101,109]

Usually the swallowing sequence is initiated voluntarily. A locus for this obvious involvement of the cerebral cortex in swallowing is present in the frontal area.[11,101] Subcortical structures are also linked to the swallowing center and can elicit or facilitate activity there.[11,101] Finally, there is close interconnection and interplay between the swallowing center and other medullary centers, the most apparent being with the respiratory center,[12,101] where protection of the airway is of importance.

Sensory information from the entire esophagus including its sphincters is carried in the vagus.[11,101,110,111] The cell bodies for sensory fibers are in the nodose ganglion.[110] In a number of species, including the nonhuman primates, the information arising in the region of the UES and upper cervical esophagus is carried to the vagus in the superior laryngeal nerve,[11,101,112] while in the remaining distal esophagus, sensory data enter the vagus via the recurrent laryngeal nerve above and the esophageal branches of the thoracic vagi lower down.[11,101] There is likely some overlap in the high cervical esophagus between the distribution of the superior laryngeal and recurrent laryngeal nerves.[111,113,114] Similar physiological information in humans is not available, but on the basis of anatomical studies the sensory patterns are presumably similar to those in other species.[111,112] The proximity of the cervical esophagus to the airway may dictate doubling the sensory protection.

The Organizing or Internuncial Center. This portion of the swallowing center is the computer placed between the afferent reception center and the motor neurons. It is composed of a complex of interconnecting neurons, which programs the successive excitation of motor neurons and governs the entire motor sequence of deglutition.

A number of important features of this organizing system dictate whether all or part of the sequence of deglutition will be initiated, and the characteristics of the peristaltic contraction, including its polarity, velocity, and magnitude. (a) There are neurons or sets of neurons specific to each anatomical region along the deglutition pathway from bucopharynx to distal esophagus, including the smooth muscle esophagus and the LES. Afferent information from each region appears to impinge on the neurons specific to the site of origin of the stimulus. Similarly, motor neurons destined to excite specific regions are directed by specific corresponding neurons in the organizing system. (b) Once initiated, the system functions in a stereotyped fashion with progression of excitation through the neurons representative of sequentially more distal anatomical regions. (c) The system serves both primary peristalsis (initiated by a voluntary swallow) and secondary peristalsis (initiated by local stimulation in the periphery). With primary peristalsis, the chain of neurons is excited from its beginning, while during secondary peristalsis the excitation starts at some level within the chain and progresses from there. (d) Within this system is an effective mechanism for inhibition of neurons. Stimulation of proximal neurons in the chain inhibits interneurons controlling more distal portions of the deglutition complex. Jean has also argued that this inhibition provides a potential mechanism for activation of swallowing interneurons along the chain through postinhibitory rebound.[105] (e) Although there was initial controversy,[101] it is now apparent that this system is sensitive to afferent sensory input from the periphery, which can result in excitation, inhibition, and/or alterations in timing of the sequential motor discharges.[6,11]

The functional results of these characteristics are many. For example, afferent information can be utilized to initiate a peristaltic sequence at various levels depending on the origin of the stimulus, and to augment the firing of motor neurons through sensory feedback from the esophageal bolus. The inhibitory features within the system provide one central mechanism for "distal inhibition," that is, absence of excitation. To date, there has been no isolation of separate central neurons responsible for direct activation of peripheral intramural inhibitory neurons of the esophageal body. However, vagal fibers have been identified that fire at the time of active relaxation of the LES in the dog.[115]

Efferent Connections. As pointed out above, motor fibers to various regions along the deglutition pathway originate in motor neurons of a number of cranial nerves. The vagal nuclei are responsible for all the muscles of the esophagus, including the upper esophageal sphincter and the smooth muscle esophagus.[11,116] In the dog, the UES and a significant portion of the cervical esophagus are innervated by the pharyngoesophageal branch of the vagus nerve with some minor pathways in nerves of the deep pharyngeal plexus and the superior laryngeal nerve.[12,112,115,117] The cat is apparently similar.[12] In the human, no discrete nerve is present to the UES.[11,12,101,111,112] Clasically in the human, the cervical esophagus is innervated by the recurrent laryngeal nerves and the esophagus distally by the branches from the thoracic vagal trunks.[1] In the upper cervical esophagus of other species, there is overlap between the motor distribution of the recurrent laryngeal nerves and that of either the pharyngoesophageal nerves or branches of the superior laryngeal nerves.[101,111,112,115] This has not been investigated in humans although Lund and Adrian presented evidence that there is no extension of the recurrent laryngeal nerve motor influence to the UES of humans.[112]

The Lower Esophageal Sphincter (LES). As pointed out by Doty, there is some basis for considering central control of the LES as separable.[101] On one hand, the LES maintains tone while the rest of the esophagus is quiet. On the other, the LES is inhibited at the time the remainder of the esophagus is active with a peristaltic contraction. Further, LES relaxation can occur in isolation when an intraesophageal distension is below the threshold for induction of an esophageal contraction.[101]

The resting LES tone in many species, including the human, has a significant neural component.[65,66] There is evidence for a central vagal excitatory influence as a major contributor to this tone in the dog, where tonically firing vagal fibers cease their activity during LES relaxation[115] and cervical vagal interruption is associated with an immediate decrease in LES tone.[66,118] Contraction of the LES is associated with increased firing of the excitatory vagal fibers.[115]

LES relaxation in the dog is also associated with the firing of other vagal fibers, presumably destined to mediate active inhibition of the LES.[15] In addition, stimulation of the distal cut end of the vagus can cause LES inhibition in many species.[6,11,12,119] It is assumed that the vagal fibers concerned synapse directly on intramural inhibitory neurons in the LES region but this has not been confirmed. Therefore, at least in the dog and perhaps in other species, there is also provision for central participation in control of LES relaxation. Both removal of excitation and active inhibition are operative.

There are extrinsic nonvagal excitatory nerves to the LES that can be activated by central stimulation in the opossum[119] and dog.[118] These apparently operate through the sympathetic nervous system, since in the opossum, the activity can be abolished by α adrenergic blockade.[119] The relevance of this pathway is yet to be determined, and its central origin is unknown.

In several species, including the human, there is reason to suspect that efferent vagal fibers subserving both LES excitation and relaxation enter the esophagus at some point above the LES.[18,120-124] Truncal vagotomy and more recently selective vagotomy,[125,126] which may vagally[118,120-124] denervate up to 8–9 cm of the lower esophagus, have virtually no effect on LES tone, relaxation, or responsiveness to cholinergic stimulation. However, vagotomy variably reduces the reflex increase of LES tone with an increase in intra-abdominal pressure. This is likely due to interruption of the afferent pathway.[124,127,128]

The Sympathetic Nervous System.   The esophagus receives an abundant sympathetic innervation exiting from the thoracic spinal cord.[11,12,102] The post-ganglionic fibers leave the sympathetic chain to reach the esophagus with the blood vessels, or a few fibers join the vagus nerves to the esophagus.[11,12,14] In the cat there is evidence for sympathetic LES innervation via the sphlanchnic nerves.[129-131] The participation of sympathetic nerves in central control of the peristaltic sequence and LES function seems unlikely, unless they can function to modulate features such as contraction amplitude and LES tone. For example, there is a nonvagal excitatory nerve pathway to the LES susceptible to α adrenergic blockade,[119] and β adrenergic blockers can increase LES tone in the opossum[131] and the human,[132] and increase amplitude and duration of the esophageal contraction in the human.[132] Peristalsis and LES relaxation continue despite adrenergic blockade in these species, while splanchnic stimulation can reduce neurally mediated LES relaxation in the cat.[129] Gonella et al. have demonstrated convincingly that the excitatory effect of splanchnic stimulation on the cat LES is due to release of acetylcholine from cholinergic axon endings by an α adrenergic mechanism.[133]

Intramural

Striated Muscle.   It is generally held that postganglionic vagal fibers pass directly to innervate the striated muscle fibers through cholinergic nicotinic receptors. Vagally induced twitch contractions of the striated muscle are prevented by neuromuscular blocking agents, such as curare and succinylcholine, but striated muscle contraction is not altered by atropine.[4,11,12,81,134-136] The motor end plates in man and other primates tend to be of the "en-grappe" type rather than the "en-plaque" type.[137] The functional significance of this is unclear. In many species, the same motor fiber can lead to more than one end plate on a muscle fiber.[28,137,138] However, a single muscle fiber does not apparently receive innervation from more than one nerve fiber. In the sheep, a few muscle fibers show innervation through small multiple nerve endings along the fiber.[28] These muscle fibers, usually occurring in the inner muscle layer near the distal esophagus, resemble the frog slow muscle fibers.[29] They perhaps relate in some way to sphincter function. Similar fibers have not been described in the human.

There is a well-developed myenteric plexus in the striated muscle that presumably serves primarily a sensory function.[14] Sensory endings of various types are found in the striated muscle.[137-139] One study of the dog suggested that there may be an intramural interneuron in the pathway of some excitatory vagal fibers to the striated muscle.[134] Mann et al. provided evidence for an intramural pathway within the striated muscle esophagus of the guinea pig *in vitro* for mediating LES relaxation.[140] However, in the dog, this intramural pathway does not seem to be present.[66] Therefore, certain evidence for a motor function of the myenteric plexus in striated muscle remains to be established.

Sympathetic innervation within the myenteric plexus of the striated muscle esophagus has been demonstrated by fluorescent histochemical methods in the dog, cat, rabbit, and rhesus monkey.[141-143] At present, there is no reason to suspect a motor function for this innervation in this region of the esophagus.

Smooth Muscle. The relationships between morphology and function of the nerve plexuses in the smooth muscle portion of the esophagus are yet to be determined. The various neuronal types described within the plexuses[137,143,144] speak of the complexity of this neural network. It no doubt corresponds in many ways to the enteric nervous system in the more distal gut.[103,145,146] There are two important effector neurons within the system, one capable of mediating cholinergic excitation of both longitudinal and circular layers of smooth muscle, and the other mediating nonadrenergic, noncholinergic (NANC) inhibition mainly of the circular muscle layer.[6,11,41,42,48,51,77,81,82,85,94,147] The neurotransmitter released by the latter neuron(s) is unknown although purine nucleotides and/or peptide hormones, such as vasoactive intestinal polypeptide (VIP), have been among the substances proposed.[6,11,12,148] Both types of neurons are excited by cholinergic input from preganglionic vagal fibers and intramural interneurons. The cholinergic excitation of the neurons is nicotinic, and occasionally muscarinic in addition.[12,148] Both types of neurons innervate the body and LES. At the LES, the dominance of the inhibitory effect and lack of a specific blocking agent for this effect makes demonstration of the cholinergic excitation difficult, especially with vagal or electrical field stimulation of the muscle.[147]

Within the muscle layers nerve fibers of different types are noted, at times in close apposition to the muscle cells. Although not entirely satisfactory, the cholinergic, NANC and adrenergic nerves have been described in terms of the vesicles in the terminal varicosities.[35,103,149] In the human esophagus, both cholinergic and NANC nerves are found, as well as a few adrenergic nerves.[35] Especially in the region of the LES, cholinergic, and less frequently, NANC nerves, make close contact (60 Å) with the tightly coupled muscle cells.[35] Daniel et al. point out that close nerve–muscle contact in combination with tightly coupled cells provides a mechanism for easy neuronal control of muscle activity of the region.[35] Nerve fibers and muscle cells may make mutual contact with "glial"-like or "fibroblast"-like interstitial cells.[35,150,151] These have been described in the human and opossum esophagus.[35,150] Daniel et al. have proposed that the interstitial cell could take part in the release of inhibitory neurotransmitter, or even be a potential source of inhibitory mediator substance.[150]

Mechanisms for effective distal inhibition are present within the intramural neural network. *In vivo* with the vagi sectioned in the neck, or *in vitro,* proximal balloon distension in the smooth muscle esophagus induces hyperpolarization of the muscle membrane distally, reduction of motor activity distal to the balloon, and relaxation of the LES.[40,42,94,140,147] These phenomena have been noted in a number of species, and evidence points to the operation of at least two neural mechanisms, activation of distal NANC neurons to the muscle,[94] and neuronal inhibition of the more distal excitatory cholinergic neurons.[147] Similar mechanisms are known to operate in the small intestine.[146]

From the sensory point of view, at least stretch receptors in the smooth muscle esophagus react with other intramural neural elements as well as with the central control mechanism.[41,42,78] Both rapidly and slowly adapting receptors are present in the smooth muscle esophagus.[110] The slowly adapting receptors seem most physiological and respond to both distension and esophageal contraction. It is not known whether other esophageal receptors sensitive to pH[114,152,153] or temperature[154] also react locally, but it is assumed they can.

Sympathetic nerves are abundant in the smooth muscle esophagus. In the monkey they make both axo-somatic and axo-axonic contact with neurons of the plexuses, but only sparse contact with the smooth muscle cells themselves.[142,35] Presumably, the human is similar.[35] Therefore, it seems that, as elsewhere in the gut,[103] sympathetic nerves serve mainly to modulate the activity of other neurons and the release of their respective neurotransmitters. At the LES of the cat, for example, sympathetic influence may affect both excitatory and inhibitory neuronal function by augmenting release of acetylcholine from the former and inhibiting release of inhibitory neurotransmitters from the latter.[130,133] These are α adrenergic effects. At the muscle level in the body and the LES there are excitatory α and inhibitory β adrenergic receptors. The functional importance of these is not established. However, as noted above, the effect of β adrenergic blocking agents on increasing LES tone and the amplitude of peristaltic contraction in humans, suggests that a small degree of tonic sympathetic activity (β adrenergic) may be present.[132]

It is apparent both *in vivo* and *in vitro* that esophageal smooth muscle, especially in the region of the LES, is sensitive to the action of virtually every conceivable peptide hormone and most drugs, as well as to other substances, such as histamine, prostaglandins, dopamine, serotonin, and opiates.[4,6,10,104,148,150,151] This is true in most species, including the human. The majority of these agents can act on muscle, nerve or both. Recent studies indicate that nerves with enkephalin-like immunoreactivity are present within the myenteric plexus and the smooth muscle of the esophageal body of the opossum, cat, pig, monkey, and human.[155] There is no conspicuous activity in the region of the LES. It is only a matter of time before other peptides are identified in esophageal neural tissues and the various types of plexus neurons are characterized by their pharmacological, electrophysiological, and morphological properties. Only then can their function be adequately contemplated and their physiological significance properly established. At the moment there is no convincing reason to consider other than the cholinergic excitatory neuron and the NANC inhibitory neuron, whatever its neurotransmitter(s), as the basic effector machinery of the smooth muscle esophagus. The nature of the interneurons and the interaction of other modulating factors await elucidation.

As pointed out above, the contractions of the longitudinal and circular smooth muscle layers have been defined by their responses to neural stimulation. The neural basis for the contractions has also been characterized. The "duration response" of the longitudinal layer[4,77] and the neural "on-contraction" of circular muscle are both cholinergic.[44,81,82,85,147] The "off-response" of circular muscle has a cholinergic[4,44,79,84] and noncholinergic[4,44,79] component and is preceded by a period of active inhibition.[6,43,48,51] Exictatory cholinergic neurons are given responsibility for the cholinergic contractions, while the inhibition preceding the "off-response" is attributed to the activation of the NANC inhibitory neuron(s). In the opossum, the "off-response" is selectively depressed by some neurotropic veratrum alkaloids. This suggests that the active neurogenic component of this response affected by the alkaloids is different from that mediating cholinergic excitation of the longitudinal "duration response," and presumably different from the cholinergic component of the "off-response."[47]

COORDINATED MOTILITY

The relationships of structure, physiological properties, and function become evident in the coordinated motility of the esophagus and its sphincters. Nevertheless, lack of understanding of the underlying mechanisms of control has generated considerable controversy, especially over control of the smooth muscle esophagus.

UES

At rest the UES is tonically closed due to continuous neural excitation, and in addition there is a small passive component to the tone.[11,12,22,101] The slit-like structure of the UES gives marked radial assymetry to the profile of intraluminal pressure. Pressures are higher anteriorly and posteriorly corresponding to the position of the cricopharyngeus muscle sling and its action.[12,156,157] Excitatory discharge to the UES and UES pressure increases with each inspiration,[8,22,158] providing extra protection for the airway. In addition, distension and acid in the upper esophagus cause a reflex increase in UES pressure,[114,159] as do a Valsalva maneuver, gagging,[12] and secondary peristalsis.[8]

On swallowing, excitatory discharge to the UES ceases transiently in exquisite coordination with the rapid sequence of muscle activity in the bucopharyngeal phase of swallowing.[11,12,22,101] This is entirely controlled by the central control mechanism.[101] Both cessation of neural excitation to the UES and elevation and forward movement of the cricoid cartilage act together to decrease the UES resting pressure and to open the sphincter on swallowing.[12,101] A short burst of excitation and contraction follows.[12,22,101]

Striated Muscle Esophagus

Peristalsis in the striated muscle is directed by sequential excitation along the esophagus through vagal fibers programmed by the central control mechanism.[6,11,12,101] In the dog only, afferent sensory input from an intraluminal bolus in the cervical esophagus is necessary to adequately excite the central program for the more distal thoracic esophagus.[11,160,8] Deviation of the swallowed bolus at the cervical level eliminates peristalsis below the level of deviation. This does not occur to any extent in the rabbit, opossum, or rhesus monkey, nor does it occur with bolus deviation in the thoracic region of the dog.[8,11] Therefore, in most species, a swallow can adequately excite the entire central program regardless of the presence of an intramural bolus. However, afferent information from the esophagus and elsewhere has a significant effect on the central program to alter the force and velocity of the peristaltic contraction in both the striated and smooth muscle esophagus (see above and below). Deglutitive inhibition in the striated muscle esophagus results from cessation of the excitatory discharges from the central program.[8,108]

It is of interest to consider whether the local neuromuscular anatomy of the striated muscle contributes to the nature of peristalsis in the striated muscle esophagus. This has not been investigated in any species. The apolar-screw orientation of the fiber bundles[14,16] and the network of fibro-elastic connections between muscle fibers[25] may provide a mechanism to mechanically link contraction of longitudinal fibers with circular fibers at a distance, the latter usually being more distally placed. The usefulness of an interneuron in the pathway of occasional vagal fibers to the striated muscle, if there presence is confirmed, is open for investigation.[134] Finally, the function of cholinesterase-positive junctions between striated muscle fibers is unknown.[27,28] They could serve to chemically couple striated muscle fibers during excitation.

Smooth Muscle Esophagus

There are at least four different potential mechanisms for the production of peristalsis in the smooth muscle esophagus:

(1) the central neural program sends sequential excitatory discharges to this region,[11,116]

(2) there is an intramural neural mechanism that can be excited to produce

peristalsis near the onset of vagal stimulation or intraluminal balloon distension—the "on-contraction,"[41,42,81,82,89,161]

(3) there is an intramural neural mechanism that can be excited to produce peristalsis onsetting after the vagal or balloon stimulus is terminated—the "off-response" or "off-contraction,"[42,78,80–82,89,161]

(4) there is some type of mechanism for myogenic propagation of a contraction.[39,52] It is not clear whether the repetitive propagating contraction produced by carbachol in the cat[44] is similar to the neurally mediated activity induced by balloon or vagal stimulation,[41,42] or is myogenic like that described in the opossum[52] or chicken.[39]

The use of simultaneous stimulation of all efferent and afferent fibers in the vagus nerves has led some to question the wisdom and validity of extrapolating results from these types of experiments to the control mechanism for primary and secondary peristalsis in the intact animal or human.[6,8,11] Similarly, the presence of a tetrodotoxin-insensitive propagating contraction in the esophagus of the heavily anaesthetized or agonal opossum,[52] or of contraction in the *in vitro* nerve-blocked, over-distended chicken esophagus[39] does not translate easily into a normal mechanism for peristalsis under ordinary circumstances. Therefore, controversy has arisen when results of these types of experiments are difficult to reconcile with those experiments where primary and secondary peristalsis are assessed in the intact animal.[6,8,11,12] Differences among species have compounded the confusion.

The controversy and confusion have been highlighted by four major questions: (1) Is final neurally mediated excitation of the muscle a direct "on-response," or is it an "off-response" following a period of muscle inhibition? (2) Do the centrally mediated vagal fibers exert a dominant coordinating control over peristalsis, or do they serve only to facilitate excitation of the intramural neurons within an intramural coordinating mechanism? (3) What is the mechanism of distal inhibition? At the central level is cessation of excitatory vagal discharges accompanied by firing of other vagal fibers destined to synapse on NANC inhibitory neurons? Within the intramural network, is inhibition due to activation of inhibitory NANC neurons to the muscle, neuronal inhibition of excitatory neurons, or a combination of these? (4) Are there myogenic coordinating mechanisms that take part in peristalsis and/or distal inhibition?

The "On-response" - "Off-response" Controversy.   The "off-response" has generated interest as a potential mechanism of excitation (and also coordination) of the peristaltic contraction under normal circumstances—that is, of primary and secondary peristalsis in the intact animal. However, most evidence to date favors direct muscle excitation by the intramural cholinergic neurons as the likely mechanism for muscle contraction during normal peristalsis. If so, this would dictate that coordination of the excitation, and therefore of the peristaltic contraction, is primarily due to sequencing and activation of the excitatory neurons, not a function of the "off-response" and its characteristics.

Evidence in support of direct cholinergic excitation of esophageal muscle is convincing. Elsewhere in the gut, muscle contraction occurs during stimulation and as a result of direct excitation of the muscle, usually via a cholinergic mechanism.[103] In the human, cat, and monkey, swallow-induced peristalsis is usually totally atropine sensitive and therefore cholinergic.[14,65] Furthermore, the contraction is augmented by cholinergic agonists and cholinesterase inhibition.[163,164] Even in the opossum, swallow-induced peristalsis has a significant cholinergic component,[165] although an atropine-resistant component remains.[165]

As shown in Figure 1-2, Dodds et al., using vagal stimulation with selected parameters, were able to demonstrate both a peristaltic "on-contraction" and a

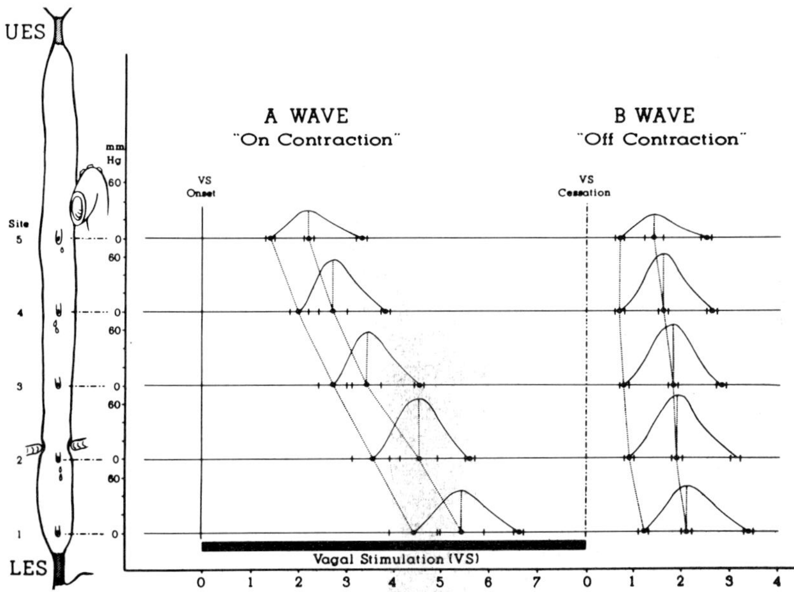

Fig. 1-2. Response of the opossum smooth muscle esophagus to vagal stimulation. The "on-contraction" (A wave) occurs shortly after the onset of stimulation, has a velocity similar to primary peristalsis, and is atropine sensitive. The "off-contraction" (B wave) appears after cessation of the stimulus, is atropine resistant, and has a propagation velocity much greater than normal peristalsis. Reprinted by permission from Dodds WJ, Christensen J, Dent J, et al.: Esophageal contractions induced by vagal stimulation in the opossum. Am J Physiol 235:E392–E401, 1978.

separate peristaltic "off-contraction" in the opossum[82] and cat.[81] In the opossum, stimulation at 1–5 Hz for 1 sec produced only the "on-contraction," while at stimulation greater than 20 Hz, only the "off-contraction" occurred. At frequencies between 5 and 20 Hz both contractions were often observed as long as the pulse train was longer than 2 sec. The apparent propagation velocity of the "on-contraction" resembled that of swallow-induced peristalsis while that of the "off-contraction" was much more rapid and corresponded to the off-response delays of serial muscle strips *in vitro.*[82] In experiments by others, where adequate vagal stimulation with parameters similar to those expected *in vivo* has produced a peristaltic contraction (freq < 8–10 Hz, pulse train duration < 3–4 sec), the velocity of the contraction has resembled that of swallow-induced peristalsis.[89,161] This is likely the case in the experiments of Mukhopadhyay and Weisbrodt,[161] and in many of the instances in the recent paper by Gidda et al.,[89] although neither confirmed the type of response being studied by adequately checking its sensitivity to atropine.[82] The "on-contraction" in both the opossum and the cat is completely abolished by atropine, while the "off-contraction" is atropine resistant.[81,82] In other experiments in opossum[4,79] and human tissues,[8,83] the "off-response" has been partially or totally atropine resistant, although in the cat, the "off-response" may at times be abolished by atropine.[44,84] Finally, the "off-response" should demonstrate a period of preceding inhibition. However, there is no firm evidence for vagal fibers that synapse directly on the inhibitory neurons in the esophageal body,[11] and during swallow-induced peristalsis electrical recording has not demonstrated clear membrane hyperpolarization before the excitatory depolarization and spiking occurs.

Therefore, at present, a cholinergic "on-contraction" seems the most likely and sensible explanation for excitation of esophageal smooth muscle during normal peristalsis in most species, including the human. If some degree of "off-response" excitation occurs, it would appear to be of much less importance.[41,42,65,165] There is no evidence that the "off-response" contributes to peristalsis in the human.

Central vs Local Neural Control of Peristalsis.   In the intact animal, the central program plays an important role in control of the smooth muscle peristalsis. In the baboon, Roman and Tiefenbach found different motor fibers that fire during primary or secondary peristalsis in a close temporal relationship with the sequential contractions along the striated and smooth muscle esophagus.[116] Afferent stimulation from an esophageal bolus increases the duration and frequency of the discharges but the experiment did not permit accurate assessment of the bolus effect on the progression velocity of the sequential discharges or the peristaltic contraction. In the sheep, both are slowed.[162] The importance of the central program is further illustrated in a careful series of experiments by Janssens.[8] In both the rhesus monkey and the opossum, peristalsis in the smooth muscle crossed a level of transection regardless of whether the ends were reanastomized, or were separated with deviation of the bolus. This was true of both primary and secondary peristalsis. In addition, secondary peristalsis induced by balloon distension below the level of transection could begin above the transection. Thus, with extrinsic nerves intact, continuity of the intramural mechanism is not an absolute requirement for primary or secondary peristalsis and the central program operates in the absence of afferent stimulation due to a bolus. This latter fact has been confirmed in the opossum, baboon, monkey, and human,[8,42,105,165] where passage of the bolus to the smooth muscle section has been prevented by abolition of striated muscle contraction with curare or succinylcholine. Peristalsis still occurred in the smooth muscle esophagus.

As in the striated muscle esophagus, it is tempting to assume that centrally programmed vagal fibers to the smooth muscle esophagus serve both an excitatory and, as a result, a coordinating role. That is, at each successive level the vagal influence is the main input to the excitatory cholinergic neurone, which then responds to produce a muscle contraction at that level. However, it is unlikely that the situation is quite so simple. The intramural mechanism is perfectly capable of producing neurally mediated peristalsis on its own in the absence of extrinsic vagal excitation,[41,42] or with experimental vagal stimulation that does not incorporate sequential excitation.[41,42,81,82,89,161] Therefore, the intramural neurons are themselves connected and programmed. As pointed out above, under the latter circumstances the cholinergic "on-contraction" most closely resembles swallow-induced peristalsis. The question still remains; How does the sequented vagal discharge interact with the local mechanism to produce normal primary and secondary peristalsis? The answer probably lies in those factors determining how and when the threshold for activation of the excitatory cholinergic neuron is reached. This would be determined by both excitatory and inhibitory influences.

There are at least three excitatory inputs to the intramural cholinergic neuron: interneurons in the local network, central vagal fibers, and local sensory neurons. In the baboon, Roman and Tieffenbach noted that the strength of stimulus required to excite peristalsis in the smooth muscle esophagus on stimulation of the cut end of the vagus was greater than that present when recording from vagal fibers presumably destined to activate the distal esophagus.[42,116] Furthermore, in the cat, subliminal local and vagal stimuli, either alone insufficient to induce peristaltic activity, added to produce a coordinated contraction.[42] This led these authors and others to suggest that the excitatory neuron may frequently require more than one input to reach threshold and induce a contraction.[6,11,42,116] The inability of a swallow to always induce primary peristalsis without a bolus is one example of this phenomenon. With a bolus, either central or local sensory reinforcement would facilitate the vagal excitation of the cholinergic neurone.[11,116] This reinforcement would be even more positive if the vagal influence or local sensory influence also activated the intramural peristaltic mechanism rather than just facilitated the excitation at each local level.[116] Furthermore, since the muscle probably has receptors sensitive to contraction, the contraction itself could be a source of sensory input, varying with the magnitude of contraction.[110]

Janssens' experiments are of interest in this regard.[8] After a delay, peristalsis appeared below the level of transection even without propulsion of a bolus into the distal segment. The delay could represent the extra time required for vagal impulses alone to activate the excitatory neuron in the absence of reinforcement from the bolus or from activity within the intramural neural network. It is not clear whether some variation on this theme will explain the delay at the striated muscle–smooth muscle junction after atropine administration in the human.[65]

Roman and Tieffenbach proposed that for primary peristalsis the central mechanism dictated sequential excitation and therefore coordination of peristalsis with added sensory reinforcement from the bolus; while for secondary peristalsis the intramural mechanism was the determining mechanism of excitation and coordination, with the central discharges facilitating the plexus activity.[116] There is a potential alternative relationship between the central and peripheral mechanism during primary peristalsis. Since we consider the same central program to function for both primary and secondary peristalsis, it may be justified to consider that the peripheral intramural program does so as well; that is, for both primary and secondary peristalsis within the smooth muscle the peripheral mechanism is the fundamental coordinating mechanism once excited to activity. Under these circumstances, the central mechanism would function to initiate the peripheral mechanism at least proximally, to facilitate the activation of excitatory neurons as sequential vagal excitation passed along the esophagus in tandem with that of the peripheral mechanism, and to modulate other characteristics of the peripheral program such as the contraction amplitude, duration, and velocity of propagation. Some reflection of this central effect independent of sensory feedback from a bolus is seen during raised intra-abdominal pressure, which increases the contraction amplitude and duration and slows the peristaltic progression.[116] Insight into a possible mechanism for the central program to alter propagation velocity may be present in the experiments of Gidda et al.[89] These authors described a marked effect of different vagal stimulus parameters on the velocity and direction of the propagated contraction in the smooth muscle esophagus. They were, of course, stimulating all fibers simultaneously. Some of the changes were very noticeable when the stimulus current intensity was submaximal. The findings would be pertinent if these studies were mainly of the "on-contraction" rather than the "off-contraction." Unfortunately, as pointed out above, the two types of contractions were not identified by their differential sensitivity to atropine.

The Mechanisms for Distal Inhibition. The potential local mechanisms for distal inhibition within the smooth muscle esophagus have been described above. Both activation of inhibitory neurons to the muscle and neuronal inhibition of excitatory neurons can operate within the esophageal body and LES. Daniel et al. have demonstrated a third potential mechanism in the opossum. They found a tetrodotoxin-insensitive LES relaxation and proposed a role of prostaglandins and the "glial-like" interstitial cells in this mechanism.[150] These latter findings and their functional importance have not been assessed in humans.

Most controversy has arisen over the mechanism of deglutitive inhibition. Repetitive swallowing inhibits all esophageal activity until after the last swallow.[8,14,167] A second swallow during the progression of peristalsis induced by a pervious swallow temporarily inhibits central excitation to the striated muscle esophagus.[11,14,105] In the smooth muscle esophagus, the ongoing contraction is not inhibited, but further progression of the first swallow-induced contraction is prevented.[8,14,167,168] Janssens has argued that since the intramural mechanism is already activated by the first swallow, cessation of active vagal excitation cannot account for disappearance of the distal contraction, and therefore vagally mediated active inhibition must be present.[8] However, such a vagal firing pattern to the esophageal body has not yet been identified. Furthermore, if passage of the peristaltic wave along the esophagus requires adequate excitation of the cholinergic neuron by integration of more than one input, absence of one or more of these inputs (e.g., vagal excitation) could then prevent distal progression of the waves. Further experimentation is required to resolve the issue. The effect of deglutitive inhibition lasts for up to 15–20 sec, as evidenced by decreased amplitude of a subsequent muscle contraction within this time period.[167,168] Although Meyer et al. suggested the diminished response represents muscle refractoriness,[167] this is not established. It is just as possible that either central or peripheral neural mechanisms are less active.

Myogenic Contribution to Peristalsis. The suggestion has been made that peristalsis can occur in the smooth muscle esophagus independent of an intrinsic or extrinsic neural coordinating mechanism.[52] However, the role of such a mechanism in normal primary or secondary peristalsis has not been established. As discussed above, there are potential morphological and physiological characteristics of the smooth muscle (e.g., cell–cell contacts and oscillator properties) that provide a basis for a coordinated propagating myogenic contraction under the proper conditions of excitation. A single peristaltic contraction would be viewed as the activation of a series of connected "excitable oscillators," with the conditions of excitation dictating a single or "one-shot" oscillation.[52] Whether an extrinsic or intrinsic neural wave of excitation along the esophagus could normally serve to activate such a myogenic mechanism is yet to be determined.

Since the longitudinal and circular muscle layers are connected in the apolar-screw systems of fiber bundles, a potential myogenic mechanism is present to coordinate activity between the two muscle layers. The longitudinal layer contracts in advance of the circular layer in a number of species including the human.[41,42,169] Myogenic coupling of more proximal external muscle cells of the longitudinal layer with more distal circularly oriented cells of the same fiber bundle would produce this result.

LES

Mechanisms for control of the LES have been discussed in preceding sections. Resting tone is due to a combination of myogenic properties and active tonic neural excitation, modulated by a complex interaction of numerous other neurohumoral and hormonal factors. Swallow-induced inhibition includes both active inhibition of the muscle and cessation of tonic neural excitation. The contraction of the LES at the end of a peristaltic sequence has an active excitatory component. However, this is the one occasion where the conditions for an "off-response" contribution occur—that is, preceding active inhibition of the muscle followed by some active cholinergic excitation.

The anatomy of the LES provides a potential explanation for some of the radial assymetry in the LES pressure profile. The thicker left-lateral portion of the LES contains gastric string fibers[26] and is also the location of highest pressure.[170] This portion of the LES also shows greater decrease in pressure with atropine. Richardson and Welch suggest that these findings are due to greater cholinergic sensitivity of the gastric muscle fibers.[171]

REFERENCES

1. Inglefinger FJ: Esophageal motility. Physiol Rev 38:533–584, 1958.
2. Winship DH, Zboralske FF, Weber WN, Soergel KH: Esophagus in rumination. Am J Physiol 207:1189–1194, 1964.
3. Palmer ED: Disorders of the cricopharyngeus muscle: a review. Gastroenterology 71:510–519, 1976.
4. Christensen J: Effects of drugs on esophageal motility. Arch Int Med 136:532–537, 1976.
5. Weisbrodt NW: Neuromuscular organization of esophageal and pharyngeal motility. Arch Int Med 136:524–531, 1976.
6. Diamant NE, El-Sharkawy TY: Neural control of esophageal peristalsis. A conceptual analysis. Gastroenterology 72:546–556, 1977.

7. Snape WJ Jr.,Cohen S: Control of esophageal and lower esophageal sphincter function: neurohumoral and myogenic factors. Front Gastrointest Res 3:76–94, 1978.
8. Janssens J: The Peristaltic Mechanism of the Esophagus. Acco, Leuven, 1978.
9. Roed-Petersen K: The pharyngoesophageal sphincter. A review of the literature. Dan Med Bull 26:275–281, 1979.
10. Rozé C; Régulation de la motricité oesophagienne et gastrique. Aspects physiologiques et pharmacologiques récents (Première partie: Oesophage). Gastroenterol Clin Biol 4:486–496, 1980.
11. Roman C, Gonella J: Extrinsic control of digestive tract motility. In Johnson LR (ed): Physiology of the Digestive Tract, Raven Press, New York, 1981:289–333.
12. Goyal RK, Cobb BW: Motility of the pharynx, esophagus, and esophageal sphincters. In Johnson LR (ed): Physiology of the Digestive Tract, Raven Press, New York, 1981:359–391.
13. Dent J: What's new in the esophagus. Dig Dis Sci 26:161–173, 1981.
14. Vantrappen G, Hellemans J: Diseases of the Esophagus, Springer-Verlag, New York, 1974.
15. Lerche W: The esophagus and pharynx in action. A study of structure in relation to function. Charles C Thomas, Springfield, 1950.
16. Kaufmann P, Lierse W, Stark K, Stelzner F: Die muskelanordnung in der speiserohre. Ergebn Anat Entwickl-Gesch 40:H3, 1968.
17. Botha GSM: The Gastro–Oesophageal Junction. Clinical Applications to Oesophageal and Gastric Surgery. J. and A. Churchill, London, 1962.
18. Brash JC (ed): Cunningham's Textbook of Anatomy, Oxford, London, 1951.
19. Zaino C, Jacobson HG, Lepow H, Ozturk CH: The Pharyngo–Esophageal Sphincter. Charles C Thomas, Springfield, 1970.
20. Andrew BL: The nervous control of the cervical esophagus of the rat during swallowing. J Physiol (Lond) 134:729–740, 1956.
21. Inouye T: Electromyographic investigation of the esophagus in animals. Laryngoscope 76:1502–1519, 1966.
22. Car A, Roman C: L'activité spontanée du sphincter oesophagien supérieur chez le mouton. Ses variations au cours de la déglutition et de la rumination. J Physiol (Paris) 62:505–511, 1970.
23. Asoh R, Goyal RK: Manometry and electromyography of the upper esophageal sphincter in the opossum. Gastroenterology 74:514–520, 1978.
24. Monges H, Sladucci J, Roman C: Étude électromyographique de la contraction esophagienne chez l'homme normal. Arch Fr Mal App Digestif 57:545–560, 1968.
25. Rohen J: Ülber den function ellen zusammenhang zurschen glatter und quergestreifter muskulatur im menschlichen oesophagus (oesophagustudien I). Anat Anz 102:210–216, 1955.
26. Liebermann-Meffert D, Allgower M, Schmid P, Blum AL: Muscular equivalent of the lower esophageal sphincter. Gastroenterology 76:31–38, 1979.
27. Gruber H: Uber stukter und innervation der quergestreiften muskulatur des oesophagus der ratte. Zeitsch fur Zellforschung 91:236–247, 1968.
28. Floyd K: Cholinesterase activity in sheep esophageal muscle. J Anat 116:357–373, 1973.
29. Hess A: Vertebrate slow muscle fibers. Physiol Rev 50:40–62, 1970.
30. Diamant NE: In-vitro characteristics of dog esophageal striated muscle. Rendic R Gastroenterol 3:138, 1971.
31. Floyd K, Morrison JFB: The mechanical properties of esophageal striated muscle in the cat and sheep. J Physiol (Lond) 248:717–724, 1975.

32. Jackson AJ: The spiral constrictor of the gastroesophageal junction. Am J Anat 151:265–269, 1978.
33. Friedland GO: Historical review of the changing concepts of lower esophageal anatomy: 430 B.C.–1977. Am J Roentgenol 131:373–386, 1978.
34. Cassella RR, Ellis FJ Jr, Brown AL Jr: Fine-structure changes in achalasia of the esophagus. II. Esophageal smooth muscle. Am J Pathol 46:467–475, 1965.
35. Daniel EE, Bowes KL, Duchon G: The structural basis for control of gastrointestinal motility in man. In Vantrappen G (ed): Proceedings of the Fifth International Symposium on Gastrointestinal Motility, Typoff-Press, Herentals, 1975:142–151.
36. Harman JW, O'Hegarty MT, Byrnes CK: The ultrastructure of human smooth muscle. 1. Studies of cell surface and connections in normal and achalasia esophageal smooth muscle. Exp Mol Pathol 1:204–228, 1962.
37. Gonella J, Condamin M, Roman C: Relation between the amount of nexuses in digestive smooth muscle and the amplitude of spikes recorded by extracellular electrodes. In Vantrappen G (ed): Proceedings of the Fifth International Symposium on Gastrointestinal Motility, Typoff-Press, Herentals, 1975:152–157.
38. Bortoff A: Digestion: motility. Annu Rev Physiol 34:261–290, 1972.
39. Bartlet AL: Myogenic peristalsis in isolated preparations of chicken esophagus. Br J Pharmacol 48:36–47, 1973.
40. Weisbrodt NW, Christensen J: Gradients of contractions in the opossum esophagus. Gastroenterology 62:1159–1166, 1972.
41. Roman C, Tieffenbach L: Electrical activity of esophageal smooth muscle in vagotomized and anesthetized cats. J Physiol (Paris) 63:733–762, 1971.
42. Tieffenbach L, Roman C: The role of extrinsic vagal innervation in the motility of the smooth-muscled portion of the esophagus: electromyographic study in the cat and the baboon. J Physiol (Paris) 64:193–226, 1972.
43. Chan WW-L, Diamant NE: Electrical off-response of cat esophageal smooth muscle: an analogue simulation. Am J Physiol 230:233–238, 1976.
44. El-Sharkawy TY, Diamant NE: Contraction patterns of esophageal circular smooth muscle induced by cholinergic excitation. Gastroenterology 70:111 (abstr), 1976.
45. Nelson DO, Mangel AW: Acetylcholine induced slow-waves in cat esophageal smooth muscle. Gen Pharmacol 10:19–20, 1979.
46. Sarna SK: Relaxation oscillators. In Duthie HL (ed): Gastrointestinal Motility in Health and Disease, MTP Press, Lancaster, 1978:659–668.
47. Christensen J, Iskandarani M: Neuromuscular functions in esophageal smooth muscle of opossums as differently affected by veratrum alkaloids. Gastroenterology 81:866–871, 1981.
48. Diamant NE, Chan WW-L: The electrical off-response of cat circular esophageal smooth muscle: the effect of stimulus frequency on its timing. In Vantrappen G (ed): Proceedings of the Fifth International Symposium on Gastrointestinal Motility, Typoff-Press, Herentals, 1975:158–163.
49. Schulze K, Conklin J, Christensen J: A potassium gradient in smooth muscle segment of the opossum esophagus. Am J Physiol 223:E270–E273, 1977.
50. Christensen J, Arthur C, Conklin J: Some determinants of latency of off-response to electrical field stimulation in circular layer of smooth muscle of opossum esophagus. Gastroenterology 77:677–681, 1979.
51. Dektor DL, Ryan JP: Trans membrane voltage of oppossum esophageal smooth muscle and its response to electrical stimulation of intrinsic nerves. Gastroenterology 82:301–308, 1982.

52. Sarna SK, Daniel EE, Waterfall WE: Myogenic and neural control systems for esophageal motility. Gastroenterology 73:1345–1352, 1977.
53. Christensen J: Pharmacologic identification of the lower esophageal sphincter. J Clin Invest 49:681–691, 1970.
54. Lipshutz W, Cohen S: Physiological determinants of lower esophageal sphincter function. Gastroenterology 61:16–24, 1971.
55. Christensen J, Conklin JL, Freeman BW: Physiologic specialization at esophagogastric junction in three species. Am J Physiol 225:1265–1270, 1973.
56. Christensen J, Freeman BW, Miller JK: Some physiological characteristics of the esophagogastric junction in the opossum. Gastroenterology 64:1119–1125, 1973.
57. El-Sharkawy TY, Chan WW-L, Diamant NE: Neural mechanism of lower esophageal sphincter relaxation: a pharmacological analysis. In Vantrappen G (ed): Proceedings of the Fifth International Symposium on Gastrointestinal Motility, Typoff-Press, Herentals, 1975:176.
58. Goyal RK, Rattan S: Genesis of basal sphincter pressure: effect of tetrodotoxin on lower esophageal sphincter pressure on opossum in vivo. Gastroenterology 71:62–67, 1976.
59. DeCarle DJ, Szabo AC, Christensen J: Temperature dependence of responses of esophageal smooth muscle to electrical field stimulation. Am J Physiol 232:E432–E436, 1977.
60. DeCarle DJ, Christensen J, Szabo AC, Templeman DC, McKinley DR: Calcium dependence of neuromuscular events in esophageal smooth muscle of the opossum. Am J Physiol 232:E547–E552, 1977.
61. Mukhopadhyay AK, Kunneman M: Effect of KCL depolarization on and Ca^{++} sensitivity of esophageal smooth muscle Gastroenterology 76:1206 (abstr), 1979.
62. Weisbrodt NW, Tague LL: Relationships between contractile and metabolic activities in esophageal muscle. In Christensen J (ed): Gastrointestinal Motility, Raven Press, New York, 1980:51–57.
63. Biancani P, Zabinski M, Kerstein M, Behar J: Lower esophageal sphincter mechanics: anatomic and physiologic relationships of the esophagogastric junction of cat. Gastroenterology 82:468–475, 1982.
64. Daniel EE, Taylor GS, Holman ME: The myogenic basis of active tension in the lower esophageal sphincter. Gastroenterology 70:874 (abstr), 1976.
65. Dodds WJ, Dent J, Hogan WJ, Arndorfer RC: Effect of atropine on esophageal motor function in humans. Am J Physiol 240:G290–G296, 1981.
66. Price LM, El-Sharkawy TY, Mui HY, Diamant NE: Effect of bilateral cervical vagotomy on balloon-induced lower esophageal sphincter relaxation in the dog. Gastroenterology 77:324–329, 1979.
67. Richter JE, Sinar DR, Cordova CM, Castell DO: Calcium antagonists-potent inhibitors of esophageal peristalsis. Z Gastroenterologie 19:443 (abstr), 1981.
68. Rattan S, Goyal RK: Influence of verapamil on the stimulated lower esophageal sphincter pressure. Gastroenterology 74:1082 (abstr), 1978.
69. Dent J, Dodds WJ, Arndorfer RC: Effect of nitroprusside and verapamil on esophageal smooth muscle contractility in the opossum. Gastroenterology 74:1119 (abstr), 1978.
70. Golenhofen K: Theory of p and t systems for calcium activation in smooth muscle. In Bulbring E, Sherba MF (eds): Physiology of Smooth Muscle, Raven Press, New York, 1976:197–202.
71. Snyder N, Hughes W: Basal and calcium-stimulated gastroesophageal sphincter pressure in patients with Zollinger-Ellison syndrome. Gastroenterology 72:1240–1243, 1977.
72. Danielides IC, Mellow MH: Effect of acute hypercalcemia on human esophageal motility. Gastroenterology 74:1115–1119, 1978.

73. Bortolotti M, Labo G: Clinical and manometric effects of nifedipine in patients with esophageal achalasia. Gastroenterology 80:39–44, 1981.

74. Arimori M, Code DF, Schlegel JF, Sturm RE: Electrical activity of the canine esophagus and gastroesophageal sphincter: its relation to intraluminal pressure and movement of material. Am J Dig Dis 15:191–208, 1970.

75. Asoh R, Goyal RK: Electrical activity of the opossum lower esophageal sphincter in vivo. Gastroenterology 74:835–840, 1978.

76. Ellis FG, Kauntze R, Trounce JR: The innervation of the cardia and lower esophagus in man. Br J Surg 47:466–472, 1960.

77. Christensen J, Daniel EE: Electric and motor effects of autonomic drugs on longitudinal esophageal smooth muscle. Am J Physiol 211:387–394, 1966.

78. Christensen J, Lund GF: Esophageal responses to distension and electrical stimulation. J Clin Invest 48:408–419, 1969.

79. Lund GF, Christensen J: Electrical stimulation of esophageal smooth muscle and effects of antagonists. Am J Physiol 1369–1374, 1969.

80. Christensen J: Patterns and origin of some esophageal responses to stretch and electrical stimulation. Gastroenterology 59:909–916, 1970.

81. Dodds WJ, Steff JJ, Stewart ET, Hogan WT, Arndorfer RC, Cohen EB: Responses of feline esophagus to cervical vagal stimulation. Am J Physiol 235:E63–E73, 1978.

82. Dodds WJ, Christensen J, Dent J, Wood JD, Arndorfer RC: Esophageal contractions induced by vagal stimulation in the opossum. Am J Physiol 235:E392–E401, 1978.

83. Burleigh DE: The effects of drugs and electrical field stimulation on the human lower oesophageal sphincter. Arch Int Pharmacodyn 340:169–176, 1979.

84. DeCarle DJ, Templeman DL, Christensen J: The cat esophagus: responses of the circular layer of smooth muscle from the body to electrical field stimulation. In Duthie HL (ed): Gastrointestinal Motility in Health and Disease, MTP Press, Lancaster, 1978:513–521.

85. Diamant NE, El-Sharkawy TY: The "on-response" contraction in esophageal circular smooth muscle. Clin Res 23:620 (abstr), 1975.

86. Cohen S, Green F: The mechanics of esophageal muscle contraction. Evidence of an inotropic effect of gastrin. J Clin Invest 52:2029–2040, 1973.

87. Christensen J, Dons RF: Regional variations in response of cat esophageal muscle to stimulation with drugs. J Pharmacol Exp Ther 161:55–58, 1968.

88. Cohen S: Force velocity characteristics of oesophageal muscle: interaction of isoproterenol and calcium. Europ J Clin Invest 5:259–265, 1975.

89. Gidda JS, Cobb BW, Goyal RK: Modulation of esophageal peristalsis by vagal efferent stimulation in opossum. J Clin Invest 68:1411–1419, 1981.

90. Dodds WJ, Hogan WJ, Reid DP, Stewart ET, Arndorfer RC: A comparison between primary esophageal peristalsis following wet and dry swallows. J Appl Physiol 35:851–857, 1973.

91. Biancani P, Zabinski MP, Behar J: Pressure, tension, and force of closure of the human lower esophageal sphincter and esophagus. J Clin Invest 56:476–483, 1975.

92. Humphries TJ, Castell DO: Pressure profile of esophageal peristalsis in normal humans as measured by direct intraesophageal transducers. Dig Dis 22:641–645, 1977.

93. Cohen S, Green F: Force–velocity characteristics of esophageal muscle: effect of acetylcholine and norephinephrine. Am J Physiol 226:1250–1256, 1974.

94. Diamant NE: Electrical activity of the cat smooth muscle esophagus: a study of hyperpolarizing responses. In Daniel EE (ed): Proceedings of the Fourth International Symposium on Gastroentestinal Motility, Mitchell Press, Vancouver, 1974:593–605.

95. Christensen J, Lund GF: Atropine excitation of esophageal smooth muscle. J Pharmacol Exp Ther 163:287–289, 1968.
96. Christensen J, Daniel EE: Effects of some autonomic drugs on circular esophageal smooth muscle. J Pharmacol Exp Ther 159:243–249, 1968.
97. Kramer P, Ingelfinger FJ: I. Motility of the human esophagus in control subjects and in patients with esophageal disorders. Am J Med 7:168–173, 1949.
98. Creamer B, Schlegel J: Motor responses of the esophagus to distension. J Appl Physiol 10:498–504, 1957.
99. Winship DH, Zboralske FF: The esophageal propulsice force: esophageal response to acute obstruction. J Clin Invest 46:1391–1401, 1967.
100. Goyal RK, Gidds JS: Relation between electrical and mechanical activity in esophageal smooth muscle. Am J Physiol 240:G305–G311, 1981.
101. Doty RW: Neural organization of deglutition. In Code CF (ed): Handbook of Physiology, Sec 6, Alimentary Canal; Vol 4, American Physiological Society, Washington, D.C., 1968:1861–1902.
102. Goyal RK, Rattan S: Neurohumoral, hormonal, and drug receptors for the lower esophageal sphincter. Gastroenterology 74:598–619, 1978.
103. Gershon MD, Erde SM: The nervous system of the gut, Gastroenterology 80:1571–1594, 1981.
104. Roze C: Neurohumoral control of gastrointestinal motility. Reprod Nutr Develop 20:1125–1141, 1980.
105. Jean A: Localization and activity of medullary swallowing neurons. J Physiol (Paris) 64:227–268, 1972.
106. Sumi T: Role of pontine reticular formation in the neural organization of deglutition. Jap J Physiol 22:295–314, 1972.
107. Niel JP, Gonella J, Roman C: Localization par la technique de marquage á la péroxydase des corps cellulaires des neurones ortho et parasympathiques innervant le sphincter oesophagièn inférieur du chat. J Physiol (Paris) 76:591–599, 1980.
108. Jean A: Controle bulbaire de la deglutition et de la motricite oesophagienne. PhD thesis, Faculty of Sciences, Marseille, 1978.
109. Pommerenke WT: A study of the sensory areas eliciting the swallowing reflex. Am J Physiol 84:36–41, 1928.
110. Nei N: Anatomical arrangement and electrophysiolical properties of sensitive vagal neurones in the cat. Exp Brain Res 11:465–479, 1970.
111. Lemere F: Innervation of the larynx. Anat Rec 54:389–407, 1932.
112. Lund WS, Adrian GM: The motor nerve supply of the cricopharyngeal sphincter. Ann Otol 73:599–612, 1964.
113. Roman C, Car A: Deglutition et contractions oesophagiennes reflexes obtenus par la stimulation des nerfs vagues et la larynge superieur. Exp Brain Res 11:48–74, 1970.
114. Freiman J, El-Sharkawy TY, Diamant NE: Effect of bilateral vagosympathetic nerve blockade on response of the dog upper esophageal sphincter (UES) to intraesophageal distension and acid. Gastroenterology 81:78–84, 1981.
115. Miolan JP, Roman C: Activite des fibres vagales efferentes destinees a la musculature lisse du cardia du chien. J Physiol (Paris) 74:709–723, 1978.
116. Roman C, Tieffenbach L: Enreqistrement de l'activité unitaire des fibres motrices vagales destinées à l'oesophage du babouin. J Physiol (Paris) 64:479–506, 1972.
117. Hwang K, Grossman MI, Ivy AC: Nervous control of the cervical esophagus. Am J Physiol 154:343–357, 1948.
118. Jennewein HM, Hummelt H, Meyer U, Siewert R, Koch A, Waldek F: The effect of vagotomy on the resting pressure and reactivity of the LES in man and dog. In

Vantrappen G (ed): Proceedings of the Fifth International Symposium on Gastrointestinal Motility, Typoff-Press, Herentals, 1975:186–189.
119. Rattan S, Goyal RK: Neural control of the lower esophageal sphincter. Influence of the vagus nerves. J Clin Invest 55:899–906, 1974.
120. Carveth SW, Schlegel JF, Code CF, Ellis FH Jr: Esophageal motility after vagotomy, phrenicotomy, myotomy, and myomectomy in dogs. Surg Gynecol Obstet 114:31–42, 1962.
121. Greenwood RK, Schlegel JF, Code CF, Ellis FH, Jr: The effect of sympathectomy, vagotomy and esophageal interruption on the canine gastroesophageal sphincter. Thorax 17:310–319, 1962.
122. Cohen S, Kravitz JJ, Snape WJ Jr: Vagal control of lower esophageal sphincter function. In Duthie HL (ed): Gastrointestinal motility in Health and Disease, MTP Press, Lancaster, 1978:505–512.
123. Higgs RH, Castell DO: The effect of truncal vagotomy on lower esophageal sphincter pressure and response to cholinergic stimulation. Proc Soc Exp Biol Med 153:379–382, 1976.
124. Angorn IB, Dimopoulos G, Hegarty MM, Moshall MG: The effect of vagotomy on the lower esophageal sphincter: a manometric study. Br J Surg 64:466–469, 1977.
125. Csendes A, Oster M, Moller J, Brandsborg O, Brandsborg M, Amdrup E: The effect of extrinsic denervation of the lower part of the esophagus on resting and cholinergic stimulated gastroesophageal sphincter in man. Surg Gynecol Obstet 148:375–379, 1979.
126. Temple JG, Goodall RJR, Hay DJ, Miller D: Effect of highly selective vagotomy upon the lower oesophageal sphincter. Gut 22:368–370, 1981.
127. Crispin JS, McIver DK, Lind JF: Manometric study of the effect of vagotomy on the gastro-oesophageal sphincter. Can J Surg 10:299–303, 1967.
128. Csendes A, Oster M, Brandsborg O. Moller JT, Overgaard H, Brandsborg M, Funch-Jensen P, Amdrup E: The effect of vagotomy on human gastroesophageal sphincter pressure in the resting state and following increases in intra-abdominal pressure. Surgery 85:419–424, 1979.
129. Fournet J, Snape WJ Jr, Cohen S: Sympathetic control of lower esophageal sphincter function in the cat. Action of direct cervical and splanchnic nerve stimulation. J Clin Invest 63:562–570, 1979.
130. Gonella J, Niel JP, Roman C: Sympathetic control of lower oesophageal sphincter motility in the cat. J Physiol (Lond) 287:177–190, 1979.
131. Di Marino AJ, Cohen S: The adrenergic control of lower esophageal sphincter function. J Clin Invest 52:2264–2271, 1973.
132. Thorpe JAC: Effect of propanalol on the lower esophageal sphincter in man. Curr Med Res Opin 7:91–95, 1980.
133. Gonella J, Niel JP, Roman C: Mechanism of the noradrenergic motor control on the lower esophageal sphincter in the cat. J Physiol (Lond) 306:251–260, 1980.
134. Toyama T, Yokoyama I, Nishi K: Effects of hexamethonium and other ganglionic blocking agents on electrical activity of the esophagus induced by vagal stimulation in the dog. Eur J Pharmacol 31:63–71, 1975.
135. Bartlett AL: The effect of vagal stimulation and eserine on isolated guinea-pig oesophagus. Q J Exp Physiol 53:170–174, 1968.
136. Kantrowitz PA, Siegel CI, Hendrix TR: Differences in motility of the upper and lower esophagus in man and its alteration by atropine. Bull Johns Hopkins Hosp 118:476–491, 1966.
137. Yamamoto T: Histologic studies on the innervation of the esophagus in Formosan macaque. Arch Hist Jap 18:545–564, 1960.

138. Cecio A, Califano G: Neurohistological observations on the oesophageal innervation of rabbit. Z Zellforsch 83:30–39, 1967.

139. Nonidez JF: Afferent nerve endings in the ganglia of the intermuscular plexus of the dog oesophagus. J Comp Neurol 85:177–189, 1946.

140. Mann CV, Code CF, Schlegel JF, Ellis FH Jr: Intrinsic mechanisms controlling the mammalian gastro-oesophageal sphincter deprived of extrinsic nerve supply. Thorax 23:634–639, 1968.

141. Jacobowitz P, Nemir P Jr: The autonomic innervation of the esophagus of the dog. J Thorac Cardiovasc Surg 58:678–684, 1969.

142. Baumgarten HG, Lange W: Adrenergic innervation of the oesophagus in the cat (felix domestica) and rhesus monkey (macaccus rhesus). Z Zellforsch 95:529–545, 1969.

143. Nishimina T, Takasu T: The adrenergic innervation in the esophagus and respiratory tract of the rabbit. Acta Otolaryngol 67:444–452, 1969.

144. Von Jabonero V: Mikroskopische studien uber die innervation des verdauungstraktes. I. Osophagus. Acta Neuroveg 17:308–353, 1958.

145. Hirst GDS, Holman ME, McKirdy HC: Two descending nerve pathways activated by distension of guinea-pig small intestine. J Physiol (Lond) 244:113–127, 1975.

146. Wood JD: Physiology of the enteric nervous system. In Johnson LR (ed): Physiology of the Gastrointestinal Tract, Raven Press, New York, 1981:1–37.

147. Gonella J, Niel JP, Roman C: Vagal control of lower esophageal sphincter motility in the cat. J Physiol (Lond) 273:647–664, 1977.

148. Goyal RK, Rattan S: Neurohumoral, hormonal, and drug receptors for the lower esophageal sphincter. Gastroenterology 74:598–619, 1978.

149. Burnstock G: Ultrastructure of autonomic nerves and neuroeffector junctions; analysis of drug action. In Daniel EE, Paton DM (eds): Methods in Pharmacology, Vol 3, Smooth Muscle, Plenum Press, New York, 1975:113–137.

150. Daniel EE, Sarna S, Crankshaw J: Mechanism of tetrodotoxin-insensitive relaxation of opossum lower oesophageal sphincter. In Duthie HL (ed): Gastrointestinal Motility in Health and Disease, MTP Press, Lancaster, 1978:525–535.

151. Daniel EE, Crankshaw J, Sarna S: Prostaglandins and tetrodotoxin-insensitive relaxation of opossum lower esophageal sphincter. Am J Physiol 235:E153–E172, 1979.

152. Harding R, Titchen DA: Chemosensitive vagal endings in the oesophagus of the cat. J Physiol (Lond) 247:52–53P, 1979.

153. Waterfall WE, Lewis TD, Fox JET, Daniel EE: pH as a determinant of lower esophageal sphincter tone. Gastroenterology 76:1267 (abstr), 1979.

154. Winship DH, Viegas de Andrade SR, Zboralske FF: Influence of bolus temperature on human esophageal motor function. J Clin Invest 49:243–250, 1970.

155. Uddman R, Alumets J, Hakanson R, Sundler F, Walles B: Peptidergic (enkephalin) innervation of the mammalian esophagus. Gastroenterology 78:732–737, 1980.

156. Winans CS: The pharyngoesophageal closure mechanism: a manometric study. Gastroenterology 63:768–777, 1972.

157. Welch RW, Luckmann K, Ricks PM, Drake ST, Gates GA: Manometry of the upper esophageal sphincter and its alteration in laryngectomy. J Clin Invest 63:1036–1041, 1979.

158. Goyal RK, Sangree MH, Hersh T: Pressure inversion point at the upper high pressure zone and its genesis. Gastroenterology 59:754–759, 1970.

159. Gerhardt DC, Shuck TJ, Bordeaux RA, Winship DH: Human upper esophageal sphincter. Response to volume, osmotic and acid stimuli. Gastroenterology 75:268–274, 1978.

160. Longhi EH, Jordan PH Jr: Necessity of a bolus for propagation of primary peristalsis in the canine esophagus. Am J Physiol 220:609–612, 1971.

161. Mukhopadhyay AK, Weisbrodt NW: Neural organization of esophageal peristalsis: role of vagus nerve. Gastroenterology 68:444–447, 1975.
162. Roman C: Controle nerveux du peristaltisme oesophagien. J Physiol (Paris) 58:79–108, 1966.
163. Hollis JB, Castell DO: Effects of cholinergic stimulation on human esophageal peristalsis. J Appl Physiol 40:40–43, 1976.
164. Humphries TJ, Castell DO: Effect of oral bethanecol on parameters of esophageal peristalsis. Dig Dis Sci 26:129–132, 1981.
165. Dodds WJ, Christensen J, Dent J, Arndorfer RC, Wood JD: Pharmacologic investigation of primary peristalsis in smooth muscle portion of opossum esophagus. Am J Physiol 237:E561–E566, 1979.
166. Dodds WJ, Hogan WS, Stewart ET, Stef JJ, Arndorfer RC: Effects of intra-abdominal pressure on esophageal peristalsis. J Appl Physiol 37:378–383, 1974.
167. Meyer GW, Gerhardt DC, Castell DO: Human esophageal response to rapid swallowing: muscle refractory period or neural inhibition? Am J Physiol 241:G129–G136, 1981.
168. Ask P, Tibbling L: Effect of time interval between swallows on esophageal peristalsis. Am J Physiol 238:G485–G490, 1980.
169. Bortolotti M, Labo G, Bragaglia RB, Mattioli S, Possati L: Electromyographic study in diffuse esophageal spasm and achalasia. In Weinbeck M (ed): Eighth International Symposium on Gastrointestinal Motility, Koenigstein, 1981 (In Press).
170. Winans, CS: Manometric asymmetry of the lower esophageal high pressure zone. Am J Dig Dis 22:348–354, 1977.
171. Richardson BJ, Welch RW: Differential effect of atropine on rightward and leftward lower esophageal sphincter pressure. Gastroenterology 81:85–89, 1981.

2 Esophageal Pharmacology

Konrad Schulze-Delrieu

INTRODUCTION

Esophageal pharmacology[1,2] is a young discipline that is concerned with the effect of drugs and biologic agents on esophageal functions. Rapid and irreversible transport of ingested material from the pharynx to the stomach is the main function of the esophagus. Most nonmalignant diseases of the esophagus originate in the motor apparatus of the distal esophagus.[3,4] Accordingly, most studies have attempted to define the role of various agents on esophageal motor functions, on esophageal smooth muscle, and on the lower esophageal sphincter.[5] Such studies have rapidly expanded the understanding of esophageal drug receptors and have led to the introduction of one conventional cholinergic agent (bethanechol) and another that has recently been developed (metoclopramide) into the treatment of gastroesophageal reflux.[6] Progress has been fast because esophageal manometry has provided a simple tool to obtain quantitative data on esophageal motor functions. The task of defining drug actions has also been facilitated by the availability of in vitro tests of intrinsic neuromuscular functions of the lower esophageal sphincter and the circular and longitudinal muscle layers.[7-9] Unfortunately, interest in the functions of esophageal smooth muscle has led to neglect of the pharmacology of the esophageal mucosa and of the striated muscle.

This review concentrates on those drugs and biologic agents that have important effects on normal esophageal motor functions or that have diagnostic and therapeutic value in esophageal motor disorders. The review does not detail the actions of these agents outside the esophagus, nor of other drugs that improve esophageal disease by actions outside the esophageal motor apparatus.

THE UPPER ESOPHAGEAL SPHINCTER AND THE ESOPHAGEAL STRIATED MUSCLE

Maintenance of a baseline pressure by the upper esophageal sphincter depends on tonic nerve impulses that reach the cricopharyngeal muscle through vagal nerve fibers from the dorsal motor nucleus and the nucleus ambiguus. Swallowing leads to a temporary relaxation of the sphincter by central inhibition of the tonic motor discharge.[10-13] Swallowing also elicits contraction of sequential parts of the esophagus by serial excitation of motor nerves to the esophagus, a process known as primary peristalsis. Primary peristalsis in the esophageal striated muscle is abolished by curare and succinylcholine.[14,15] This finding implies that primary peristalsis in the proximal esophagus is mediated by acetylcholine acting on nicotinic receptors as it is in other types of striated muscle. Nicotinic receptors have also been identified in esophageal smooth muscle and the lower esophageal sphincter. Since esophageal smooth muscle has many muscarinic receptors and since cholinergic excitation in the esophageal smooth muscle seems to be mediated by those receptors, these nicotinic receptors seem redundant.[15]

Motor problems in the proximal esophagus generally arise as part of systemic neuromuscular disorders. Polymyositis, myasthenia gravis, and midbrain strokes can all cause dysphagia by interfering with the development of proper peristaltic contractions.[3,4] No attempt has been made to alter esophageal striated muscle dysfunctions by drug treatment, presumably because they generally resolve with treatment of the underlying disorder.

CHOLINERGIC EFFECTS ON ESOPHAGEAL FUNCTIONS

Primary esophageal peristalsis is a programmed sequential contraction of the esophageal body that follows swallowing. Primary peristalsis is mediated by cholinergic fibers in the vagus nerve. In the distal esophagus these nerve fibers act primarily through muscarinic receptors: atropine depresses peristalsis in the distal esophagus, as curare does in the proximal esophagus. However, depression of nerve-mediated peristalsis by atropine is often incomplete.[15] This incomplete inhibition may indicate that primary peristalsis is also mediated by nervous mechanisms other than cholinergic impulses on muscarinic receptors. It remains, nevertheless, that muscarinic agonists like bethanechol strikingly enhance esophageal peristalsis: the amplitude of contractions is increased and the progression of the peristaltic wave is slowed so that the duration of peristaltic activity in the esophagus is prolonged.[16] Atropine has opposite effects: contractions become weak and the duration of the entire peristaltic sequence is shortened. It is also clear that the longitudinal layer of the esophageal muscle coat and most of the mucosal muscle are innervated by cholinergic neurons that act through muscarinic receptors.[17] Acetylcholine and its analogues produce contraction of these muscular structures, and the effect of these substances is simulated by stimulating the intrinsic nerves and is inhibited by atropine. In contrast, stimulation of the intrinsic nerves to the lower esophageal sphincter (LES) leads to muscle relaxation.[7,8] Sphincter relaxation is not mediated by one of the classical neurotransmitters of the autonomic nervous system, e.g., acetylcholine, noradrenaline, or dopamine.[18] Hence, the inhibitory nerves to the LES are noncholinergic and nonadrenergic, and it has been suggested that vasoactive intestinal polypeptide is their neurotransmitter.[19]

Differences in the innervation of various muscular structures, however, do not imply differences in the density of specific receptors.[5] The density of muscarinic receptors is about the same in the longitudinal and circular muscle layers as it is in the sphincter and in segments of small intestine.[20] Most of these muscarinic receptors are located directly on smooth muscle cells, and their activation causes muscle contraction. Some muscarinic receptors, however, are located on the non-adrenergic inhibitory nerves. Activation of these receptors by a cholinergic agonist leads to a paradoxic relaxation of smooth muscle.[5]

DRUG TREATMENT OF GASTROESOPHAGEAL REFLUX

Much work on esophageal pharmacology was motivated by the search for drugs that would benefit patients with gastroesophageal reflux. Cholinergic agents appeared to be a logical choice. They increase the baseline pressure of the LES, thereby presumably increasing gastroesophageal competence. Cholinergic agonists also increase the amplitude and decrease the speed of peristaltic contractions. These changes in peristalsis improve its acid-clearance capacity.[6,21] Thus, if reflux occurs, a cholinergic compound should reduce the contact time of noxious material with the esophageal mucosa. Unfortunately, traditional cholinergic agonists also increase acid secretion by the stomach. The acidity of refluxed material is one factor in reflux damage, since antacids and antisecretory drugs improve esophagitis.[22] This drawback of cholinergic agonists can be overcome by combining the use of a conventional cholinergic agent such as bethanechol with that of antacids or cimetidine. Alternatively, a drug like metoclopramide, which stimulates only esophagogastric motor activity but not secretory activity, can be used.[23]

Bethanechol decreases heartburn and antacid consumption in patients with reflux esophagitis. Acute inflammatory lesions in the esophagus are also improved after a course of treatment.[24] Bethanechol is given in daily doses of 10 to 30 mg p.o. q.i.d.

Metoclopramide is a potent anti-emetic. It is a dopamine antagonist in the central nervous system, and it enhances gut motor activity primarily either by releasing endogenous acetylcholine or by sensitizing muscarinic muscle receptors to the actions of acetylcholine. Enhancement of the peristaltic reflex through actions on serotoninergic neurons has also been proposed.[25] Metoclopramide in a dose of 10 mg p.o. q.i.d. also improves symptoms in patients with reflux esophagitis.[26]

Clinical results with both bethanechol and metoclopramide are encouraging. Still, these drugs may do little to change the long-term prognosis of gastroesophageal reflux and may not be needed to control symptoms in the majority of patients presenting with reflux. It has been recommended that elevation of the head of the bed, weight reduction, the avoidance of irritant foods, and the use of antacids should be fully tried in all patients before resorting to pharmacotherapy.[6] It is probably also wise to determine the nature and extent of morphologic changes in the esophagus before embarking on prolonged, perhaps fruitless, drug administration. Radiographic, endoscopic, or histologic evidence for chronic esophagitis provides a reasonable indication for operative treatment.

Anticholinergic agents such as atropine are contraindicated in reflux esophagitis. They are likely to increase the risk of reflux by somewhat depressing pressure in the LES and reducing peristaltic activity. The baseline pressure of the LES has been credited with providing the major barrier to gastroesophageal reflux, and the effectiveness of cholinergic agonists against reflux has been explained mostly by their generation of a greater baseline sphincter pressure. Both assumptions are simplistic and may be wrong. It is true that devastating gastroesophageal reflux is common if sphincter action is abolished, as it is in many patients with systemic sclerosis. Beyond that, however, baseline sphincter pressure is a poor predictor for the likelihood of reflux. Individual episodes of reflux are better correlated with temporary relaxation of the sphincter than with a low baseline pressure.[27] It is not known if cholinergic drugs decrease the frequency of spontaneous sphincter relaxations.

Furthermore, decreased sphincter pressure may be a consequence rather than a cause of gastroesophageal reflux. Inflammation of the esophageal mucosa depresses sphincter activity,[28] and the sphincter can be rendered competent by cholinergic and other pharmacologic stimuli. Poor gastric emptying has also been claimed to be a common pathogenetic factor in reflux esophagitis,[29] but attempts to relate the beneficial effects of cholinergic agonists to their gastrokinetic effects have failed so far.[30] Cholinergic agonists may benefit reflux esophagitis by mechanisms altogether unrelated to motility. These drugs also increase salivation,[31] and saliva may protect the esophagus by enhancing primary peristalsis or by neutralizing esophageal contents.

DRUGS ACTING ON HISTAMINE AND SEROTONIN RECEPTORS

Histamine was discovered at the same time as acetylcholine and shares many actions with the latter. Both histamine and acetylcholine have powerful actions on gastric secretion and on the mechanical activity of smooth muscle: hypotension resulting from relaxation of smooth muscle in small blood vessels is the most striking effect of both agents in the cardiovascular system, whereas stimulation of motility is their most common effect in gut smooth muscle.

Contraction of the LES occurs as part of the histamine test for gastric secretion. To avoid headaches, hypotension, and dyspnea during histamine tests of acid secretion, an antihistamine such as diphenhydramine must be administered. Some histamine analogues, such as betazole, preferentially stimulate gastric acid secretion without causing many of the untoward effects of histamine administration. This finding indicates that histamine acts on two different receptors. The one that mediates the systemic reactions and is blocked by conventional antihistamines is called the H_1 receptor; the other mediates gastric acid secretion and is known as the H_2 receptor.

Histamine causes contraction of the LES and this effect is simulated by the selective H_2 agonist betazole.[32,33] This observation implies that the actions of histamine on esophageal smooth muscle are preferentially mediated by excitatory H_2 receptors. However, additional histamine receptors have been identified: inhibitory H_2 receptors and inhibitory and excitatory H_1 receptors.[34]

The identification of the various histamine receptors is one important step towards an understanding of how histamine and histaminergic drugs affect the esophagus. The identification of such receptors per se does not imply, however, that histamine plays a role in normal esophageal motility or that stimuli that release histamine will also activate all of these receptors. Rather, endogenous histamine should primarily affect receptors in the vicinity of its storage sites. Histamine receptors exist on both nerves and muscle in the esophagus,[5] but which receptors are closer to the histamine-releasing cells is not known.

Histamine receptors are believed to be located on cell membranes, but their molecular structure is not known. The action of histamine seems to reside in alterations of the ionic permeability of the receptor cell membrane and in changes in adenylate-cyclase activity. Contraction and relaxation of visceral smooth muscle by histamine are at least in part independent of membrane potential, and the LES is no exception.[35] The histamine receptors that are located directly on muscle cells and mediate relaxation appear to be of the H_2 group. The muscle relaxation is preceded by accumulation of cyclic AMP. Most H_1 receptors on smooth muscle mediate contraction, perhaps by accumulation of cyclic GMP. H_1 receptors that relax the lower esophageal sphincter are located on inhibitory nerves. The exact location of the ₊excitatory H_2 receptors mediating histamine contraction of the LES remains to be determined.[5]

A knowledge of the various receptors is helpful when considering the effect of drugs on esophageal functions.[2,5] A drug effect is the sum of individual actions on various receptor sites, and variable and even opposite drug reactions are more easily explained if the involved receptors are known. Knowledge of existing receptors also allows one to explain the actions of many different drugs and biologic agents by actions through comparatively few well-defined mechanisms. It has for instance been suggested that paradoxic inhibition of the LES by gastrin is mediated by H_2 receptors.[35]

The H_2 blocking agents currently used to inhibit gastric acid secretion in patients with peptic ulcers and reflux esophagitis do not notably affect esophageal motor functions.[32] A course of cimetidine treatment that alleviates the symptoms of gastroesophageal reflux is not followed by an increase in baseline pressure of the LES.[36] Nevertheless, histamine may play a pathogenetic role in reflux esophagitis. Trauma and corrosive reflux are likely to release histamine from the numerous mast cells present in the esophagus.[33] This histamine release could well contribute to the esophageal motor changes that occur early in esophageal injury.

Serotonin is suspected of acting as a neurotransmitter in the myenteric plexus and some of the effects of metoclopramide have been attributed to serotinergic mechanisms.[37] Serotonin contracts the LES by directly activating both cholinergic neurons and muscle cells. These actions mask the presence of serotonin receptors on inhibitory nerves that by themselves cause sphincter relaxation.[38]

ADRENERGIC COMPOUNDS

Esophageal functions are primarily controlled by vagal activity: peristalsis is initiated by cholinergic neurons, and relaxation of the LES is mediated by inhibitory neurons that are neither cholinergic nor adrenergic.[7,39] Adrenergic nerves from the sympathetic system reach the esophagus mostly through perivascular plexuses and only modulate esophageal motor functions. Stimulation of splanchnic nerves contracts the lower esophageal sphincter,[40] and this effect results from release of acetylcholine by noradrenaline.[41]

Adrenergic receptors of the α-type mediate contraction, and those of the β-type inhibit esophageal smooth muscle.[2] Thus, phenylephrine typically contracts the LES and isoproterenol relaxes it. Selective adrenergic blocking agents such as propranolol and phentolamine by themselves, however, have little effect on esophageal functions.[1,2] Dopamine relaxes the LES and decreases the amplitude of circular muscle contractions, but a physiologic role for dopamine in esophageal functions cannot be implied.[42]

CALCIUM ANTAGONISTS AND SMOOTH MUSCLE RELAXANTS

Calcium ions are essential for neurotransmitter release and for activation of contractile proteins. Calcium withdrawal reduces the baseline tension of the LES and interferes with the contractions of circular smooth muscle.[43] Calcium is thought to activate smooth muscle by two different mechanisms. The first, which operates in muscle from the gastric antrum, generates phasic contractions that are selectively blocked by verapamil. The second mechanism generates the baseline tension of muscle from the gastric fundus; this tension is selectively blocked by nitroprusside.[44] Differences in calcium activation systems are less distinct in the esophagus than in the stomach. Still, verapamil is more effective than nitroprusside in reducing the amplitude of esophageal contractions, and nitroprusside relaxes the LES more promptly than does verapamil. These esophageal effects occur at drug doses that also produce arterial hypotension but are not caused by poor tissue perfusion.[45]

Hypercalcemia can cause dysphagia. Acute hypercalcemia produces opposite motor effects in the striated and in the smooth muscle segments of the human esophagus: the amplitude of contractions is decreased in the former and increased in the latter. The velocity of peristalsis is not affected.[46] The clinical uses of calcium antagonists will be discussed below in the sections on achalasia and esophageal spasm.

PROSTAGLANDINS, NEUROPEPTIDES, AND HORMONES

Prostaglandins

The baseline tension that is maintained by muscle from the gastric fundus is intimately linked to prostaglandin synthesis. The LES shares with muscle from the gastric fundus the intrinsic ability to maintain a high baseline tension. Still, maintenance of that tension by the sphincter is not dependent on prostaglandin synthesis. Rather, inhibition of prostaglandin synthesis by indomethacin increases sphincter pressure.[5] This suggests that prostaglandins, if anything, tonically inhibit sphincter muscle.[47] Also, it has been proposed that increased tissue prostaglandin levels during inflammation are responsible for the depression of sphincter pressure that occurs with various forms of esophagitis.[48] The prostaglandins involved are probably muscle inhibitors like PGE_1, PGE_2, and PGA_2. $PGF_{2\alpha}$ cannot be invoked since it contracts sphincter muscle.[49]

Neuropeptides

Polypeptides of the gastrin family have mostly positive inotropic effects on esophageal smooth muscle.[5] Those of the secretin family have largely negative inotropic effects. Gastrin contracts the LES and increases the amplitude of esophageal contractions, but this finding does not imply that those activities are part of its usual physiologic role. Most effects of gastrin are mediated by excitatory receptors directly on smooth muscle cells,[50] but actions on cholinergic neurons, histamine receptors, and inhibitory muscle receptors have also been proposed.[5] Multiple attempts to make use of pentagastrin in the diagnosis of esophageal motor disorders have failed.[51,52]

Vasoactive intestinal polypeptide (VIP) is a member of the secretin family and is a candidate neurotransmitter for the inhibitory neurons that mediate sphincter relaxation. It is found in high concentrations around the intrinsic nerves of sphincter muscle and is a powerful inhibitor of the sphincter.[19,53]

Hormones

The progestational hormones alter esophageal smooth muscle function along with their effects on uterine and vascular smooth muscle. Heartburn is frequent during pregnancy, and gastroesophageal reflux may aggravate esophagitis particularly during the third trimester. Progesterone in combination with estrogen depresses esophageal motor functions, and oral contraceptives may increase the risk of gastroesophageal reflux.[54-56]

Table 2-1 lists effects of additional neuropeptides and hormones (cholecystokinin,[57] secretin,[53] gastric inhibitory polypeptide,[58] substance P,[59] and the enkephalins[60]) on the esophageal motor apparatus.

Table 2-1. Effect of selected neuropeptides and hormones on esophageal function

Compound	Receptor Type and Location	Effect on LES	Effect on Esophageal Body	Comments
Cholecystokinin[57]	Inhibitory—neurons	Relaxation	Repetitive contractions	Net result LES relaxation; (LES contraction only in patients with achalasia)
	Excitatory—sphincter muscle	Contraction		
Secretin[53]	Inhibitory—sphincter muscle	Relaxation	Unknown	
Gastric inhibitory polypeptide[58]	Not identified	Relaxation	Unknown	
Substance P[59]	Muscarinic cholinergic receptors	Contraction	Unknown	Physiologic significance unknown
Enkephalins[60]	Presynaptic adrenergic nerves		Decrease of esophageal contractions	?Role of enkaphalins in sympathetic neurotransmission to esophagus
	Inhibitory—neurons Excitatory—sphincter muscle	Relaxation		

DRUG RESPONSES IN ESOPHAGEAL MOTILITY DISORDERS

Drugs are used to diagnose and to treat esophageal motor disorders. Untoward drug reactions are rare in the normal esophagus but have to be considered in the diseased esophagus.

Achalasia and Chagas' Disease

Achalasia is characterized by weak contractions of the esophageal smooth muscle and an excessively contracted LES that fails to relax on swallowing ("cardiospasm"). Similar esophageal dysfunctions occur in Chagas' disease when at least half of the nerve cells in the myenteric plexus are destroyed by trypanosomes. This denervation leads to an increased sensitivity to exogenous agents (Cannon's law). Testing for cholinergic hypersensitivity of the esophagus is a useful adjunct to the diagnosis of achalasia.[61] Acetyl-β-methylcholine (Mecholyl) typically produces contraction of the esophageal body and sphincter and causes chest pain. From 2 to 8 mg of the drug are given subcutaneously in successive 1-mg doses until a response occurs. The esophageal response is recorded by cine-esophagography, expulsion of air from an esophageal balloon or manometry.

The cardiospasm of patients with achalasia has been explained by hypersensitivity to circulating gastrin.[62] Such a phenomenon would not extend to patients with Chagas' disease whose lower esophageal sphincter is fairly insensitive to gastrin.[63] The primary effect of cholecystokinin in achalasia is sphincter contraction, directly mediated by excitatory receptors on the muscle cells. This effect of cholecystokinin occurs in the normal esophagus, but it is masked.[57] Normally, the net effect of cholecystokinin is relaxation of the LES. This is mediated by receptors on the inhibitory nerves, which fail in achalasia.

Pneumatic dilatation or myotomy of the LES leads to excellent recovery in most cases of achalasia, and attempts to treat achalasia by pharmacologic means are open to criticism. The calcium antagonist verapamil (Nifedipine) decreases the pressure in the LES in patients with achalasia, and it does not impair any residual relaxation. Verapamil administration improves dysphagia, retrosternal discomfort, regurgitation and weight loss.[64] During a 6- to 18-month observation period up to 30 mg of verapamil were given before each meal to reduce symptoms, and no untoward effects were reported. This trial was restricted to patients with early achalasia, and the treatment is not advised in patients whose esophagus is dilated. It is not known if pneumatic dilatation or myotomy will eventually be necessary in patients who respond initially to treatment with calcium antagonists.[65]

Esophageal Spasm and Related Disorders

If esophageal spasm is defined strictly by the presence of simultaneous high-amplitude contractions of long duration that involve long segments of the esophagus and are unrelated to swallowing, this condition is rare.[66-68] One problem is that it is difficult to obtain a manometric recording precisely at the time when the motor disorder occurs. Attempts to use agents such as pentagastrin to elicit esophageal spasms in susceptible persons have generally failed.[68,69] Inadvertent provocation of esophageal spasm has been blamed for the chest pain caused by ergonovine.[70] Ergonovine is used to elicit spasm of the coronary arteries and electrocardiographic changes in patients suspected of having Prinzmetal's angina. Some patients who developed chest pain on ergonovine infusion without demonstrable cardiovascular changes were found to have abnormalities in their esophageal manometry before administration of ergonovine and an abnormal increase in esophageal pressures after its infusion.[71]

Verapamil has also been tried in patients with esophageal spasm. The trial differed from most others by its positive results rather than by its lack of controls.[64] There is one other exception, however, a trial in which patients with esophageal spasm responded well to nitroglycerin and long acting nitrates provided that they did not have underlying gastroesophageal reflux.[72]

Diabetic Esophagopathy

Poor esophageal sphincter pressure and weak peristaltic contractions are common in patients with diabetes. The esophageal response to cholinergic stimuli is normal in diabetes. This has been taken to mean that the muscular end-organ is intact, because otherwise stimulation should be ineffective. It has also been inferred that the intrinsic neurons of the esophagus function normally, since otherwise there should be denervation hypersensitivity as in achalasia.[73,74] Since the two processes should produce contrary results, normal pharmacologic responsiveness of the diabetic esophagus is probably meaningless for defining the underlying pathogenetic mechanisms.

Esophageal motor abnormalities in diabetes per se are no indication for treatment. Despite slow gastric emptying, low sphincter pressure, and poor esophageal peristalsis in many patients with diabetes, symptoms of gastroesophageal reflux are not particularly common in these patients.[74] This could mean that these motor abnormalities are less important in the pathogenesis of reflux than has been assumed. Alternatively, the reduction of gastric acid secretion by diabetes[75] could reduce the occurrence of heartburn with reflux, or the sensory neuropathy of diabetic patients may protect them from esophageal symptoms.[76]

Parkinson's Disease

Motor disorders of the esophagus often complicate the pharyngeal dysphagia of Parkinson's disease.[3,4,71,77] Approximately half the patients have findings of esophageal spasm, and gastroesophageal reflux and ineffective esophageal clearance are common in the rest. Treatment with levodopa may aggravate rather than improve esophageal functions.[77] Furthermore, administration of anticholinergics interrupts the peristaltic sequence in patients with Parkinson's disease. These findings indicate that a defect in dopaminergic neurons is not the likely cause for esophageal dysfunction in Parkinson's disease.[77,78]

ESOPHAGEAL PROBLEMS FROM SYSTEMIC DRUGS

Esophageal side effects are strikingly absent in patients receiving drugs that act on the autonomic nervous system and visceral smooth muscle.[2] One possible exception is alcohol, which commonly produces heartburn. Even moderate amounts of alcohol increase the likelihood of reflux and depress the pressure of the LES.[79] Reflux has long been suspected as an initiating factor in bleeding from esophageal varices, but a role for alcohol-induced reflux has not been specifically sought.[80] The roles of progestational hormones in heartburn and of ergonovine in esophageal pain have been discussed previously.

Diazepam, often given during endoscopic procedures, depresses the LES for a few minutes.[81] Dipyramidole and theophylline have similar effects, but probably through different mechanisms. Both inhibit the phosphodiesterase that converts cyclic AMP to AMP in muscle cells. Cyclic-AMP accumulation is held responsible for smooth muscle relaxation.[5,81] Therapeutic administration of these and other such drugs does not pose undue risks to the esophagus.[2]

CONCLUSIONS

The effects of drugs on esophageal motor functions are well studied. The esophagus is largely controlled by cholinergic mechanisms, and drugs with cholinergic actions are a useful adjunct to treating gastroesophageal reflux. Esophageal motor activity is often weak in inflammation of the esophagus, and cholinergic drugs restore it to normal. It remains to be determined, however, if cholinergic drugs prevent esophageal complications from severe and longstanding gastroesophageal reflux. These drugs are also used to demonstrate esophageal denervation as it occurs in achalasia and less often in esophageal spasm.

The use of drugs in treating achalasia and other motor disorders of the esophagus is still controversial. The calcium antagonist verapamil has been used to reduce cardiospasm and esophageal spasm, but pneumatic dilatation or myotomy remain the treatment of choice in the former and a trial of long-acting nitrates seems preferable in the latter. Drug treatment is rarely indicated in diabetic esophagopathy, and esophageal problems are more likely to deteriorate than to improve with drug control of Parkinson's disease.

Esophageal motor changes are common with drugs used to treat cardiovascular and bronchopulmonary problems, but these changes are without clinical relevance.

ACKNOWLEDGMENTS

Dr. Konrad Schulze-Delrieu is supported by Grant AM 00519 from the NIAMDD. Drs. Christensen, Gurll, and Reynolds made helpful comments on the manuscript, and B. Velázquez prepared it.

REFERENCES

1. Christensen J: Pharmacology of the esophagus. In Code CF (ed): Handbook of Physiology, Sec 6, Alimentary Canal; Vol 4, Motility; American Physiological Society, Washington, D.C., 1968: 2325–2330.
2. Christensen J: Effects of drugs on esophageal motility. Arch Intern Med 136:532–537, 1976.
3. Creamer B: Motor disturbances of the esophagus. In Code CF (ed): Handbook of Physiology, Sec 6, Alimentary Canal; Vol 4, Motility, American Physiological Society, Washington, D.C., 1968: 2331–2343.
4. Hurwitz AL, Duranceau A: Upper-esophageal sphincter dysfunction: pathogenesis and treatment. Am J Dig Dis 23(3):275–281, 1978.
5. Goyal RK, Rattan S: Neurohumoral, hormonal, and drug receptors for the lower esophageal sphincter. Gastroenterology 47:598–619, 1978.
6. Castell DO: Medical therapy of reflux esophagitis. Ann Intern Med 93:926–927, 1980.
7. Christensen J, Freeman BW, Miller JK: Some physiologic characteristics of the esophagogastric junction in the opossum. Gastroenterology 64:1119–1125, 1973.
8. Christensen J, Conklin JL, Freeman BW: Physiologic specialization at the esophagogastric junction in three species. Am J Physiol 225:1265–1270, 1973.
9. Weisbrodt NW, Christensen J: Gradients of contractions in the opossum esophagus. Gastroenterology 62:1159–1166, 1972.
10. Hellemans J, Vantrappen G: Electromyographic studies on canine esophageal motility. Am J Dig Dis 12:1240–1255, 1967.
11. Hellemans J, Vantrappen G, Valembois P, et al.: Electrical activity of striated and smooth muscle of the esophagus. Am J Dig Dis 12:320–334, 1968.
12. Car A, Roman C: L'activité spontanée du sphincter oesophagien supérieur chez le mouton. J Physiol (Paris) 62:505–511, 1970.
13. Asoh R, Goyal RK: Manometry and electromyography of the upper esophageal sphincter in the opossum. Gastroenterology 74:514–520, 1978.
14. Rattan S, Goyal RK: Effect of nicotine on the lower esophageal sphincter: studies on the mechanism of action. Gastroenterology 69:154–159, 1975.
15. Dodds WJ, Christensen J, Dent J, et al.: Pharmacologic investigation of primary peristalsis in smooth muscle portion of opossum esophagus. Am J Physiol 237(6)E561–E566, 1979.
16. Humphries TJ, Castell DO: Effect of oral bethanechol on parameters of esophageal peristalsis. Dig Dis Sci, 26(2):129–132, 1981.
17. Christensen J, Lund GF: Esophageal responses to distension and electrical stimulation. J Clin Invest 48:408–419, 1969.
18. Goyal RK, Rattan S: Genesis of basal sphincter pressure: effect of tetrodotoxin on lower esophageal sphincter pressure in opossum in vivo. Gastroenterology 71:62–67, 1976.
19. Uddman R, Alumets J, Edvinsson L, et al.: Peptidergic (VIP) innervation of the esophagus. Gastroenterology 75:5–8, 1978.
20. Rimele TJ, Rogers WA, Gaginella TS: Characterization of muscarinic cholinergic receptors in the lower esophageal sphincter of the cat: binding of [^{3}H] quinuclidinyl benzilate. Gastroenterology 77:1225–1234, 1979.
21. Miller WN, Ganeshappa KP, Dodds WJ, et al.: Effect of bethanechol on gastroesophageal reflux. Am J Dig Dis 22(3):230–234, 1977.
22. Behar J, Brand DL, Brown FC, et al.: Cimetidine in the treatment of symptomatic gastroesophageal reflux. Gastroenterology 74:441–448, 1978.

23. Jacoby HI, Brodie DA: Gastrointestinal actions of metoclopramide: and experimental study. Gastroenterology 52:676–684, 1967.
24. Thanik KD, Chey WY, Shah AN, Gutierrez JG: Reflux esophagitis: effect of oral bethanechol on symptoms and endoscopic findings. Ann Intern Med 93:805–808, 1980.
25. Schulze-Delrieu K: Metoclopramide. Gastroenterology 77:768–779, 1979.
26. McCallum R, Ippoliti A, Cooney C, et al.: A controlled trial of metoclopramide in symptomatic gastroesophageal reflux. N Engl J Med 296:354–357, 1977.
27. Dent J, Dodds WJ, Friedman RH, et al.: Mechanism of gastroesophageal reflux in recumbent asymptomatic human subjects. J Clin Invest 65:256–267, 1980.
28. Welch WW, Luckmann K, Ricks P, et al.: Lower esophageal sphincter pressure in histologic esophagitis. Dig Dis Sci 25(6):420–426, 1980.
29. McCallum RW, Berkowitz DM, Lerner E: Gastric emptying in patients with gastro-esophageal reflux. Gastroenterology 80:285–291, 1981.
30. Behar J, Ramsby G: Gastric emptying and antral motility in reflux esophagitis. Gastroenterology 74:253–256, 1978.
31. Helm JF, Dodds WJ, Pelc LR, et al.: Mechanisms of esophageal acid clearance in supine normal subject: a unifying hypothesis. Gastroenterology 80:1171 (abstr) 1981.
32. Kravitz JJ, Snape WJ, Cohen S: Effect of histamine and histamine antagonists on human lower esophageal sphincter function. Gastroenterology 74:435–440, 1978.
33. de Carle DJ, Brody MJ, Christensen J: Histamine receptors in esophageal smooth muscle of the opossum. Gastroenterology 70:1071–1075, 1976.
34. Rattan S, Goyal RK: Effects of histamine on the lower esophageal sphincter in vivo: evidence for action at three different sites. J Pharmacol Exp Ther 204:334–342, 1978.
35. Cohen S, Snape Jr WJ: Action of metiamide on the lower esophageal sphincter. Gastroenterology 69:911–919, 1975.
36. Goodall RJR, Temple JG: Effect of cimetidine on lower esophageal sphincter pressure in esophagitis. Br Med J 280:611–612, 1980.
37. Okwuasaba FK, Hamilton JT: The effect of metoclopramide on intestinal muscle responses and the peristaltic reflex in vitro. Can J Physiol Pharmacol 54:393–404, 1976.
38. Rattan S, Goyal RK: Effects of 5-hydroxytryptamine on the lower esophageal sphincter in vivo. J Clin Invest 59:125–133, 1977.
39. Burleigh DE: The effects of drugs and electrical field stimulation on the human lower oesophageal sphincter. Arch Intern Pharmacodyn 240:169–176, 1979.
40. DiMarino AJ, Cohen S: The adrenergic control of lower esophageal sphincter function: an experimental model of denervation supersensitivity. J Clin Invest 52:2264–2271, 1973.
41. Gonella J, Niel JP, Roman C: Mechanism of the noradrenergic motor control on the lower oesophageal sphincter in the cat. J Physiol (Lond) 306:251–260, 1980.
42. de Carle DJ, Christensen J: A dopamine receptor in esophageal smooth muscle of the opossum. Gastroenterology 70:216–219, 1976.
43. de Carle DJ, Christensen J, Szabo AC, et al.: Calcium dependence of neuromuscular events in esophageal smooth muscle of the opossum. Am J Physiol 232(6):E547–E552, 1977.
44. Golenhofen K: Theory of p and t systems for calcium activation in smooth muscle. In Bülbring E, Shuba MF (eds): Physiology of Smooth Muscle. Raven Press, New York, 1976.
45. Goyal RK, Rattan S: Effects of sodium nitroprusside and verapamil on lower esophageal sphincter. Am J Physiol 238:G40–G44, 1980.
46. Danielides IC, Mellow MH: Effect of acute hypercalcemia on human esophageal motility. Gastroenterology 75:1115–1119, 1978.
47. Dilawari, JB, Newman A, Poleo J, Misiewicz JJ: Response of the human cardiac sphinc-

ter to circulatory prostaglandins $F_{2\alpha}$ and E_2 and to antiinflammatory drugs. Gut 15:137–143, 1975.

48. Higgs RH, Castell DO, Eastwood GL: Studies on the mechanism of esophagitis-induced lower esophageal sphincter hypotension in cats. Gastroenterology 71:51–56, 1976.

49. Rattan S, Goyal RK: Role of endogenous prostaglandins in the regulation of lower esophageal sphincter. In Christensen J (ed): Gastrointestinal Motility. Raven Press, New York, 1980.

50. Ryan JP, Duffy KR: LES pressure response to pentagastrin: effect of cholinergic augmentation and inhibition. Am J Physiol 234(3):E301–E305, 1978.

51. Wexler RM, Kaye MD: Pentagastrin in diffuse oesophageal spasm. Gut 22:213–216, 1981.

52. Orlando RC, Bozymski EM: The effects of pentagastrin in achalasia and diffuse esophageal spasm. Gastroenterology 77:471–477, 1979.

53. Behar J, Field S, Marin C: Effect of glucagon, secretin, and vasoactive intestinal polypeptide on the feline lower esophageal sphincter: mechanisms of action. Gastroenterology 77:1001–1007, 1979.

54. Schulze K, Christensen J: Lower sphincter of the opossum esophagus in pseudopregnancy. Gastroenterology 73:1082–1085, 1977.

55. Fisher RS, Roberts GS, Grabowski CJ, Cohen S: Altered lower esophageal sphincter function during early pregnancy. Gastroenterology 74:1233–1237, 1978.

56. Van Thiel DH, Gavaler JS, Stremple JF: Lower esophageal sphincter pressure during the normal menstrual cycle. Am J Obstet Gynecol, 134:64–67, 1979.

57. Dodds WJ, Dent J, Hogan WJ, et al.: Paradoxical lower esophageal sphincter contraction induced by cholecystokinin-octapeptide in patients with achalasia. Gastroenterology 80:327–333, 1981.

58. Sinar DR, O'Dorisio TM, Mazzaferri EL, et al.: Effect of gastric inhibitory polypeptide on lower esophageal sphincter pressure in cats. Gastroenterology 75: 263–267, 1978.

59. Mukhopadhyay AH: Effect of substance P on the lower esophageal sphincter of the opossum. Gastroenterology 75:278–282, 1978.

60. McCallum RW, Dodds J, Osborne HP, Biancani P: Effect of enkephalin and other opiates on opossum lower esophageal sphincter. In Christensen J (ed): Gastrointestinal Motility. Raven Press, New York, 1980.

61. Kramer P, Ingelfinger FY: Esophageal sensitivity to Mecholyl in cardiospasm. Gastroenterology 19:242–251, 1951.

62. Cohen S, Lipshutz W, Hughes W: Role of gastrin supersensitivity in the pathogenesis of lower esophageal sphincter hypertension in achalasia. J Clin Invest, 50:1241–1247, 1971.

63. Padovan W, Godoy RA, Dantas RO, et al.: Lower oesophageal sphincter response to pentagastrin in chagasic patients with megaoesophagus and megacolon. Gut 21:85–90, 1980.

64. Weiser HF, Lepsien G, Golenhofen K, Siewert R: Clinical and experimental studies on the effect of nifedipine on smooth muscle of the esophagus and LES. In Christensen J (ed): Gastrointestinal Motility. Raven Press, New York, 1980.

65. Bortolotti M, Labò G: Clinical and manometric effects of nifedipine in patients with esophageal achalasia. Gastroenterology 80:39–44, 1981.

66. Mellow M: Symptomatic diffuse esophageal spasm: manometric follow-up and response to cholinergic stimulation and cholinesterase inhibition. Gastroenterology 73:237–240, 1977.

67. Brand CL, Martin D, Pope II CE: Esophageal manometrics in patients with angina-like chest pain. Dig Dis Sci. 22:300–304, 1977.

68. Wexler RM, Kaye MD: Pentagastrin in diffuse oesophageal spasm. Gut 22:213–216, 1981.
69. Orlando RC, Bozymski EM: The effects of pentagastrin in achalasia and diffuse esophageal spasm. Gastroenterology 77:472–477, 1979.
70. Gravino FN, Perloff JK, Yeatman LA, Ippolitti AF: Coronary arterial spasm versus esophageal spasm: response to ergonovine. Am J Med 70:1293–1296, 1981.
71. London RL, Ouyang A, Snape WJ, Jr., et al.: Provocation of esophageal pain by ergonovine or edrophonium. Gastroenterology 81:10–14, 1981.
72. Swamy N: Esophageal spasm: clinical and manometric response to nitroglycerine and long acting nitrites. Gastroenterology 72:23–27, 1977.
73. Stewart IM, Hosking DJ, Preston BJ, Atkinson M: Oesophageal motor changes in diabetes mellitus. Thorax, 31:278–283, 1976.
74. Hollis JB, Castell DO, Braddner RL: Esophageal function in diabetes mellitus and its relation to peripheral neuropathy. Gastroenterology 73:1098–1102, 1977.
75. Feldman M, Corbett DB, Ramsey EJ, et al.: Abnormal gastric function in longstanding, insulin-dependent diabetic patients. Gastroenterology 77:12–17, 1979.
76. Kristensson K, Nordborg C, Olsson Y, Sourander P: Changes in the vagus nerve in diabetes mellitus. Acta Pathol Microbiol Scand 79:684–685, 1971.
77. Kaye MD, Hoehn MM: Esophageal motor dysfunction in Parkinson's disease. In Vantrappen G (ed): Proceedings of the Fifth International Symposium on Gastrointestinal Motility. Typoff-Press, Herentals, 1976.
78. Bramble MG, Cunliffe J, Dellipiani AW: Evidence for a change in neurotransmitter affecting oesophageal motility in Parkinson's disease. J Neurol Neurosurg Psychiatry 41:709–712, 1978.
79. Kaufman SE, Kaye MD: Induction of gastro-oesophageal reflux by alcohol. Gut 19:336–338, 1978.
80. Dent J: What's new in the esophagus. Dig Dis Sci 26:161–173, 1981.
81. Rushnak MJ, Leevy CM: Effect of diazepam on the lower esophageal sphincter: a double-blind controlled study. Am J Gastroenterol, 73:127–130, 1980.

3 | Radiology of the Esophagus

Marc S. Levine
Igor Laufer

INTRODUCTION

Radiologic examination of the esophagus requires evaluation of both function and morphology. The radiologic technique must therefore be adequate for both purposes; it must also be modified according to the portion of the esophagus to be examined and the specific clinical problems being posed.

TECHNIQUE

Esophageal function is assessed while the patient takes single swallows in the recumbent position. When the patient is upright, the esophagus may empty by gravity alone and therefore no assessment of peristaltic activity can be made. With the patient recumbent, however, each swallow should produce a primary peristaltic wave that results in stripping of contrast from the esophagus. With multiple swallows, the peristaltic sequence is interrupted and peristalsis cannot be evaluated. However, continuous drinking is useful for promoting maximal distention of the esophagus.

Motor Abnormalities

Motor dysfunction of the esophagus is recognized by either the absence of primary peristalsis or the presence of nonperistaltic, tertiary contractions. In both achalasia and scleroderma, function may be normal in the proximal, striated-muscle portion of the esophagus with peristalsis absent in the smooth muscle portion or distal two-thirds.[1,2] In achalasia, there is failure of the lower esophageal sphincter (LES) to relax with beak-like narrowing of the distal esophagus as it traverses the diaphragm (Fig. 3-1A). In patients with scleroderma or other connective tissue disorders affecting the esophagus, however, the LES is patulous, and there may be free gastroesophageal reflux with an associated hiatal hernia. Because peristaltic activity is absent, the refluxed material is poorly cleared from the body of the esophagus. This prolonged contact may result in a severe form of reflux esophagitis

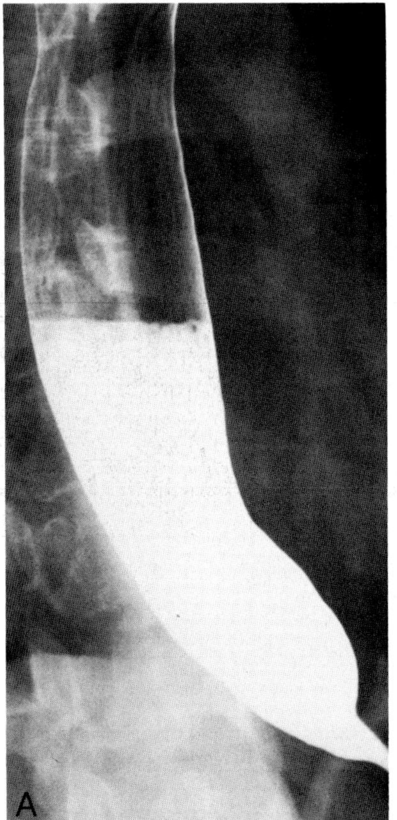
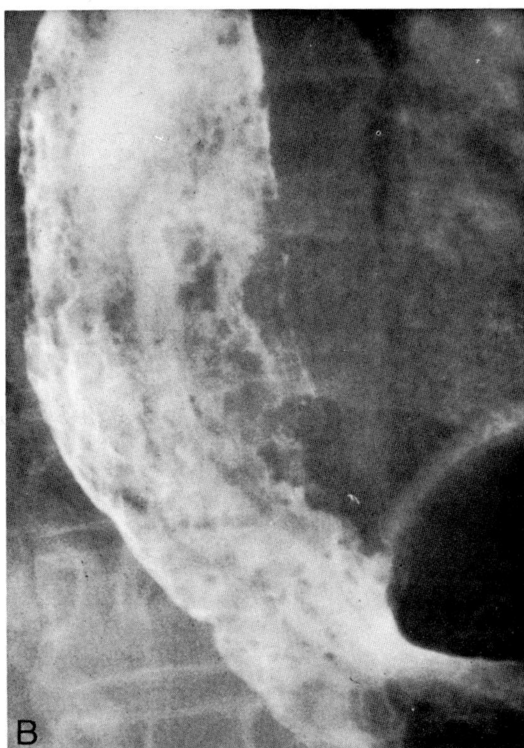

Fig. 3-1. Motility disorders. A. Typical appearance of achalasia with a barium level in the mid-esophagus and a tapered, beak-like narrowing of the distal esophagus traversing the diaphragm. At fluoroscopy, no peristalsis was apparent in the body of the esophagus, and there was intermittent relaxation of the lower esophageal sphincter (LES). B. Scleroderma with monilial infection. The esophagus is moderately dilated, and the LES is patulous, allowing for free reflux. In addition, the mucosal surface of the esophagus is covered with small plaque-like lesions representing the monilial exudate. Note also the interstitial changes in the lung base caused by scleroderma. Fig. 3-1 B. Reproduced by permission from I. Laufer: Double Contrast Gastrointestinal Radiology—With Endoscopic Correlation. WB Saunders, Philadelphia, 1979.

with eventual stricture formation in approximately 40% of patients.[1] When strictures develop, it may be difficult to distinguish radiologically between achalasia and scleroderma, although the presence of a hiatal hernia strongly favors the diagnosis of scleroderma. In either condition, esophageal stasis may lead to superinfection with *Candida albicans.*[3] This condition typically presents with nodularity, or plaque-like filling defects in the esophagus (Fig. 3-1B), which usually resolve following treatment with antifungal agents.

Diffuse esophageal spasm is characterized by tertiary, nonpropulsive contractions in the body of the esophagus.[2,4] These are seen as variable, band-like narrowings. When the condition has been long-standing, it may give rise to pulsion diverticula (Fig. 3-2). In most cases, peristaltic activity can still be detected, although normal peristaltic waves may occur less frequently. This condition is also seen in elderly patients without esophageal symptoms and is referred to as presbyesophagus. The radiologic findings are identical with those in patients with symptomatic disease.

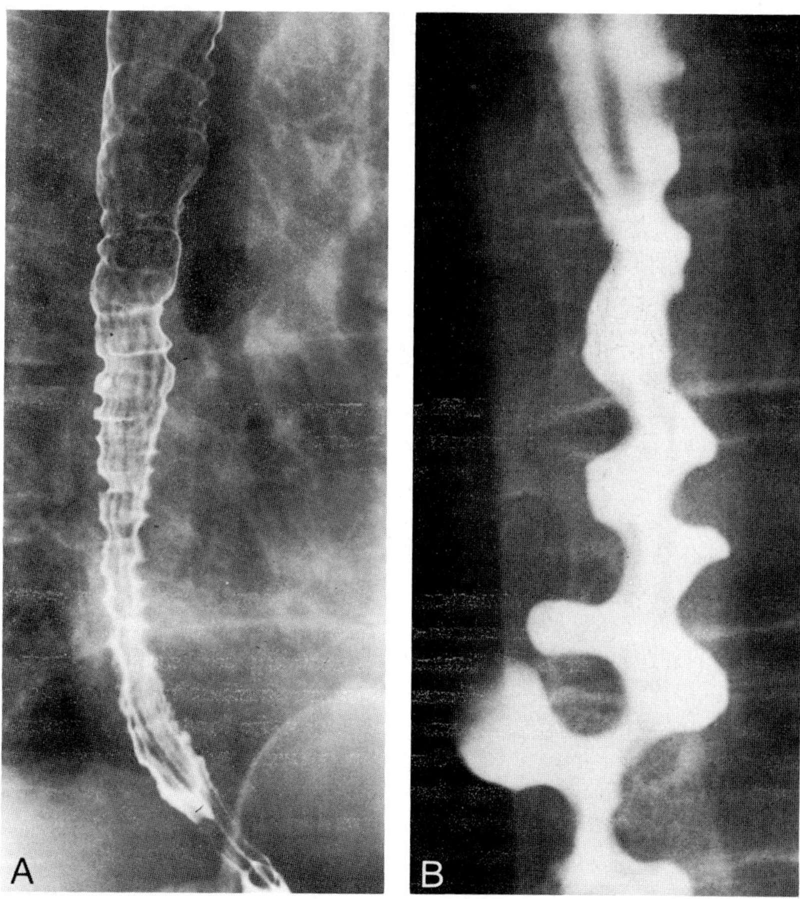

Fig. 3-2. Diffuse spasm of the esophagus. A. Multiple band-like defects representing nonpropulsive contractions in the body of esophagus. B. A more advanced case showing pulsion diverticula between the areas of muscle contraction.

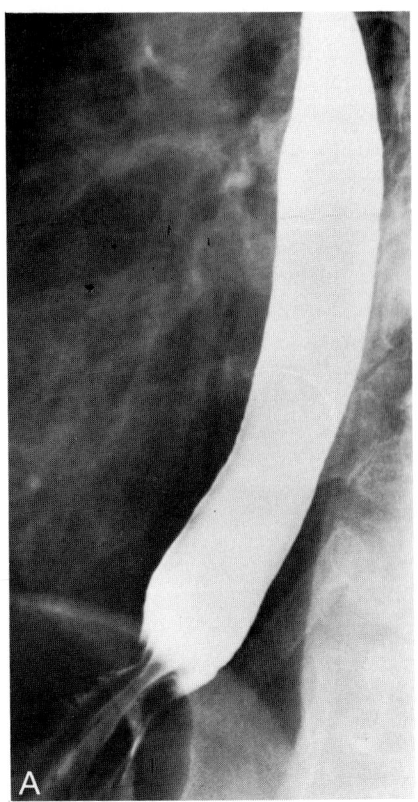

Fig. 3-3.   Normal appearances of the esophagus. A. Barium-filled view with the patient in the prone oblique position. B. Longitudinal folds seen best with the esophagus partially collapsed. C. Double-contrast view with the patient in the upright position. D. Transverse folds. Appearance of these folds is a transient phenomenon and probably results from contraction of the muscularis mucosae.

In diffuse esophageal spasm, the LES may respond normally to deglutition, or it may fail to relax, as is true in patients with achalasia. In fact, the transition from diffuse esophageal spasm to achalasia has been described in the literature.[5]

Morphologic Evaluation

Complete morphologic evaluation of the esophagus requires a combination of barium-filled, mucosal, and double-contrast views (Figs. 3-3:A,B,C). Barium-filled views may show areas of limited distensibility and contour abnormalities caused by large ulcers or tumors. Mucosal films are obtained by coating the mucosal folds in the collapsed esophagus. Such views show the longitudinal mucosal folds that may become thickened and scalloped in patients with esophageal varices or with various types of inflammatory disorders. Double contrast views are the most sensitive for demonstrating mucosal abnormalities caused by small neoplasms or early inflammatory lesions. These views are obtained by having the patient drink a high-density barium sulfate suspension while in the upright position. The normal mucosal surface is very smooth and featureless. Occasionally, delicate transverse folds are seen as a transient phenomenon (Fig. 3-3D).[6] These are believed to result

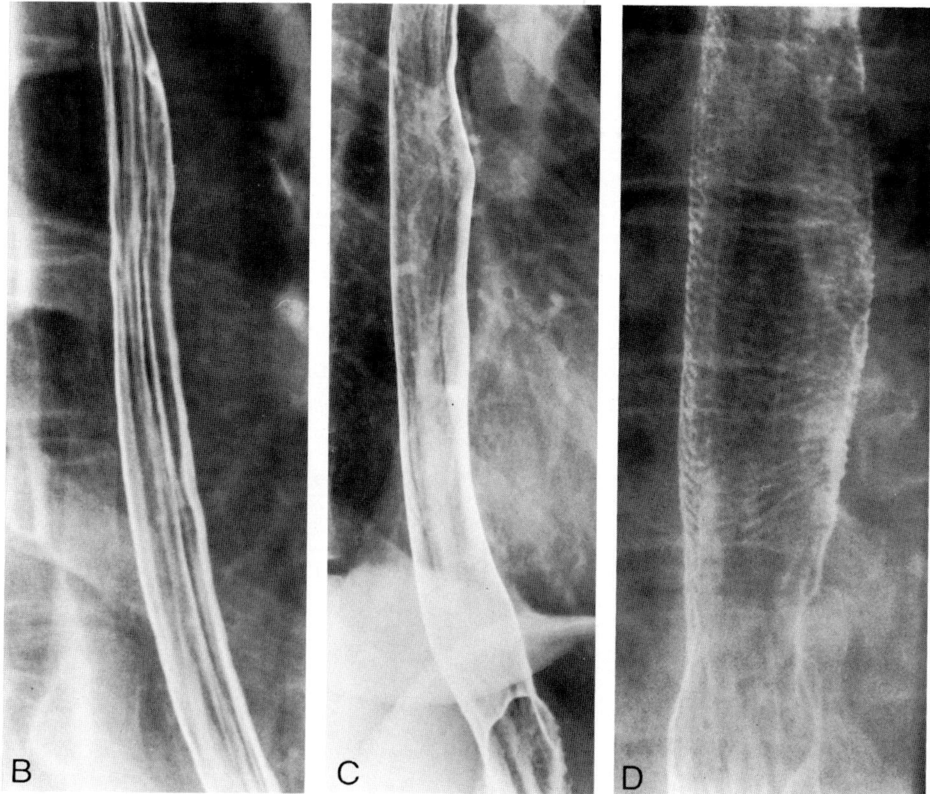

from contraction of the muscularis mucosae and are of no pathologic consequence.

In some patients, a definitive study cannot be obtained with the routine technique. In such cases, a small catheter (10–12 French) can be passed into the proximal esophagus. The patient then drinks the high-density barium suspension, and air is insufflated through the esophageal tube. Esophageal hypotonia can be induced by the intravenous administration of 15 mg of probanthine. In this way, more detailed and reproducible double-contrast views can be obtained. The tube esophagram may be performed as a primary study in patients with esophageal symptoms or as a secondary study when the routine double-contrast examination is inconclusive.

Cervical Esophagus

The pharynx and cervical esophagus are areas where physiologic events occur very rapidly. Abnormalities may be detected at fluoroscopy but may be difficult to record on standard radiographs. For this reason some form of dynamic imaging is essential in this area. This may consist of cineradiography, videotape, or rapid serial spot films at 4–6 frames/sec.

INFLAMMATORY DISORDERS

Reflux Esophagitis

Reflux esophagitis is by far the most common disorder affecting the esophagus. The traditional single-contrast esophagram is relatively insensitive in detecting inflammatory changes in the esophagus. The barium study has therefore been utilized primarily to document the presence of a hiatal hernia or gastroesophageal reflux, to rule out strictures or other complications, and to demonstrate abnormal esophageal motility.

There is controversy concerning the significance of a hiatal hernia or of gastroesophageal reflux demonstrated on barium studies. Patients with reflux esophagitis typically have a hiatal hernia, and it has been postulated that the presence of a

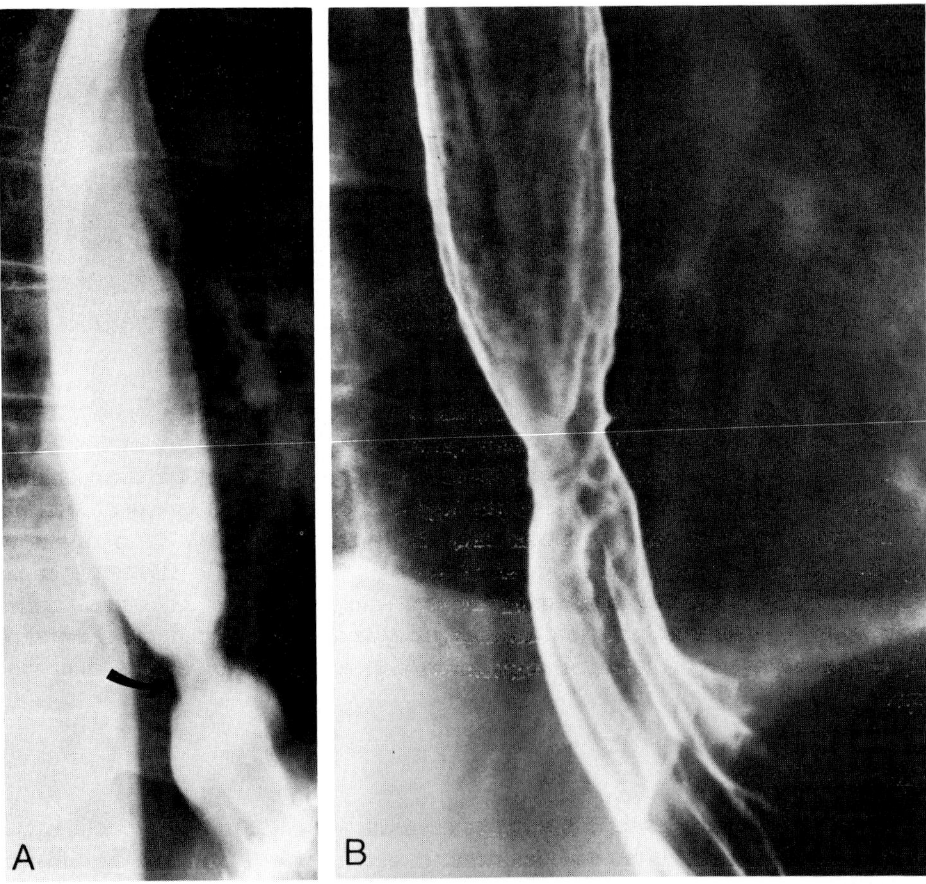

Fig. 3-4. Moderately severe reflux esophagitis. A. A single-contrast radiograph shows only a hiatus hernia with moderate narrowing at the gastroesophageal junction. B. The double-contrast radiograph shows the narrowed segment as well as multiple superficial erosions within the region of stricture.

hiatal hernia is somehow important in the pathogenesis of gastroesophageal reflux and the subsequent development of reflux esophagitis.[7,8] However, hiatal hernias are frequently observed in patients without evidence of gastroesophageal reflux or reflux esophagitis, and reflux may be demonstrated in patients without hiatal hernias. Nevertheless, it is rare to see a patient with severe reflux esophagitis in the absence of a hernia. In any event, it appears that the development of reflux esophagitis depends on multiple factors, including the frequency and duration of reflux, the potency of the refluxed material, and the intrinsic resistance of the esophageal mucosa.[9-12]

The traditional esophagram shows abnormalities only in patients with severe reflux esophagitis. The radiographic findings include abnormal esophageal motility, thickened folds, luminal contour irregularities, discrete ulceration, and segmental narrowing due to spasm or strictures (Fig. 3-4A).[13,14] More subtle mucosal abnormalities can be demonstrated on double-contrast radiographs (Fig. 3-4B). These techniques have thus expanded the role of radiology in patients with reflux.

Mild or moderate reflux esophagitis may be recognized on double-contrast views of the esophagus by thickening of the mucosal folds and by ulcerations or erosions that extend proximally from the gastroesophageal junction.[13,15] Shallow

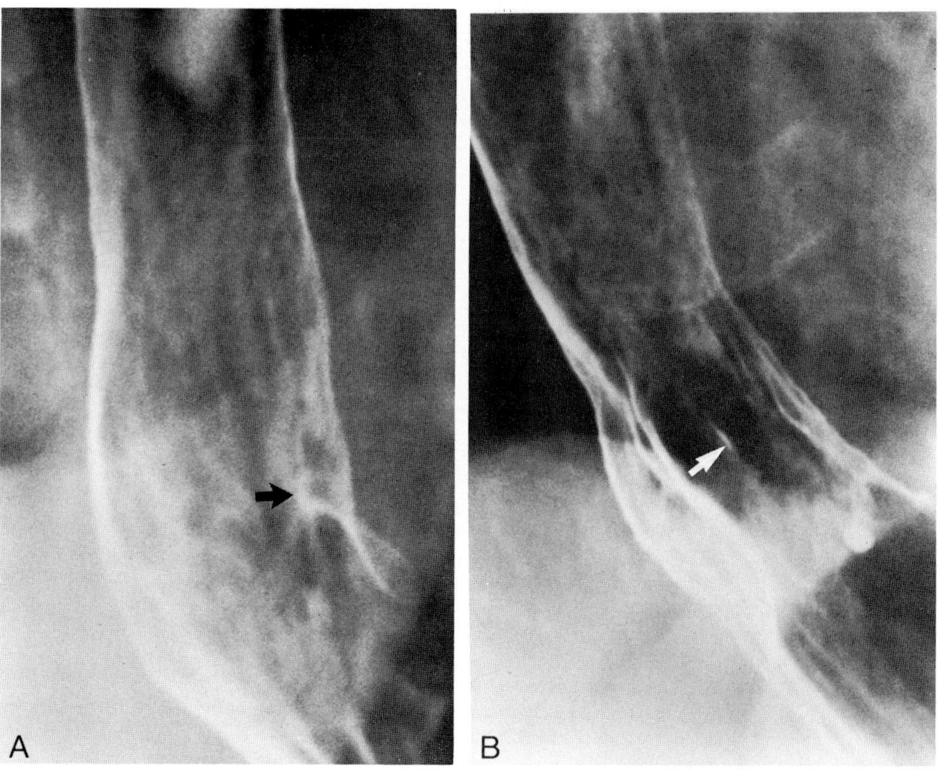

Fig. 3-5. A. Esophageal erosion due to reflux esophagitis. B. Linear ulcer in the distal esophagus caused by reflux esophagitis.

ulcers may appear as streaks or pinpoint collections of barium in the distal esophagus (Fig. 3-5A).[16] Superficial ulcers may also have a linear configuration (Fig. 3-5B), and there may be slight retraction of the adjacent esophageal wall. In chronic disease, the mucosa may acquire a finely nodular or granular appearance (Fig. 3-6). With further progression, deeper ulcers may develop (Fig. 3-7A). These are often associated with a columnar-lined or Barrett's esophagus.[17] Healing of ulcers may result in a typical peptic stricture with smooth, tapered margins and a normal mucosal surface (Fig. 3-7B). However, peptic strictures are often asymmetric, and endoscopic biopsy and cytology may be necessary to exclude carcinoma.

An unusual finding that has been described in patients with reflux esophagitis is the so-called inflammatory esophagogastric polyp and fold (Fig. 3-8).[18,19] The polyp occurs at the gastroesophageal junction and is usually associated with a prominent fold that tapers distally in the gastric fundus. The pathogenesis of the polyp–fold complex is uncertain, although it has only been observed in patients with reflux esophagitis and is presumably part of the spectrum of this disease.

Despite the variety of morphologic abnormalities associated with reflux

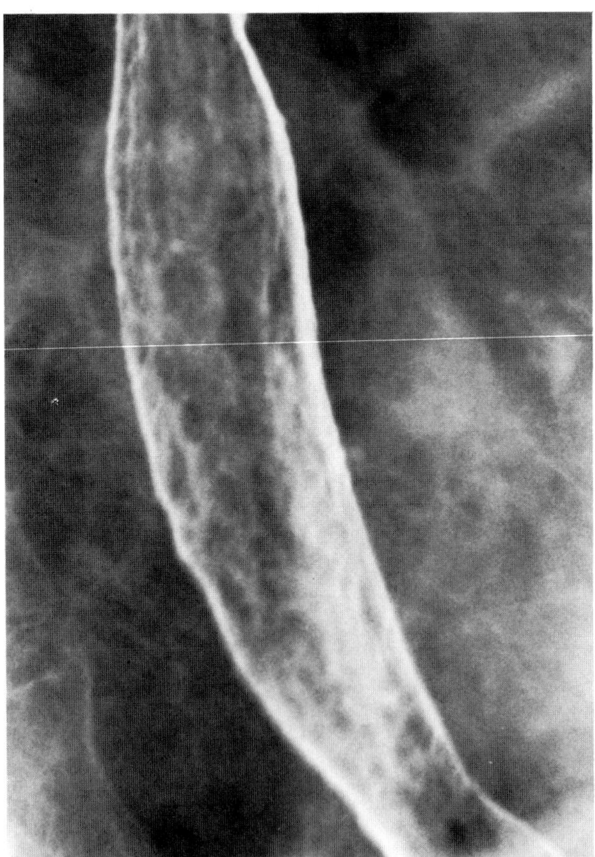

Fig. 3-6. Nodularity of the esophageal mucosa caused by chronic reflux esophagitis.

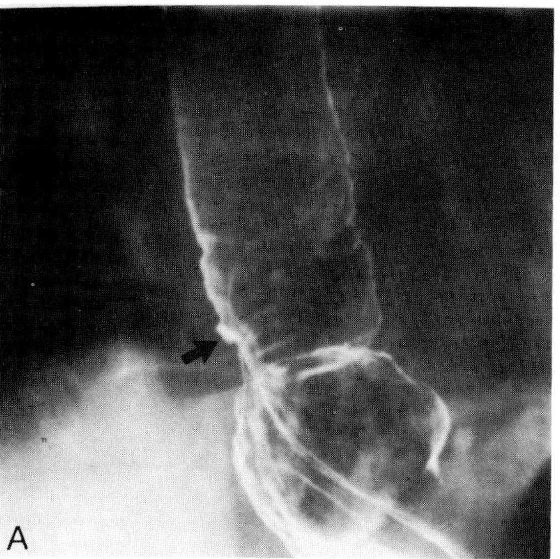

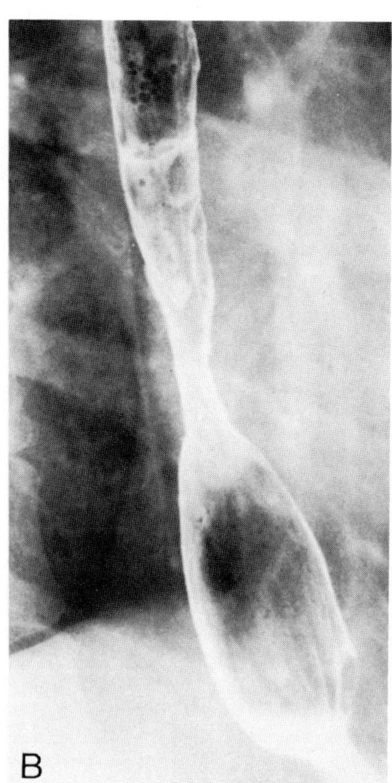

Fig. 3-7. A. Peptic ulcer of the distal esophagus caused by reflux. B. Typical benign peptic stricture with gradual tapered margins. Reproduced by permission from I. Laufer: Double Contrast Gastrointestinal Radiology—With Endoscopic Correlation. WB Saunders, Philadelphia, 1979.

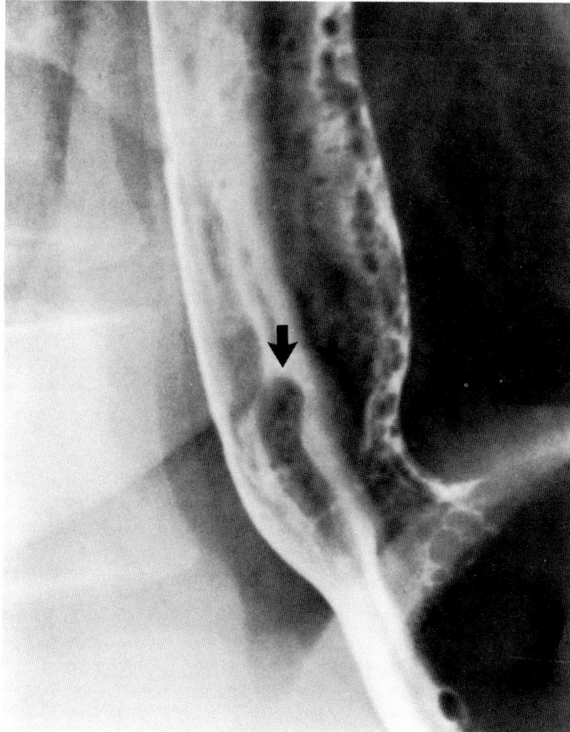

Fig. 3-8. Esophagogastric fold and polyp seen in patients with reflux. A gastric fold that extends into the distal esophagus and ends in a polypoid protuberance may be seen in this radiograph.

esophagitis, some patients have isolated motility disturbances manifested by tertiary contractions, spasm, and feeble or absent peristalsis.[20,21] In fact, aperistalsis may be the only finding in patients with severe esophagitis. This finding is probably related to neuronal damage in Auerbach's plexus secondary to direct extension of the inflammatory process. Unfortunately, abnormal motility delays esophageal emptying and exacerbates the patient's condition by prolonging exposure to the refluxed material. As a result, a vicious cycle may ensue, leading to eventual stricture formation.

Infectious Esophagitis

Although reflux esophagitis is far more common, opportunistic infection of the esophagus is an increasing problem in patients who are immunosuppressed because of underlying malignancy, debilitating illness, corticosteroid therapy, radiation, or chemotherapy. Most cases are caused by *Candida albicans* (moniliasis), although herpes simplex virus has also been recognized with increasing frequency as an opportunistic invader of the esophagus.[22]

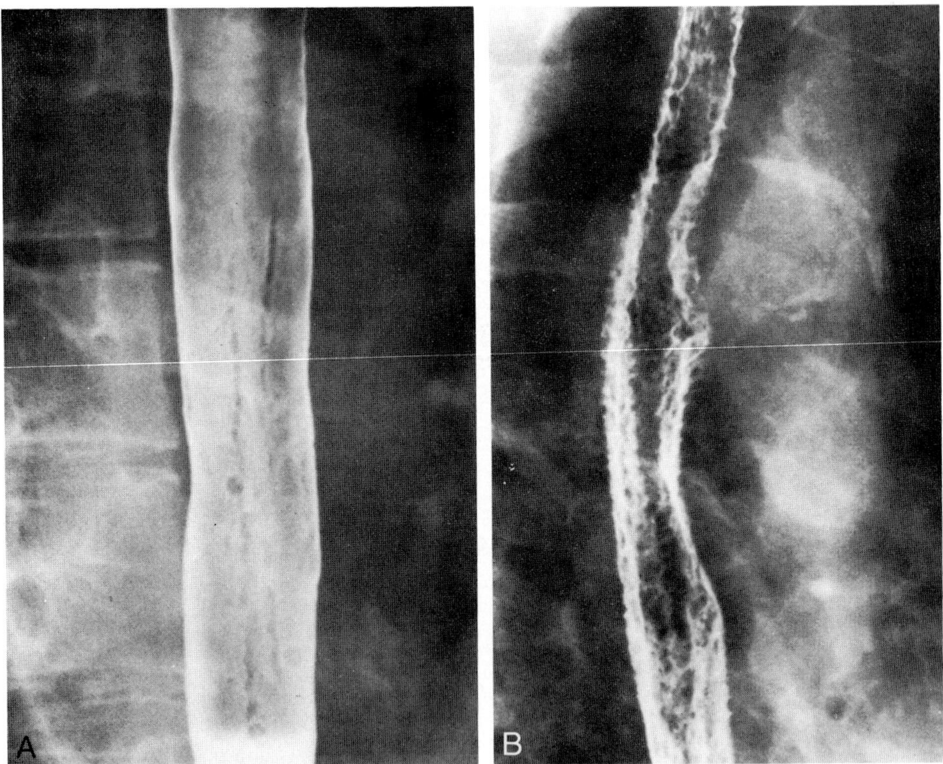

Fig. 3-9. Monilial esophagitis. A. Early changes of monilial esophagitis with linear plaques on the mucosal surface. Reproduced by permission from I. Laufer: Double Contrast Gastrointestinal Radiology—With Endoscopic Correlation. WB Saunders, Philadelphia, 1979. B. More extensive changes with a shaggy mucosal surface that is due to extensive plaque formation.

In monilial esophagitis, the double-contrast examination classically reveals the presence of multiple plaque-like defects that correspond to the small white plaques seen at endoscopy (Fig. 3-9A).[23] There may also be a "cobblestone" appearance because of submucosal edema and associated inflammatory changes.[24] In advanced cases, the esophagus can have an irregular "shaggy" contour caused by extensive plaque and pseudomembrane formation and the presence of multiple ulcerations (Fig. 3-9B).[25] Herpes esophagitis may also produce plaque-like defects in the esophagus (Fig. 3-10A). However, the presence of discrete, widely separated ulcers on an otherwise normal background mucosa appears to be characteristic of herpetic esophagitis and has not been described in patients with moniliasis (Fig. 3-10B).[22]

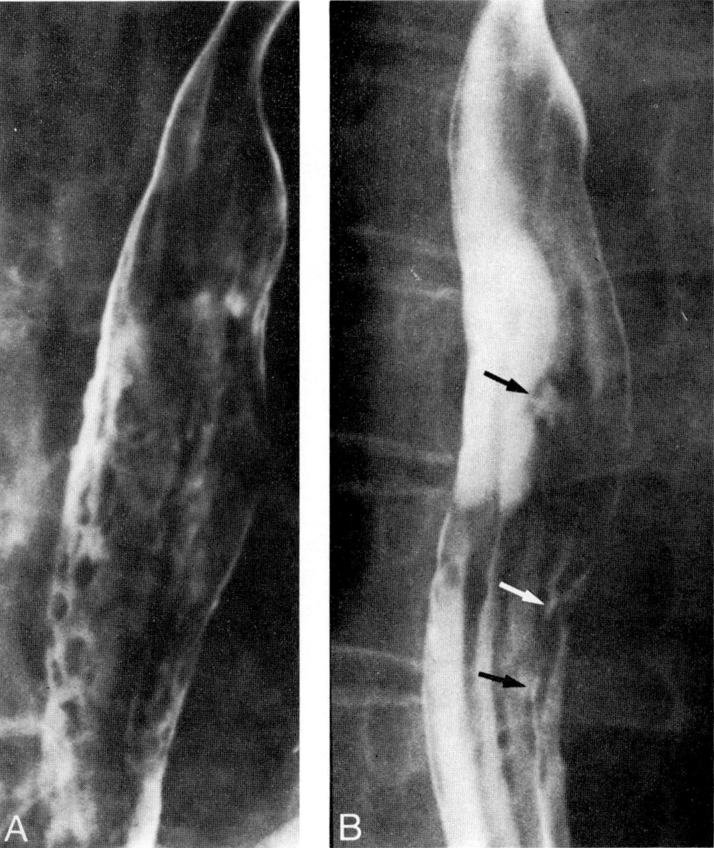

Fig. 3-10. Herpes esophagitis. A. Multiple ulcerated plaques on the mucosal surface are visible in the X-ray of patient who presented with hematemesis resulting from herpetic esophagitis. B. Characteristic appearance of multiple, discrete, separated ulcers due to herpes esophagitis. Reproduced by permission from I. Laufer: Double Contrast Gastrointestinal Radiology—With Endoscopic Correlation. WB Saunders, Philadelphia, 1979.

Other Forms of Esophagitis

Inflammatory changes in the esophagus may occasionally be due to a variety of other causes. In patients with suspected caustic ingestion,[26,27] the barium study is particularly important, since endoscopy carries the risk of perforating the esophagus. In fact, the initial radiographic study probably should be performed with water-soluble contrast in the event that perforation has already occurred. Other radiographic features associated with acute corrosive ingestion (acid or alkaline) include mucosal ulceration and sloughing, pseudomembrane formation (Fig. 3-11A), intramural dissection of barium, and persistent dilatation with intraluminal retention of barium. It has been stated that significant esophageal dilatation and atony denote widespread muscle necrosis and impending perforation analogous to toxic megacolon in patients with ulcerative colitis.[26] If the patient survives, subsequent barium studies should be performed at approximately 4 weeks, when the acute edema has subsided, in order to assess the extent of fibrosis and stricture formation and to plan appropriate therapy.

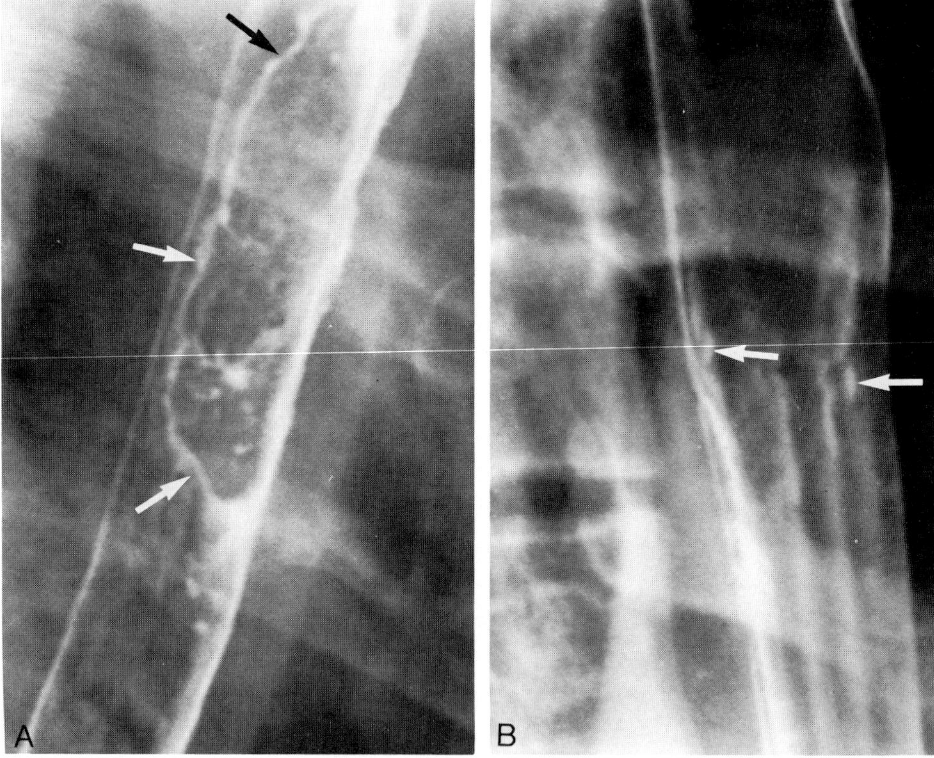

Fig. 3-11. Other forms of esophagitis. A. Lye ingestion. A large necrotic plaque in the mid-esophagus is visible in radiograph from patient who swallowed lye. B. Drug-induced ulceration. X-ray shows multiple small ulcers in the mid-esophagus of patient who had taken tetracycline immediately prior to retiring at night. Courtesy of Robert Gatenby, M.D., Philadelphia.

There have been several descriptions of esophageal ulceration in patients following ingestion of oral medications such as potassium chloride[28] and tetracycline.[29] Oral potassium chloride tablets are usually implicated in patients with mitral stenosis and left atrial enlargement, which delays passage of the tablets and exacerbates their irritant effects on the esophagus. Patients on oral tetracycline or doxycycline may also develop esophageal ulceration, probably because of the acid character of the capsules as they dissolve in the esophagus. These patients typically have a history of ingesting the capsules immediately before going to bed. This timing presumably impairs esophageal emptying and prolongs exposure to the capsules. Double-contrast views may demonstrate discrete, superficial ulcers on a normal background mucosa (Fig. 3-11B); this pattern closely resembles the appearance of herpes esophagitis. However, the latter condition is rarely seen in "immunocompetent" individuals.[30,31]

Radiation-induced esophagitis usually results from high-dose mediastinal radiation for carcinoma of the lung or breast.[32] The most frequent radiographic finding is abnormal esophageal motility. Frank ulcerations or strictures are far less common (Fig. 3-11C). Patients usually develop a self-limited esophagitis with doses of 2,000–4,500 rads, but irreversible damage with stricture or fistula formation may occur

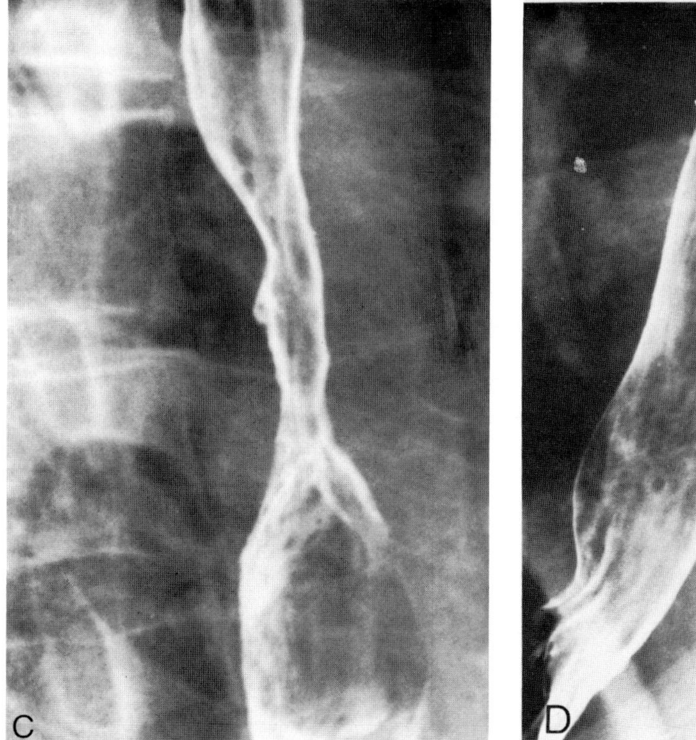
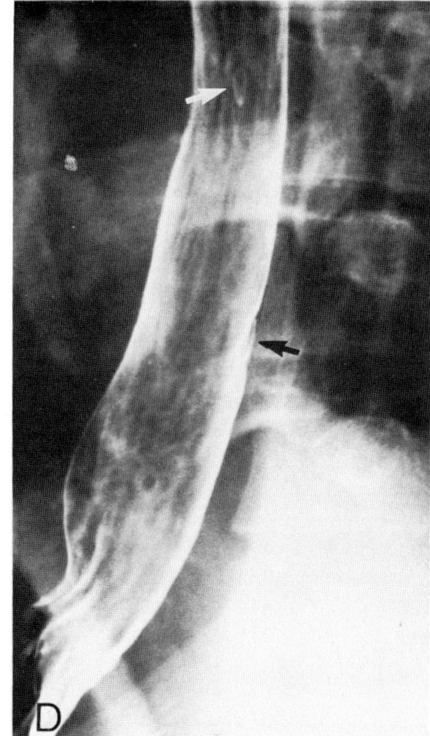

Fig. 3-11 *(continued)*   C. Radiation stricture and ulcer in patient treated with radiation for carcinoma of the esophagus. D. Aphthous ulcers in the esophagus in a patient with known Crohn's disease elsewhere in the gastrointestinal tract.

with doses of 4,500–6,000 rads. It has also been reported that patients on radiation combined with doxorubicin chemotherapy may develop esophagitis with doses as low as 500 rads.[33] Unfortunately, radiation-induced esophagitis is often indistinguishable from opportunistic esophageal infection. This entity therefore should be considered in all patients who develop dysphagia following mediastinal radiation and who show no response to appropriate treatment for moniliasis. In patients being treated with both radiation and doxorubicin, early diagnosis may prevent development of strictures by signalling for a change in chemotherapy.

Esophageal involvement by Crohn's disease is rare but should be suspected in patients known to have the disease elsewhere in the gastrointestinal tract who develop dysphagia or other esophageal symptoms. The most characteristic finding of esophageal Crohn's disease is the presence of multiple transverse and longitudinal intramural fistulous tracts.[34] Other reported findings include thickened mucosal folds, ulceration, strictures, and spontaneous fistulas to adjacent organs.[34-36] We have also encountered several cases of Crohn's disease in which double-contrast views demonstrated typical aphthous ulcers in the esophagus (Fig. 3-11D).[37] Granulomatous esophagitis has also been reported in patients with positive Kveim tests, implicating sarcoidosis rather than Crohn's disease in these individuals.[38]

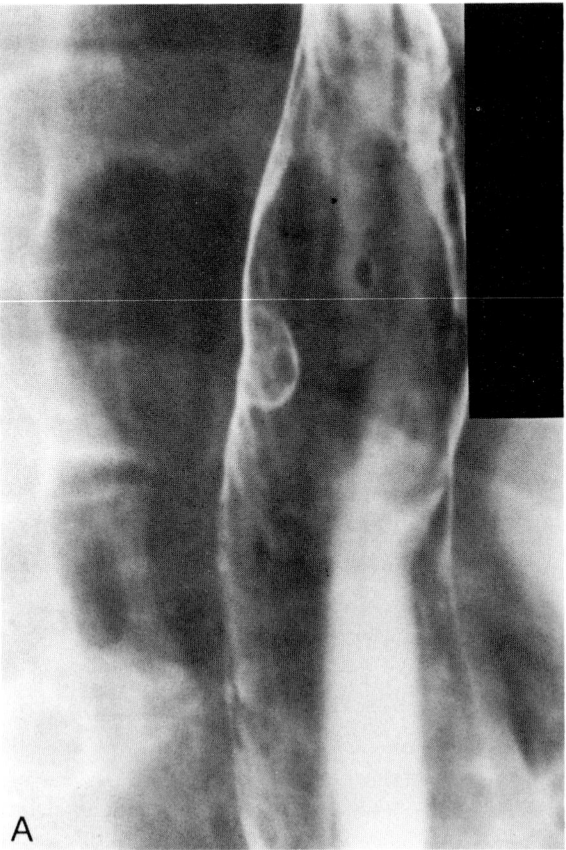

Fig. 3-12. Early esophageal cancer. A. Small polypoid cancer in the mid-esophagus as an incidental finding in a patient presenting with epigastric pain. Courtesy of Seth N. Glick, M.D., Philadelphia. B. Plaque-like lesion with a central ulcer (arrows), caused by early carcinoma. C. Superficial spreading carcinoma of the esophagus. Multiple nodular lesions on the mucosal surface represent the mucosal carcinoma. Courtesy of Akiyoshi Yamada, M.D., Tokyo.

ESOPHAGEAL TUMORS

The death rate for squamous-cell carcinoma of the esophagus has remained unchanged in the past 25 years, with an overall 5-year survival of only 5% and a rate of 20% in those who undergo radical surgery.[39] This dismal prognosis is primarily related to the advanced stage of the disease at the time of detection. In one series of 2,000 cases, fewer than 20% of patients had localized, potentially curable cancer at the time therapy was instituted.[40] These figures suggest that early diagnosis is imperative for increasing patient survival. In this regard, the double-contrast examination has tremendous potential for diagnosing esophageal cancer because of its ability to detect lesions at a far earlier stage than those previously demonstrated on single-contrast studies.

Early Cancer

Early esophageal carcinomas typically appear as plaques or flat sessile polyps (Fig. 3-12A) that frequently have areas of central ulceration (Fig. 3-12B).[39,41,42] Depressed lesions may also be recognized as shallow, irregular barium pools accom-

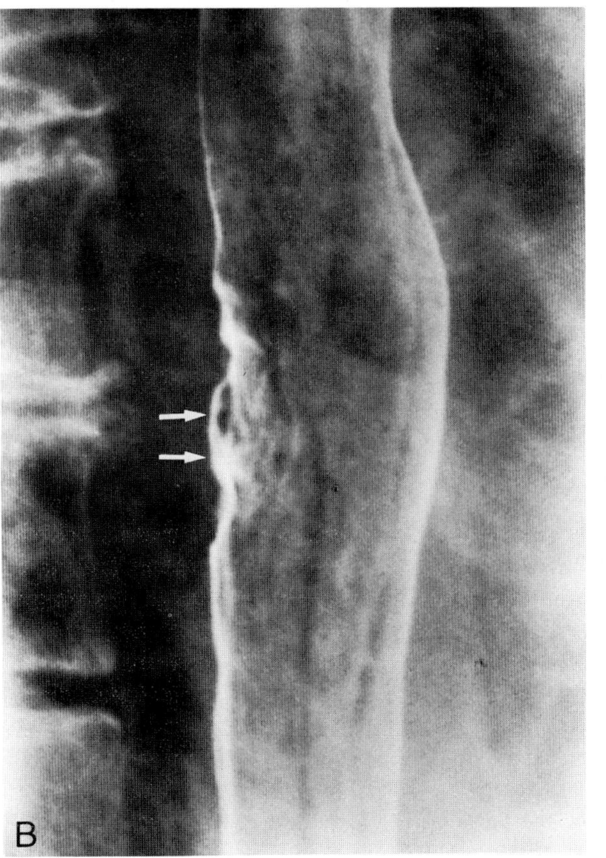

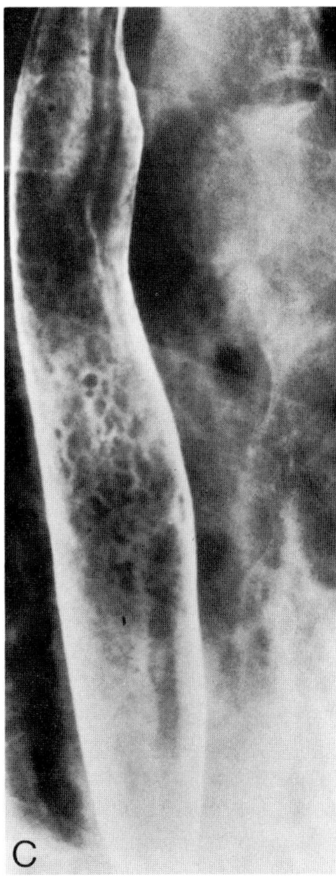

panied by various protrusions. In some cases, early lesions may be identified only as focal areas of rigidity or irregularity in a single wall of the esophagus. Double-contrast views should therefore be obtained in multiple projections to maximize the sensitivity of the examination by visualizing lesions tangentially as well as en face. Close correlation with endoscopy is also essential for any suspicious abnormalities detected by this technique. Endoscopic biopsy should yield malignant cells in 95% of early tumors.[39]

An unusual form of early esophageal malignancy is superficial spreading carcinoma.[43] This entity presents radiographically with multiple finely nodular lesions studding the esophagus, presumably resulting from the mucosal spread of the tumor (Fig. 3-12C). This appearance of diffuse nodularity has also been described in patients with monilial esophagitis, leukoplakia, and acanthosis nigricans.[43,44] Endoscopy and biopsy are required for a definitive diagnosis.

The increased sensitivity of the double-contrast examination has resulted in a lower specificity as more subtle lesions are detected and are suspected of representing cancer.[41] However, it is probably best to accept a certain percentage of false positives in order to avoid missing early lesions. The diagnosis of esophageal carcinoma therefore should be considered for any abnormality that does not have a classically benign appearance. Although benign areas of stricture, ulceration, and esophagitis may be suspected of harboring cancer, scrupulous endoscopic follow-up should clarify the diagnosis and lead to earlier detection of esophageal cancer.

Even with routine use of double-contrast techniques, the radiographic diagnosis of early esophageal carcinoma is often limited by the late onset of symptoms in patients with this disease.[41] Dysphagia, the most common presenting complaint, is often absent until the tumor is large and not resectable. However, some patients do experience dysphagia sufficiently early to permit detection while the tumor may still be resected.[42] A double-contrast examination should therefore be performed as the initial screening procedure for all patients with dysphagia or other esophageal symptoms. It is also a useful screening study for patients with conditions known to predispose to the development of carcinoma. (see ch. 12). The potential value of this technique and its ultimate role in detecting early esophageal cancer await further investigation.

Advanced Cancer

As esophageal carcinoma becomes more advanced, typical ulcerating, infiltrating, and polypoid appearances may be observed. Unfortunately, these lesions are rarely curable, and the prognosis is usually dismal at this late stage. Esophageal tumors may occasionally have an atypical appearance that is mistaken for other conditions. In particular, there is a rare infiltrating form of squamous-cell carcinoma known as "varicoid carcinoma" because it grossly resembles esophageal varices (Fig. 3-13A).[45,46] This tumor produces enlarged, tortuous folds that may appear identical to true esophageal varices (Fig. 3-13B). Unlike varices, however, the tortuous folds remain unchanged with peristalsis, respiration, and Valsalva maneuvers. Therefore, fluoroscopic examination of the esophagus should readily distinguish these entities.

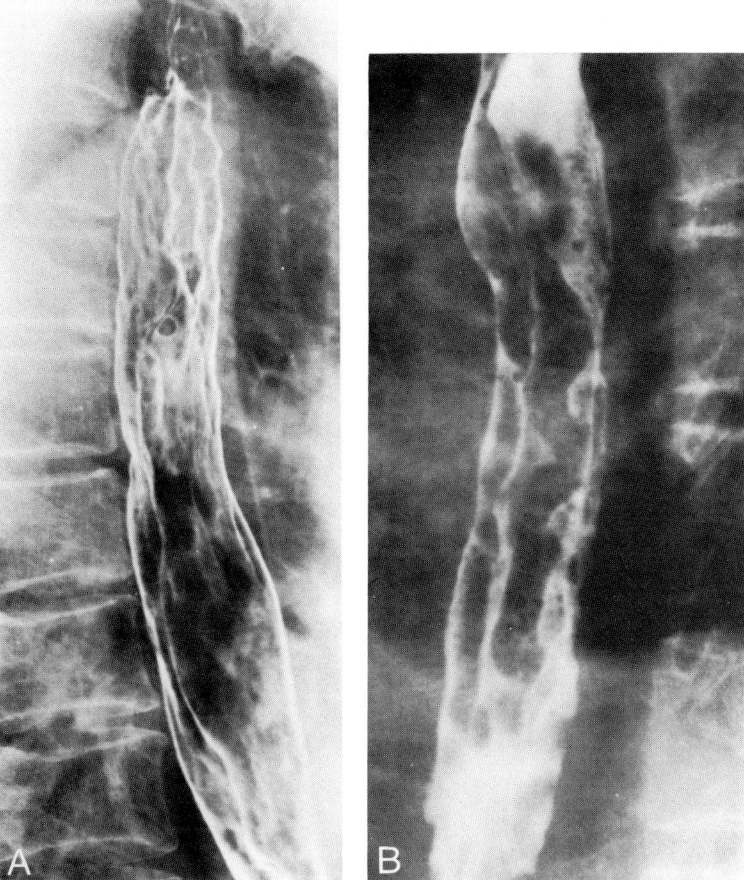

Fig. 3-13. A. Varicoid carcinoma. Multiple thickened and scalloped folds are present throughout the esophagus. These folds resemble esophageal varices, but the finding in this patient was caused by diffuse carcinoma. Courtesy of Akiyoshi Yamada, M.D., Tokyo. B. Esophageal varices. Thickened scalloped folds in the esophagus caused by esophageal varices in a patient with portal hypertension.

Another variety of malignancy occurs at the gastroesophageal junction and may be misinterpreted radiographically as benign disease resulting from reflux or achalasia. Approximately 75% of these lesions are adenocarcinomas and 25% are squamous-cell carcinomas.[47] The vast majority of adenocarcinomas arising in this location probably represent primary gastric malignancies with secondary esophageal involvement.[47,48] These tumors frequently have a fungating or ulcerating appearance that poses little diagnostic problem (Fig. 3-14). Occasionally, however, they may be infiltrating lesions with smooth narrowing and rigidity that mimic the appearance of benign strictures or achalasia (Fig. 3-15).[47] Even in these cases, certain morphologic features, such as abrupt transition, lack of symmetry, and gastric involvement favor malignancy. Nevertheless, some patients with carcinoma at the gastroesophageal junction present with the functional, radiographic, and manometric findings of achalasia, presumably because of neuronal destruction by infiltrating tumor. It is therefore critically important to examine the cardia and fundus in all patients with dysphagia, even in young patients with typical features of achalasia.

Predisposing Conditions

As mentioned above, there are a variety of known risk factors and conditions that predispose to the development of esophageal cancer. These include smoking,[49] alcohol,[49] Barrett's esophagus,[50,51] head-and-neck tumors,[52] achalasia,[53,54] lye strictures,[55] celiac disease,[56] Plummer–Vinson syndrome,[57] and tylosis.[58] Several of these entities produce so much distortion and scarring in the esophagus (i.e., Barrett's esophagus, achalasia, and lye strictures) that developing malignancies may be masked by the underlying disease until they are far advanced. Double-contrast techniques therefore may be particularly valuable in these patients to detect early tumors that are still amenable to resection.

The columnar-lined or Barrett's esophagus is felt to be related to progressive columnar metaplasia of the distal esophagus that results from chronic reflux esophagitis.[17] The typical radiographic appearance consists of a high ulcer or stricture in the esophagus associated with a hiatal hernia or reflux (Fig. 3-16A). The diagnosis should be confirmed histologically by documenting columnar metaplasia

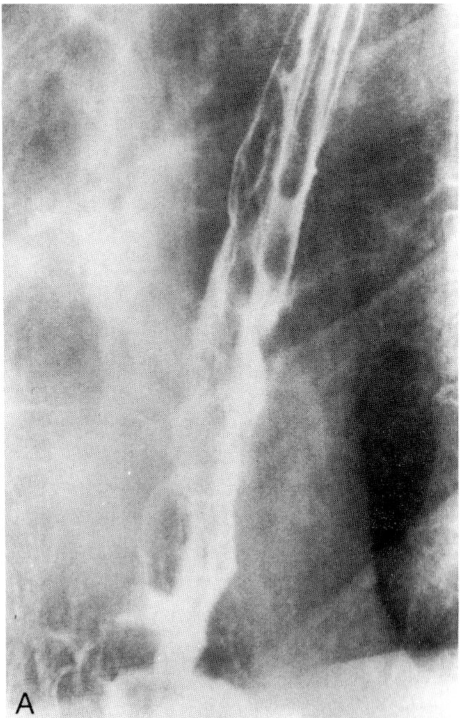

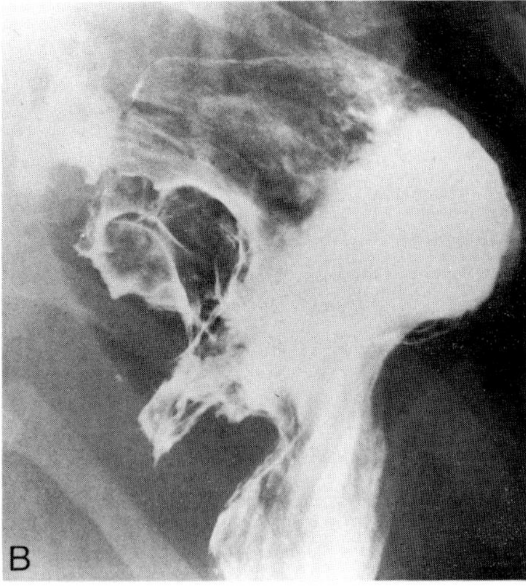

Fig. 3-14. Gastric fundal carcinoma extending into the distal esophagus. Thickened and nodular folds are visible in the distal esophagus (A). This finding was caused by extension of the patient's gastric fundal carcinoma (B).

in the esophagus. It appears that Barrett's esophagus predisposes to the development of adenocarcinoma (Fig. 3-16B) by a progressive sequence of dysplasia.[50,51] Routine surveillance with double-contrast techniques may ultimately prove useful for detecting early malignant changes. Certainly, patients with worsening dysphagia or other esophageal symptoms should undergo radiologic study and endoscopy to rule out the development of a superimposed cancer.

Achalasia is another entity that predisposes to malignancy. Patients with achalasia have an unusually high incidence of squamous-cell carcinoma of the esophagus (Fig. 3-17).[53,54] Malignant degeneration is thought to result from prolonged food retention and esophagitis with chronic irritation of the esophagus. Radiographic detection is made difficult by retained debris that may be indistinguishable from an early tumor. Esophageal lavage should therefore be performed to cleanse the esophagus prior to the barium study. Another problem is that tumors growing inside a massively dilated esophagus are usually far advanced before symptoms

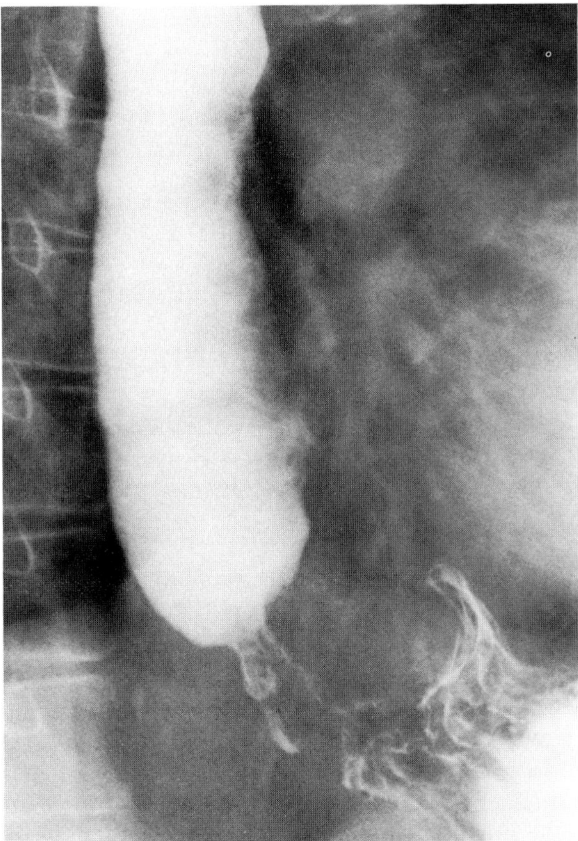

Fig. 3-15. Gastric fundal carcinoma presenting as achalasia. The appearance of the esophagus resembles that seen in achalasia. There is a long stricture with aperistalsis. However, the finding is due to a fundal carcinoma that involves the esophagogastric junction.

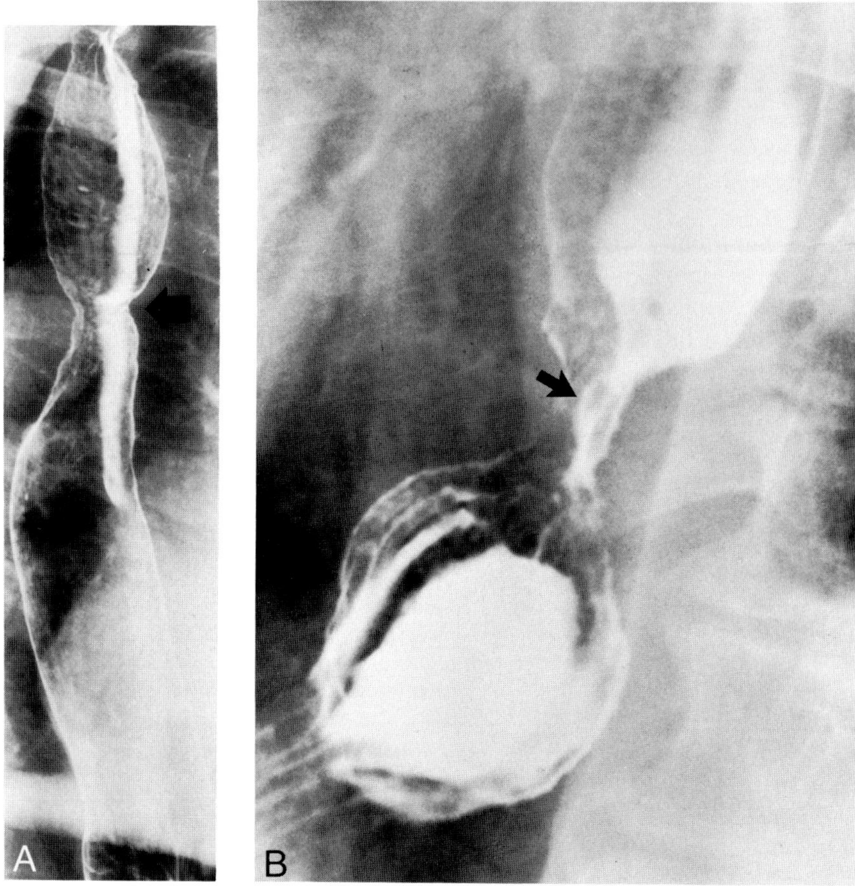

Fig. 3-16.   Barrett's esophagus. A. Typical appearance of Barrett's esophagus with a high esophageal stricture. B. Adenocarcinoma in Barrett's epithelium. Hiatal hernia with reflux esophagitis and a stricture are present. The film also shows a small polypoid lesion (arrow) within the stricture. Biopsy confirmed Barrett's esophagus with adenocarcinoma.

develop. Periodic surveillance is therefore required in the hope of detecting lesions at an early stage.

The incidence of squamous-cell carcinoma of the esophagus is also significantly increased in patients with chronic lye strictures.[55] Yet, ironically, these tumors are frequently detected while they are still amenable to resection. This is because dense scar tissue surrounding the stricture tends to prevent spread to adjacent mediastinal structures. As a result, there may be an excellent chance for survival. The development of radiographically visible ulceration, mucosal nodularity, or other changes at the site of a chronic lye stricture should be regarded with utmost suspicion. Even in the absence of symptoms, routine surveillance is probably warranted, since aggressive therapy with resection of the strictured segment will have an excellent possibility for cure.

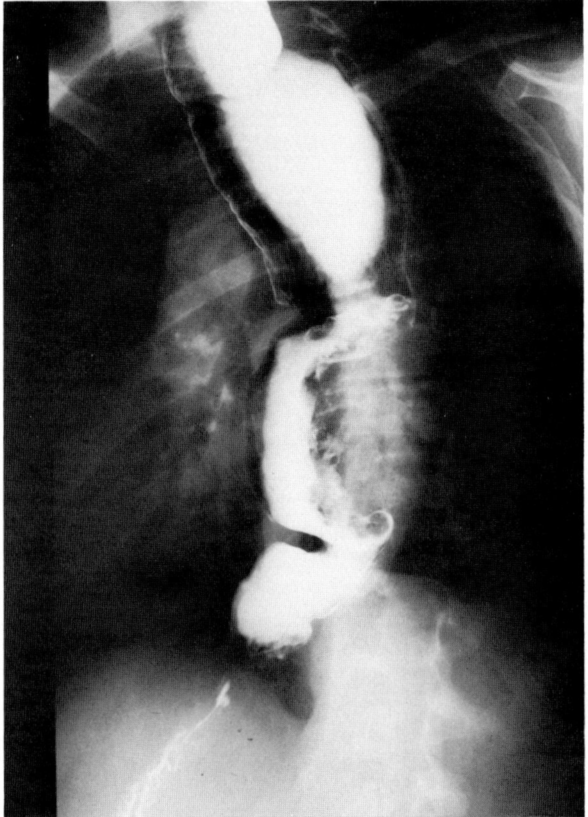

Fig. 3-17. Achalasia with squamous-cell carcinoma. The x-ray shows evidence of long-standing achalasia with marked dilatation and tortuosity of the esophagus. A large polypoid squamous carcinoma is visible in the distal third.

REFERENCES

1. Cohen S: Motor disorders of the esophagus. N Engl J Med 301:184–192, 1979.
2. Margulis AR, Koehler RE: Radiologic diagnosis of disordered esophageal motility. Radiol Clin North Am 14:429–438, 1976.
3. Gefter WB, Laufer I, Edell S, Gohel VK: Candidiasis in the obstructed esophagus. Radiology 138:25–28, 1981.
4. Gonzalez G: Diffuse esophageal spasm. Am J Roentgenol 117:251–258, 1973.
5. Castell DO: Achalasia and diffuse esophageal spasm. Arch Intern Med 136:571–579, 1976.
6. Gohel VK, Edell SM, Laufer I, Rhodes WH: Transverse folds in the human esophagus. Radiology 128:303–308, 1978.
7. Vandervelde GM, Carlson HC: Esophageal reflux. Am J Roentgenol 92:989–993, 1964.
8. Wright RA, Hurwitz AL: Relationship of hiatal hernia to endoscopically proven reflux esophagitis. Dig Dis Sci 24:311–313, 1979.
9. Dodds WJ, Hogan WJ, Miller WN: Reflux esophagitis. Am J Dig Dis 21:49–67, 1976.

10. Dodds WJ: Current concepts of esophageal motor function: clinical implications for radiology. Am J Roentgenol 128:549–561, 1977.
11. Behar J: Reflux esophagitis. Arch Intern Med 136:560–566, 1976.
12. Dodds WJ, Hogan WJ, Helm JF, Dent J: Pathogenesis of reflux esophagitis. Gastroenterology 81:376–394, 1981.
13. Ott DJ, Gelfand DW, Wu WC: Reflux esophagitis: Radiographic and endoscopic correlation. Radiology 130:583–588, 1979.
14. Rabin MS, Schmaman IB: Radiological changes of reflux esophagitis. Clin Radiol 30:187–191, 1979.
15. Koehler RE, Weyman PJ, Oakley HF: Single and double contrast techniques in esophagitis. Am J Roentgenol 135:15–19, 1980.
16. Laufer I: Double Contrast Gastrointestinal Radiology—With Endoscopic Correlation. WB Saunders. Philadelphia, 1979, pp 79–128.
17. Robbins AH, Hermos JA, Schimmel EM, et al.: The columnar-lined esophagus: analysis of 26 cases. Radiology 123:1–7, 1977.
18. Bleshman MH, Banner MP, Johnson RC, Deford JW: The inflammatory esophagogastric polyp and fold. Radiology 128:589–593, 1978.
19. Jones TB, Heller RM, Kirchner SG, Greene HL: Inflammatory esophagogastric polyp in children. Am J Roentgenol 133:314–316, 1979.
20. Olsen AM, Schlegel JF: Motility disturbances caused by esophagitis. J Thorac Cardiovasc Surg 50:607–612, 1965.
21. Simeone JF, Burrell M, Toffler R, Smith W: Aperistalsis and esophagitis. Radiology 123:9–14, 1977.
22. Levine MS, Laufer I, Kressel HY, Friedman HM: Herpes esophagitis. Am J Roentgenol 136:863–866, 1981.
23. Gonzalez B: Esophageal moniliasis. Am J Roentgenol 113:233–236, 1971.
24. Goldberg HI, Dodds WJ: Cobblestone esophagus due to monilial infection. Am J Roentgenol 104:608–612, 1968.
25. Athey PA, Goldstein HM, Dodd GD: Radiologic spectrum of opportunistic infections of the upper gastrointestinal tract. Am J Roentgenol 129:419–424, 1977.
26. Martel W: Radiologic features of esophagogastritis secondary to extremely caustic agents. Radiology 103:31–36, 1972.
27. Muhletaler CA, Gerlock AJ, de Soto L, Halter SA: Acid corrosive esophagitis: radiographic findings. Am J Roentgenol 134:1137–1140, 1980.
28. Teplick JG, Teplick SK, Ominsky SH, Haskin ME: Esophagitis caused by oral medication. Radiology 134:23–25, 1980.
29. Crowson TD, Head LH, Ferrante WA: Esophageal ulcers associated with tetracycline therapy. JAMA 235:2747–2748, 1976.
30. Deprew WT, Prentice RSA, Beck IT, et al.: Herpes simplex ulcerative esophagitis in a healthy subject. Am J Gastroenterol 68:381–385, 1977.
31. Owensby LC, Stammer JL: Esophagitis associated with herpes simplex infection in an immunocompetent host. Gastroenterology 74:1305–1306, 1978.
32. Goldstein HM, Rogers LF, Fletcher GH, Dodd GD: Radiological manifestations of radiation-induced injury to the normal upper gastrointestinal tract. Radiology 117:135–140, 1975.
33. Boal DKB, Newburger PE, Teele RL: Esophagitis induced by combined radiation and adriamycin. Am J Roentgenol 132:567–570, 1979.
34. Cynn WS, Chon HK, Gureghian PA, Levin BL: Crohn's disease of the esophagus. Am J Roentgenol 125:359–364, 1975.

35. Legge DA, Carlson HC, Judd ES: Roentgenologic features of regional enteritis of the upper gastrointestinal tract. Am J Roentgenol 110:355–360, 1970.
36. LiVolsi VA, Jaretski A: Granulomatous esophagitis. Gastroenterology 64:313–319, 1973.
37. Gohel VK, Long BW, Richter G: Aphthous ulcers in the esophagus with Crohn's colitis. Am J Roentgenol 137:872–873, 1981.
38. Weisner PJ, Kleinman MS, Condemi JJ, et al.: Sarcoidosis of the esophagus. Am J Dig Dis 16:943–951, 1971.
39. Itai Y, Kogure T, Okuyama Y, Akiyama H: Superficial esophageal carcinoma. Radiology 126:597–601, 1978.
40. Pearson JG: The value of radiotherapy in the management of squamous esophageal cancer. Br J Surg 58:794–798, 1971.
41. Moss AA, Koehler RE, Margulis AR: Initial accuracy of esophagograms in detection of small esophageal carcinoma. Am J Roentgenol 127:909–913, 1976.
42. Koehler RE, Moss AA, Margulis AR: Early radiographic manifestations of carcinoma of the esophagus. Radiology 119:1–5, 1976.
43. Itai Y, Kogure T, Okuyama Y, Akiyama H: Diffuse finely nodular lesions of the esophagus. Am J Roentgenol 128:563–566, 1977.
44. Itai Y, Kogure T, Okuyama Y, Akiyama H: Radiological manifestations of esophageal involvement in acanthosis nigricans. Br J Radiol 49:592–593, 1976.
45. Silver TM, Goldstein HM: Varicoid carcinoma of the esophagus. Am J Dig Dis 19:56–58, 1974.
46. Lawson TL, Dodds WJ, Sheft DJ: Carcinoma of the esophagus simulating varices. Am J Roentgenol 107:83–85, 1969.
47. Balthazar EJ, Goldfine S, Davidian MM: Carcinoma of the esophagogastric junction. Am J Gastroenterol 74:237–243, 1980.
48. Webb JN, Busuttil A: Adenocarcinoma of the esophagus and of the esophagogastric junction. Br J Surg 65:475–479, 1978.
49. Wynder EL, Mabuchi K: Cancer of the esophagus: Etiological and environmental factors. JAMA 226:1546–1548, 1973.
50. Haggitt RC, Tryzelaar J, Ellis FH, Colcher H: Adenocarcinoma complicating columnar epithelium-lined Barrett's esophagus. Am J Clin Pathol 70:1–5, 1978.
51. Naef AP, Savary M, Ozzello L: Columnar-lined lower esophagus: an acquired lesion with malignant predisposition. J Thorac Cardiovasc Surg 70:826–834, 1975.
52. Goldstein HM, Zornoza J: Association of squamous cell carcinoma of the head and neck with cancer of the esophagus. Am J Roentgenol 131:791–794, 1978.
53. Carter R, Brewer LA: Achalasia and esophageal carcinoma. Am J Surg 130:114–118, 1975.
54. Wychulis AR, Woolam GL, Andersen HA, Ellis FH: Achalasia and carcinoma of the esophagus. JAMA 215:1638–1641, 1971.
55. Lansing PB, Ferrante WA, Ochsner JL: Carcinoma of the esophagus at the site of lye stricture. Am J Surg 118:108–111, 1969.
56. Collins SM, Hamilton JD, Lewis TD, Laufer I: Small bowel malabsorption and gastrointestinal malignancy. Radiology 126:603–609, 1978.
57. Chisholm M: The association between webs, iron and postcricoid carcinoma. Postgrad Med J 50:215–219, 1974.
58. Harper PS, Harper RMJ, Howel-Evans AW: Carcinoma of the oesophagus with tylosis. Q J Med 39:317–333, 1970.

4 | New Diagnostic Techniques in Esophageal Disease

Richard H. Holloway
Richard W. McCallum

ESOPHAGEAL SCINTIGRAPHY

Radionuclide examination of the esophagus is the most recent technique developed to study esophageal function. It has major advantages over other methods in that it is noninvasive and involves considerably less exposure to radiation than conventional radiographic techniques. Whereas the initial studies were largely qualitative,[1] the more recent interfacing of computers to store and assess the data has enhanced quantitation. So far the technique has been applied in two main areas of esophageal function: the detection and measurement of esophageal reflux and the measurement of esophageal transit.

Gastroesophageal Reflux

Scintigraphy has been used to detect gastroesophageal reflux in both children[2-4] and adults.[5-8] In this procedure, 200–300 μCi ^{99m}Tc-sulfur colloid are swallowed in the form of an isotope-labeled liquid meal, and interval counts are measured with a gamma camera over the area of the esophagus and stomach. An abdominal binder is used to increase intra-abdominal pressure. The degree of reflux can be quantitated by expressing the counts detected over the esophagus as a percentage of those counted over the stomach—the "reflux index."[5] The technique is simple and may be reduced to a 5-min procedure.[9] In children, the test has been uniformly sensitive with positive results in 75–85% of patients with symptoms. This score was not improved by using abdominal binders or other means to increase intra-abdominal pressure. Where comparisons were made, scintigraphy was more sensitive than radiologic evaluation but less so than the standard acid-reflux test (SART).

The results in adult studies have varied. Those from one center suggest that the test is reliable and accurate with a sensitivity and specificity of 90%.[5] False-positive tests occurred in 7% of patients and false-negative in 13%. These results were appreciably better than those obtained with radiologic studies, the Bernstein test, endoscopy, or esophageal biopsy, but inferior to those obtained with SART, which was used as a reference test. Severity of gastroesophageal reflux was assessed, and showed a significant correlation between the reflux index and the symptom score.[8] A correlation was also implied between the severity of endoscopic esophagitis and the reflux index, although a direct comparison was not made. Simultaneous scanning of the lungs may detect pulmonary aspiration.[10] Studies performed after medical and surgical therapy were able to demonstrate a significant reduction in the degree of reflux.[6,8]

Hoffman et al.,[7] however, were unable to reproduce these results despite using the same technique; they reported positive scans in only 14% of patients with reflux. It is noteworthy that they also reported a similarly low rate of positive tests with SART. At our institution, we have been impressed by the method's failure to detect any consistent evidence of esophageal counts during the evaluation of gastric emptying in patients with subjective and objective evidence of gastroesophageal reflux disease. Isotope-labeled solid, semi-solid, and liquid meals were studied in patients who were supine and were monitored for 2 hours postprandially.[11] In addition, we have been unable to obtain reliable results in children using an iostope-labeled infant formula preparation when there was other objective evidence of gastroesophageal reflux.[12] In both adults and children, neither abdominal compression nor exercise were incorporated into the test.

Gastroesophageal scintigraphy offers the potential for a simple, safe, and noninvasive means of both detecting and quantitating gastroesophageal reflux. Its role in the diagnostic armamentarium would seem to be that of an alternative to SART. However, this role has not been clearly established. Future emphasis in this field should be placed in the following areas: (1) defining the contribution of the test when it is compared with other esophageal function studies, in particular defining whether it can be an indicator of subtle gastroesophageal reflux or whether it is only positive when the diagnosis would seem obvious by other methods; (2) demonstrating reproducibility of the test in a number of gastroenterology laboratories; (3) addressing the question of whether abdominal compression is critical to induction of a positive test and/or to the test's ability to discriminate between a refluxing patient and a normal subject.

Esophageal Transit

Measurement of esophageal transit was the first application of esophageal scintigraphy. Most studies have concentrated on esophageal clearance as a measure of overall esophageal transit. However, a recent report has also attempted to assess the kinetics of intraesophageal movement.

Of other currently available techniques, only barium studies address actual esophageal transit. However, even with cinerecordings, the esophagram is at its best only qualitative and entails considerable exposure to radiation. Manometry, although quantitative, measures only esophageal contractions and not the actual movement of the swallowed bolus of water. Dysphagia, especially when intermittent, may be associated with a normal manometric recording. Does a radionuclide study offer any advantage?

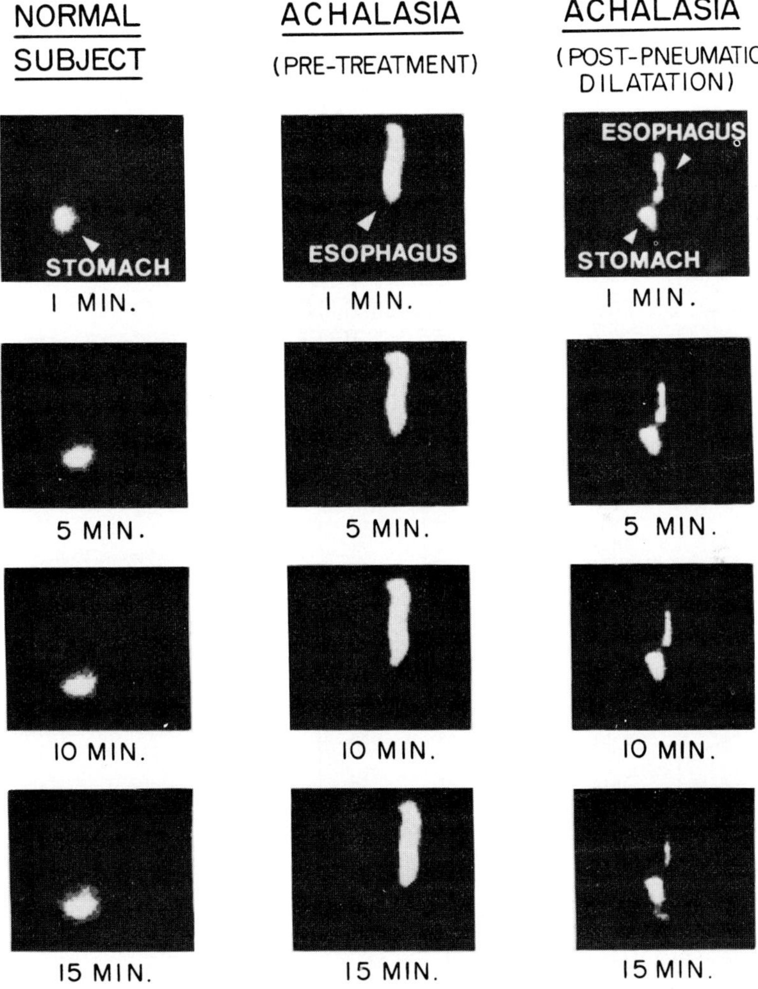

Fig. 4-1. Radionuclide esophageal emptying of a solid meal. Gastroesophageal scintiscans taken for 15 min after a normal subject and an achalasia patient ingested an egg salad sandwich meal labeled with ^{99m}Technetium-DTPA (Diethylenetriamine penta-acetic acid). A considerable amount of isotope remains in the dilated achalasia esophagus. In normal subjects, no isotope can be appreciated or scintiscans taken immediately after completion of the test meal.

The technique involves having the patient swallow a ^{99m}Tc sulfur-colloid-labeled meal while the region over the esophagus is simultaneously scanned with a gamma camera (Fig. 4-1). Either a liquid or a solid meal may be used, but a solid meal, such as an egg-salad sandwich, reproduces physiological conditions more accurately.[13] Gamma counts are measured in sequential 15-sec intervals during single or multiple swallows, and a clearance curve is plotted, as well as overall esophageal clearance time. Another method is to start monitoring counts posteriorly over the esophagus and stomach from 1–15 min after the patient completes ingesting the test meal. The latter approach is particularly appropriate for isotope-labeled solid meals.[13]

Measurement of esophageal emptying is particularly useful in assessing the effectiveness of treatment for achalasia. Studies using both liquid[13] and solid[14] meals have demonstrated significant improvement in esophageal emptying after either pneumatic dilatation or myotomy (Figs. 4-1, 4-2). We have found that the resting lower esophageal sphincter (LES) pressure in achalasia patients does not correlate with the extent of isotope retention in the esophagus prior to therapy. However, manometric studies in patients subjectively improved after pneumatic dilatation or surgical treatment indicated a marked reduction in LES pressure, and sphincter pressures of less than 15 mm Hg correlated with essentially normal

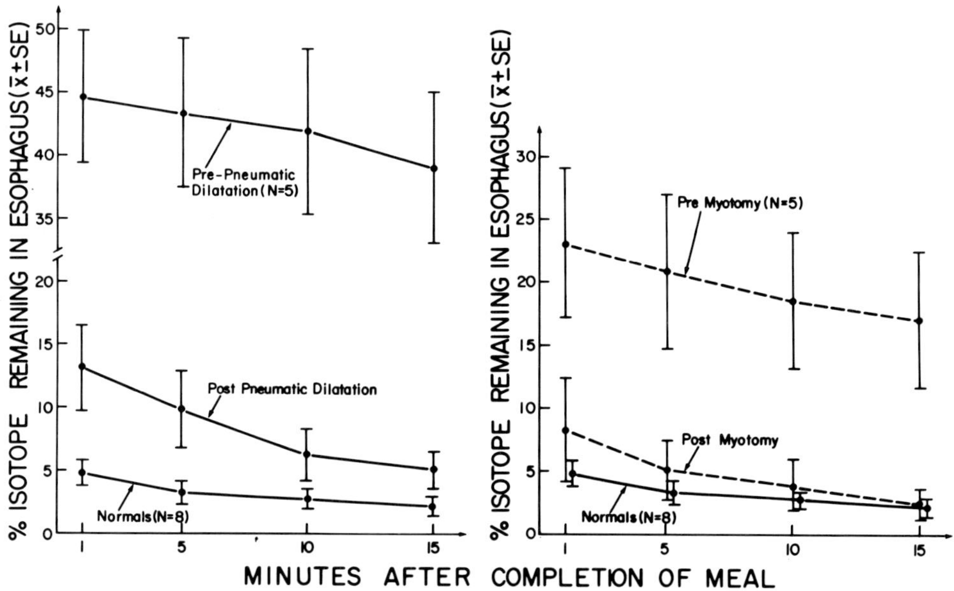

Fig. 4-2. Pre- and posttherapy mean (± SEM) esophageal retention of isotope in patients treated with pneumatic dilatation as compared with surgical myotomy with accompanying fundoplication. The test meal was an egg salad sandwich labeled with [99m]Technetium-DTPA. Patients treated by pneumatic dilatation showed significantly reduced ($p < 0.01$) isotope retention, as did the patients receiving surgical therapy ($p < 0.01$). Esophageal retention of isotope by 15 min after the test meal approaches the result obtained in normal subjects.

esophageal emptying as measured by an isotope-labeled egg-salad sandwich meal. The test tends to support the patient's assessment of symptom improvement, although many patients still have delayed clearance despite resolution of symptoms. Whether or not the finding of a normal esophageal clearance should be used to determine the end point of treatment (in particular for pneumatic dilatation) has not been assessed; however, the test does demonstrate that many patients are happy with the result of pneumatic dilatation even when esophageal emptying is still not entirely normal.

As well as providing posttreatment evaluation in achalasia patients, scintigraphy would seem to be a very useful tool to evaluate present and future treatment adjuncts or alternatives in the medical management of achalasia. Our recent experience in one patient who showed clinical and manometrically demonstrated response to therapy with the calcium antagonist, nifedipine, illustrates this point (Fig. 4-3).

In a study of both normal subjects and patients with manometrically defined abnormalities, radionuclide studies of overall esophageal transit using both single-swallow and multiple-swallow techniques demonstrated significant differences between normal subjects and patients with achalasia, diffuse spasm, and scleroderma.[15] However, the test was not applied to an unselected group of patients with symptoms of dysphagia and/or chest pain or used in patients with nonspecific motor abnormalities. In our experience, the test has been reliable and has the additional features of being inexpensive and of requiring less than 30 min; in addition, radiation exposure is several magnitudes less than that with barium radiography.

A recent study by Russell et al.[16] divided the esophagus into segments. Both

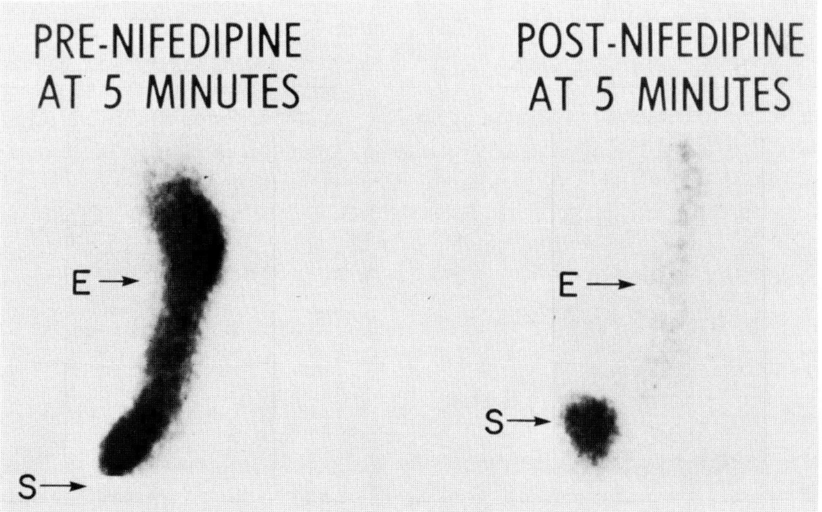

Fig. 4-3.   Esophageal scintiscans obtained 5 min after ingestion of a [99m]Technetium-DTPA-labeled egg salad sandwich meal was completed. These scintiscans demonstrate the improvement in esophageal emptying when nifedipine, 20 mg orally, was administered 30 min prior to the test meal in a patient with achalasia. E, esophagus; S, stomach.

the transit time within each segment and the total esophageal transit time could be measured. In achalasia, scleroderma, and diffuse spasm characteristic segmental transit patterns were seen that were markedly different from those seen in control subjects (Fig. 4-4). In addition, an abnormal pattern was seen in 9 of 14 patients who complained of dysphagia but had esophageal manometric findings that were regarded as being normal.

This study would suggest that radionuclide transit studies, when assessed on a segmental basis, may be more sensitive than esophageal manometry. However, although the radionuclide technique has been proposed as a screening test, unanswered questions to this approach remain. The test uses a liquid bolus that may not provide a true challenge to esophageal function. Solid-food dysphagia is generally experienced when the esophageal diameter is less than 13 mm (#40 French), a diameter at which liquids are usually swallowed with no difficulty. Thus, the currently recommended barium esophagogram, when performed with marshmallows or barium tablets, has an advantage in this respect. A particular benefit of the latter study is that the patient can state when the symptoms of dysphagia and/or chest pain are being felt and the position of the bolus can be simultaneously identified with fluroscopy. Hence, subtle areas of "hold-up" or slight narrowing can be better identified.

In any event, the final process for evaluating the esophagus, before one can decide if a motility disorder is present, is to define the anatomy and to visualize a normal mucosal outline. Hence, it would seem very important that any suggestion that the liquid-bolus technique can be a screening procedure, particularly for subtle motor abnormalities not otherwise identified, be based on a comparison with well-performed barium studies incorporating a solid bolus. Also, some consideration should be given to developing an isotope-labeled solid bolus (e.g., a chicken-liver cube) to compare with the liquid bolus.

Another question is what is the value of a negative scintiscan. The study by Russell et al. implies that a negative test virtually excludes an esophageal motor abnormality.[16] However, this conclusion has yet to be tested specificly on a large unselected patient population. Answering this question is of prime importance if scintigraphy is to justify a role as a true screening test.

Despite these criticisms, this latest technique is an exciting development in the study of esophageal motor disease and should prove a most useful addition to tests already available.

GASTRIC EMPTYING

Measurement of gastric emptying may not seem to qualify as a test of esophageal function. However, since up to 57% of patients with gastroesophageal reflux have delayed gastric emptying of an isotope-labeled solid meal,[11,17] measuring the rate of gastric clearance is relevant to their management. Symptoms suggestive of delayed emptying include postprandial epigastric bloating and fullness, early satiety, nausea, and vomiting. In patients with reflux who are not responding to

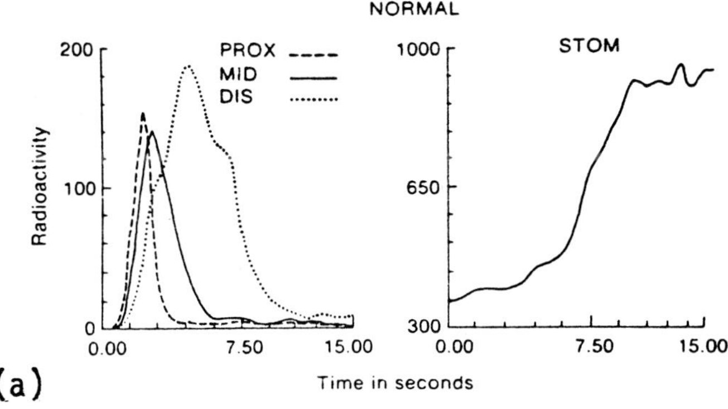

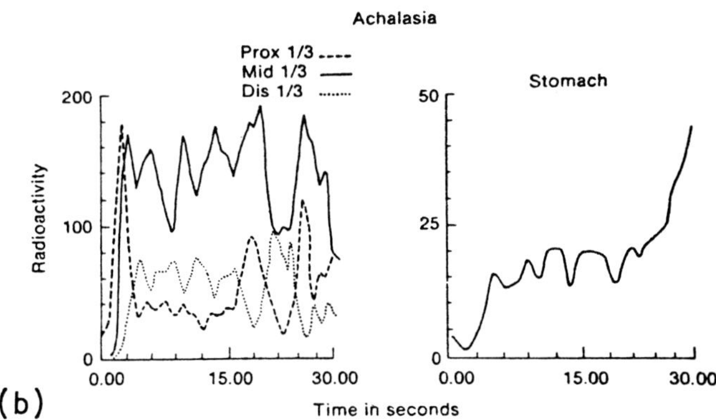

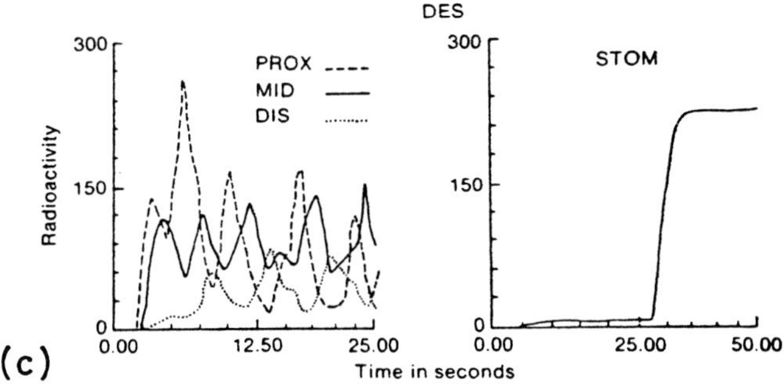

Fig. 4-4. Radionuclide transit graphs from a) a normal volunteer; b) a patient with achalasia; and c) a patient with diffuse esophageal spasm. In the graph from the normal volunteer note the sequential peaks from the three segments with early complete entry into the stomach. This is compared with the disorganization of this pattern of esophageal emptying in the patients with achalasia and with diffuse esophageal spasm. Reprinted by permission of the publisher from Radionuclide transit: a sensitive screening test for esophageal dysfunction, by Russell COH, Hill LD, Holmes ER III, et al., Gastroenterology 80:887–892. Copyright 1981 by the American Gastroenterological Association.

initial conventional treatment, especially when these symptoms are present, measurement of gastric emptying may be valuable when deciding on therapeutic options.

Gastric emptying of solids is largely independent of liquids and is controlled by a separate mechanism. Thus, separate markers are needed for each phase. Since the abnormality in gastroesophageal reflux is specific for the solid component of the meal[17] (Fig. 4-5), suggesting that an antral motility disturbance is present, only a solid-phase marker need be incorporated into the meal. The most accurate solid-phase marker, with least desorption into the liquid phase, is in vivo intracellularly ^{99m}Tc-labeled chicken liver.[18] However, this labeling technique is impractical for routine use, and a ^{99m}Tc-labeled egg-salad sandwich, although less accurate, is acceptable as a screening test for gastric emptying. After the labeled meal is

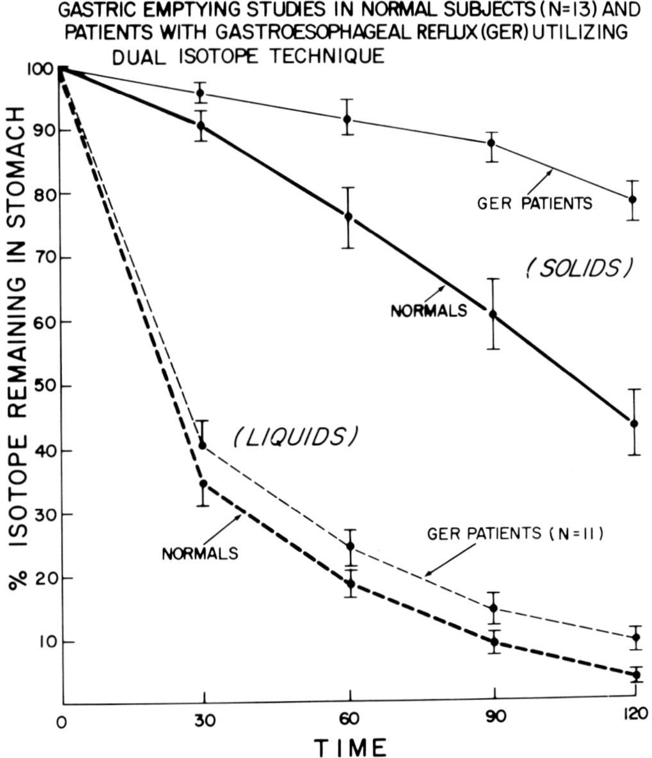

Fig. 4-5. Gastric emptying of solids and liquids simultaneously measured by the dual isotope technique in 13 normal subjects and 11 patients with gastroesophageal reflux. Gastric emptying is expressed as the percent of isotope remaining in the stomach at 30, 60, 90 and 120 min after ingestion of the solid-meal component (consisting of chicken liver intracellularly labeled with [99m]Technetium-sulfur colloid as a specific solid-food marker) and 100 cc of water labeled with [111]Indium-DTPA as the marker for the liquid component of the meal. Data are expressed as mean ± 1 SEM. Gastric emptying was significantly slower for the solid phase marker in the gastroesophageal reflux patients as compared with the normal subjects at 60 ($p < 0.05$), 90 ($p < 0.05$), and 120 min ($p < 0.01$), while the empyting of water was similar to that in normal subjects.

eaten, the patient lies under a gamma camera, and counts are made over the region of the stomach for 2 hours. Normal patients have less than 70% of isotope remaining in the stomach after 2 hours.[11] As with the other radionuclide studies, the technique is simple and noninvasive, and it can be performed in any institution where the equipment is available and "normal" values defined.

Gastric emptying studies may become routine in assessing or managing gastroesophageal reflux. It is important to appreciate that patients with reflux are not pathophysiologicly homogeneous. Thus, knowledge of the gastric emptying rate in a particular patient will allow treatment to be tailored specifically to fit the major pathophysiologic contribution. Neutralization of gastric contents may not be appropriate as the single approach to therapy, but rather a "mechanical" approach to enhance LES pressure and accelerate gastric emptying. This is in light of the great potential offered by smooth-muscle-stimulating agents that increase LES pressure and enhance gastric emptying. The dopamine antagonist metoclopramide has significantly improved gastroesophageal reflux in a number of studies. A new-generation selective peripheral dopamine antagonist, domperidone, also addresses the central concept that delayed gastric emptying is a significant contributor to the pathophysiology and etiology of gastroesophageal reflux.

ESOPHAGEAL pH MEASUREMENT

Measurement of intraesophageal pH was first proposed by Tuttle in 1958.[19] Since then the technique has expanded to include the standard acid-reflux test,[20,21] the acid-clearance test,[22] and 24-hour pH monitoring.[23]

Standard Acid-Reflux Test

The standard acid-reflux test (SART) involves measuring intraesophageal pH, 5 cm above the manometrically defined LES, before and after instillation of 300 ml 0.1N HC1 into the stomach. Reflux is measured both basally and during maneuvers, such as the Valsalva maneuver, leg raising, and coughing, that are designed to increase intra-abdominal pressure. Reflux is considered to be present if the pH falls to 4 or below (Fig. 4-6). The severity of reflux may be quantitated by measuring both the number of reflux episodes and the total duration of reflux. Some workers have reported good discrimination between control subjects and those with reflux esophagitis.[24,25] However, in other series, the test was less impressive, although still more accurate than barium studies.[21,26,27] The number of positive tests in asymptomatic subjects ranges from 4%–20%. It is possible that these represent true asymptomatic refluxers. However, this interpretation is open to question, since intragastric instillation of HC1 lowers LES pressure[28] and the relationship of the various maneuvers used in testing to physiologic conditions is not clear.

To remove some of the doubt concerning the physiologic nature of SART, future consideration should be given to an acid-reflux test that meets the following criteria: (1) It should be based on physiologic and clinical concepts that gastroesophageal reflux occurs in the immediate postprandial period; (2) it should be

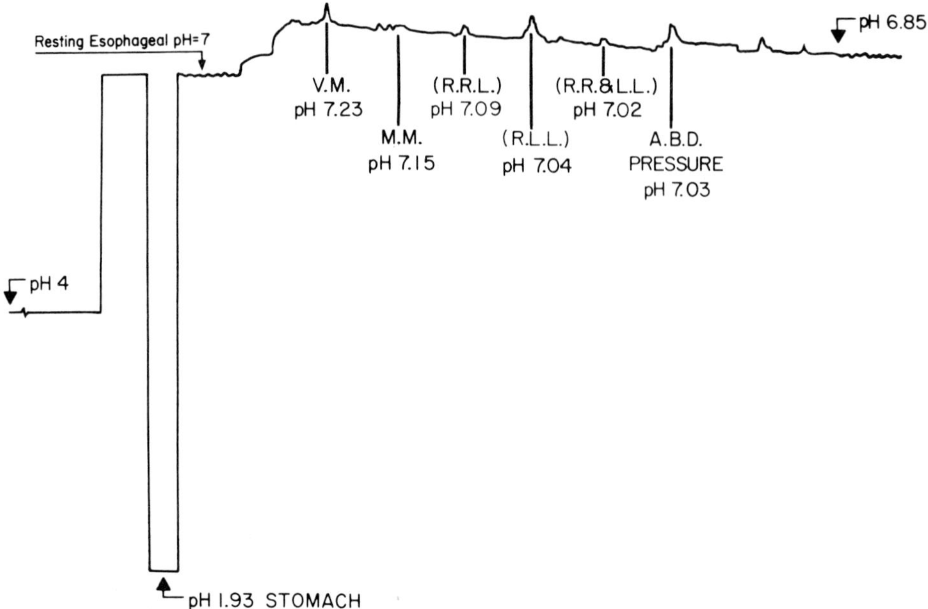

Fig. 4-6. A tracing from a patient with a normal acid-reflux test. Note the resting esophageal pH of 7 (normal > 5) and the absence of reflux (esophageal pH < 4) during various maneuvers. VM, Valsalva maneuver; MM, Moeller maneuver; RRL, raised right leg; RLL, raised left leg; RR&LL, raised right and left leg; ABD, abdominal compression.

acceptable to both patients and technicians; (3) it should have a role both in the diagnosis of gastroesophageal reflux and as a model for predicting the efficacy of planned treatment regimens or new therapeutic approaches.

Our group has carried out a postprandial acid-reflux test on a series of patients with symptoms of gastroesophageal reflux (GER) and a positive SART (*unpublished observations*). Basal reflux was evaluated preprandially in both the sitting (1-hour) and lying positions (2-hours). The subject then ingested an egg-salad sandwich and 250 ml of milk (a standard meal), and esophageal pH was monitored as before. No maneuvers were performed and no acid was instilled.

Preprandial reflux time was 14.0 ± 6.1 (SEM) min for patients with reflux as compared with 0.3 ± 0.2 min for normal subjects. However, 7 of the 15 reflux patients had a total reflux time in the basal period of less than the upper range of the normal subjects. Mean 3-hour postprandial reflux time was 44.6 ± 6.7 min in patients with GER as compared with 4.0 ± 1.2 min in normal subjects. Fourteen of the patients with GER had postprandial reflux times greater than the maximal reflux time demonstrated in normal persons (Fig. 4-7). The value of postprandial exaggeration of differences between patients with reflux and normals—differences that may not be adequately appreciated under basal conditions or in nonphysiologic settings—is clearly demonstrated in such a test. Similarly, the maximum length of reflux episodes is also increased in the postprandial period (Fig. 4-8).

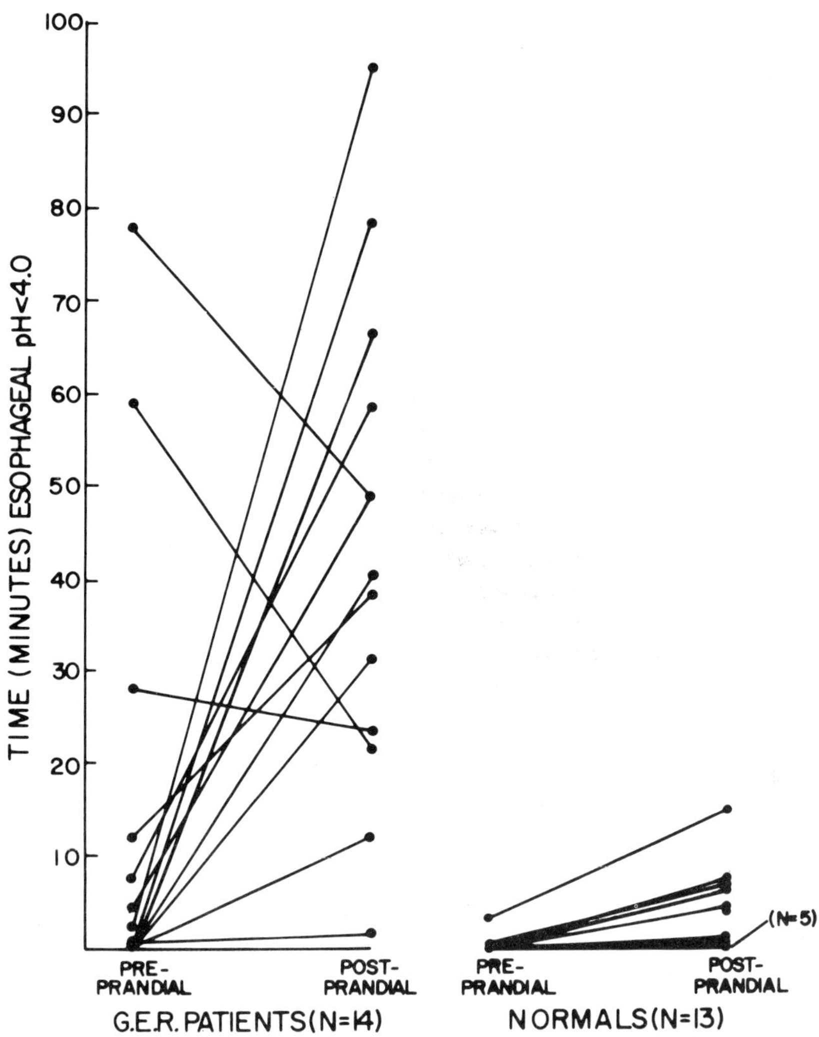

Fig. 4-7. The influence of a standard meal on the duration of gastroesophageal reflux has been measured by continuous pH probe monitoring in 13 normal subjects and in 14 patients with symptomatic gastroesophageal reflux (GER). Esophageal pH was monitored for 3 hours pre- and 3 hours postprandially. The total time during which the esophageal pH was less than 4.0 was calculated as "reflux time" in minutes. In the 3-hour preprandial period, total reflux time in the GER patients overlaps, in many cases, with that in normal subjects. However, postprandial total reflux time in GER patients is markedly different from the corresponding time in normal individuals, indicating the role of a standard meal in provoking differences between normal function and that in reflux patients.

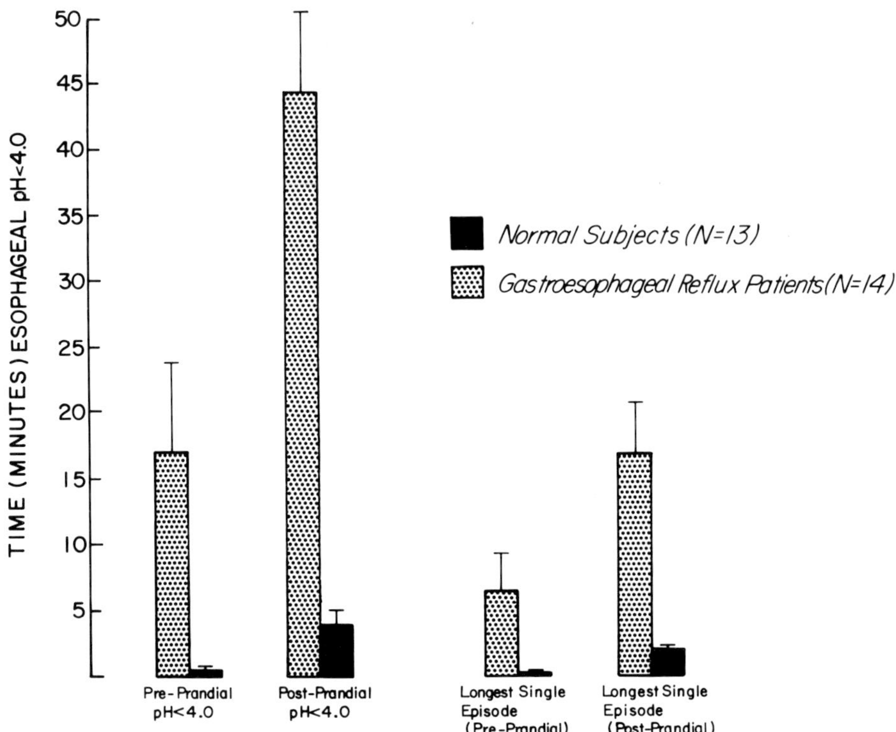

Fig. 4-8. Pre- and postprandial 3-hour esophageal pH monitoring studies in normal subjects and gastroesophageal reflux patients. Data are expressed as mean ($\pm$ SEM), summarizing the influence of a meal on both the total duration of reflux and the time of the longest episode when the pH is less than 4.0 in the esophagus.

A technique such as this postprandial reflux test has great potential. Double-blind randomized clinical trials are time-consuming, difficult, and limited because they cannot address the efficacy of combinations of medications in managing gastroesophageal reflux. A model such as this one could be a predictor of the need to pursue a clinical trial of a new medication based on its ability to decrease postprandial reflux time significantly as compared with a placebo or a validated competitor.

Acid-Clearance Test

The acid-clearance test introduced by Booth in 1968[22] is based on the concept that acid-induced changes in the esophagus lead to disordered peristalsis that results in impaired clearance of refluxed acid.[29,30] Esophageal pH is measured 5 cm above the manometrically defined LES. Following ingestion of 15 ml of 0.1N HCl, the number of swallows required to raise the intraesophageal pH to 5 or above is determined; normally less than 12 swallows are needed (Fig. 4-9). Normal subjects

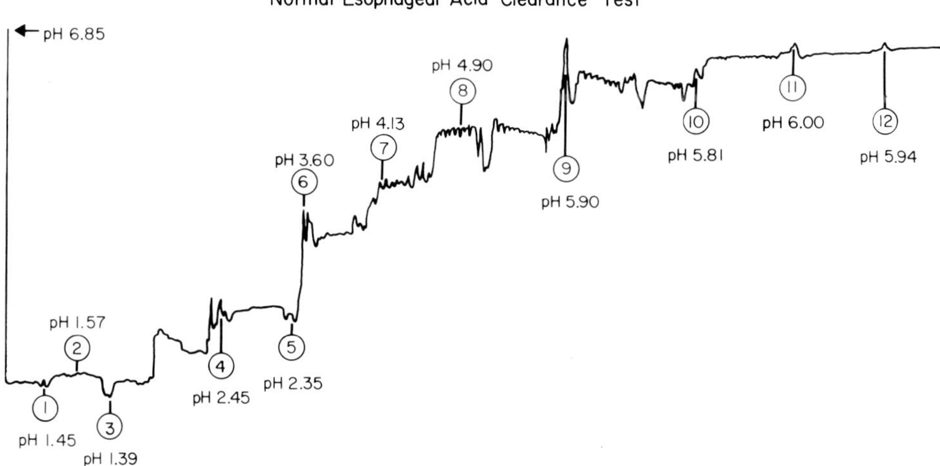

Fig. 4-9. A tracing from a patient with a normal acid-clearance test. Note the fall in esophageal pH from a resting value of 6.9 to a value of 1.5 after the patient has swallowed 15 ml 0.1N HC1. The esophageal pH is restored to normal (pH > 5.0) within 12 swallows. Swallows are indicated by the numbers within the circles.

are a well-defined group with only one study[26] reporting any positive tests in this group. The rate of positive tests in symptomatic patients ranges from 53% to 100%,[22,26,31,32] and is more often positive in those with endoscopic and/or histologic evidence of esophagitis than in patients in whom such findings are absent.[31] In one series,[32] the acid-clearance time correlated positively with the severity of the esophagitis. One pitfall in the test is that positive results may be recorded in patients with primary motility disorders,[32] and these should be excluded with esophageal manometry. In comparison with other tests for esophageal reflux,[26,31] acid clearance is at least as discriminatory as SART and more so than any other individual test, although it has not been compared with 24-hour pH monitoring.

24-Hour pH Monitoring

The most recent application of pH measurement, 24-hour monitoring has made valuable contributions to our understanding of the pathophysiology of gastroesophageal reflux, in particular the importance of nighttime reflux with episodes of prolonged duration[33] and the concepts of upright and supine reflux.[34] However, as a diagnostic test in clinical practice, its role is less clear. It would appear to be the most sensitive available indicator of reflux when compared with any other single test.[35,36] False negative rates ranging from 10%–20% have been reported, although some of these may represent bile reflux. The use of pH measurement to detect bile reflux[37] warrants more careful study. The pH of bile ranges from 5.9–7.4[38] and overlaps the normal resting esophageal pH. In addition, complete achlorhydria is uncommon, and it is presumed that the damaging agent in most patients with bile reflux is a combination of acid and bile that may result in overall masking of true "alkaline" reflux patients. Future considerations may include application of isotope-labeled (HIDA) studies of duodenogastric reflux.

Despite the sensitivity of prolonged pH monitoring for detecting acid reflux, such monitoring is probably not useful as a routine diagnostic test, although it may detect a small number of reflux patients that are not identified by other investigations. A major drawback is that it requires hospitalization for at least 24 hours where the setting and activities pursued by the patient are not necessarily comparable with those of daily life. The future in this area may involve ambulatory monitoring, either with a device akin to a Holter monitor or by telemetry with a central monitoring station. This would permit assessment of patients in their normal environment, as well as allowing them to continue their daily activities including work.

ACID-INFUSION (BERNSTEIN) TEST

Instillation of acid into the esophagus to reproduce the symptom of heartburn was first proposed as a test for reflux esophagitis by Bernstein in 1958.[39] This study and others[24,25] have suggested good correlation between a positive test and reflux symptoms; however, other studies have reported less impressive results.[21,31] The reproduction of pain correlates best with symptoms. False-positive tests occur in approximately 15% of control subjects, although this level may be reduced by excluding late-positive tests.[40] Positive tests are seen in approximately 85% of patients with symptoms, but in up to 15% of asymptomatic patients.[25]

Recently, it has become common practice to include relief of acid-induced heartburn by normal saline as a criterion for a positive Bernstein test,[25,41] although this was not part of the original test. A recent study[42] showed that 52% of patients with reflux esophagitis and acid-induced heartburn did not obtain relief by cessation of acid and institution of a saline infusion. Also relief of pain was not dependent on either elevation of esophageal pH above 4 or the use of antacids (Fig. 4-10). Thus, whereas reproduction of heartburn by acid infusion may be a reliable test, the relief of such pain is not.

Overall, the Bernstein test is a useful test to determine if thoracic symptoms are the result of gastroesophageal reflux. For the patients with atypical chest pain or chest pain that is a mixture of heartburn and pressure and/or squeezing, the possibility of esophageal spasm as an etiology is always raised. The clinical history usually includes a previous negative cardiac work-up. It is in this setting that the Bernstein test is invaluable. In some patients, pressure-like or squeezing chest pain can be induced by acid infusion while the simultaneously monitored esophageal motility remains unchanged and peristaltic with a normal contraction amplitude. This presentation is an important component of the spectrum of gastroesophageal reflux disease and in our experience is much more common than true diffuse esophageal spasm in explaining pressure-like chest pain of noncardiac origin. On rare occasions, acid infusion does provoke both pressure-type chest pain and a change in the normal baseline motility so that manometricly it resembles diffuse esophageal spasm. This condition could then qualify as a rare case of true "secondary" esopha-

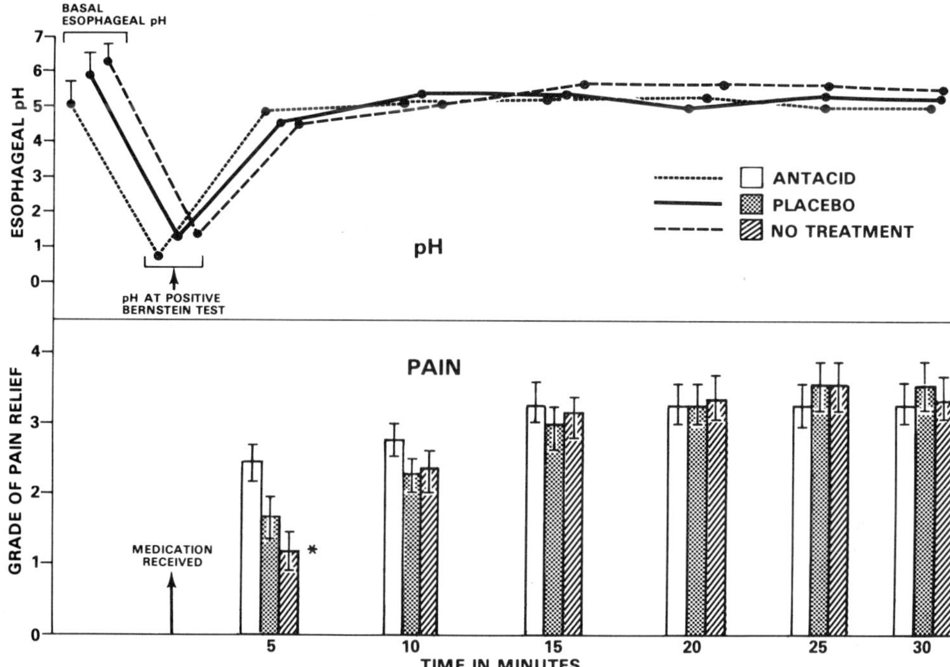

Fig. 4-10. Esophageal pH and chest pain relief (mean ± SEM) observed in six patients who received an esophageal saline infusion, ingested 30 ccs of either antacid or an antacid–placebo, or had no treatment for a positive Bernstein test. Esophageal pH was recorded basally and during the induction of chest pain by acid infusion (corresponding to "Treatment Received"). The grade of relief of the chest pain and the corresponding esophageal pH are presented at 5 min intervals for 30 min after the treatments were administered. Reproduced by permission from Winnan GR, Meyer CT, McCallum RW: A reappraisal of criteria for the interpretation of the Bernstein test. Ann Intern Med 96:320–322, 1982.

geal spasm induced by gastroesophageal reflux. The more usual setting is that of a pressure-like chest pain—alone or combined with heartburn—either in the presence of normal esophageal manometrics or with decreased contraction amplitudes that are consistent with chronic gastroesophageal reflux.

PROVOCATIVE TESTS IN ESOPHAGEAL MANOMETRY

Standard esophageal manometry does not always provide a firm diagnosis. If one accepts the concept of a spectrum of esophageal motility abnormalities ranging from diffuse spasm to achalasia,[43] the individual patient may not be easily defined. Also, patients with symptomatic diffuse spasm may be asymptomatic during the motility test and/or have a normal tracing. In an attempt to make manometry more sensitive, several provocative tests have been proposed.

Bethanechol

Heightened sensitivity of the achalasic esophagus to cholinergic agents was demonstrated several years ago.[44] Initially, methacholine was used. However, since it causes a number of possible cardiac complications, it has been withdrawn from use, and bethanechol (5–10 mg subcutaneously) is now recommended. A positive response is denoted by a rise of 25 mm Hg or more in basal intraesophageal pressure that is accompanied by chest pain. Unfortunately, a positive test is sometimes confusing because it may also occur in 25%–80% of patients with diffuse spasm. The reason for the heightened sensitivity is not clear. In achalasia, it has been attributed to cholinergic hypersensitivity. However, since the major nerves responsible for esophageal contraction do not appear to be cholinergic,[45] this explanation needs clarification. In diffuse spasm, Auerbach's plexus is intact and the sensitivity may be due to hypertrophy of the smooth muscle. A positive response to methacholine or betanechol in an aperistaltic esophagus is good confirmatory evidence for the diagnosis of achalasia. However, a negative test carries no weight by itself. The significance of the test in diffuse spasm is less clear. A negative test has no diagnostic importance. A positive test, especially associated with the reproduction of chest pain, is useful supportive evidence towards the diagnosis.

Pentagastrin

Based on the effect of gastrin on LES pressure[46] and the effect of pentagastrin on esophageal contractions in patients with diffuse spasm,[47] pentagastrin has been studied as a possible diagnostic test for diffuse spasm. Bolus doses of pentagastrin (6 μg/kg) significantly increase the amplitude and duration of esophageal contractions in both diffuse spasm and achalasia.[48,49] This response was not seen during intravenous infusions of pentagastrin or gastrin-17 designed to mimic the postprandial serum gastrin concentration, and thus the findings do not support a pathophysiologic role for gastrin in diffuse esophageal spasm.[50-52] The responses in patients with achalasia and in those with diffuse spasm to single-dose i.v. pentagastrin have been reported as similar, but we have identified differences between the two groups by using dosages normally injected for esophageal stimulation (0.4 μg/kg) rather than for gastric acid stimulation (6 μg/kg) (Fig. 4-11).[51,52] However, manometric abnormalities could not be produced in patients suspected on clinical grounds of having diffuse spasm in whom the initial manometry was normal.[49]

The response of the esophagus to pentagastrin is interesting from the viewpoint of esophageal physiology. However, for most workers familiar with esophageal manometry and manometric features of esophageal motor disorders, a diagnosis can usually be made from the standard tracing with the addition of the Bernstein test and/or bethanechol stimulation. Pentagastrin does not seem to offer any substantial advantage.

Ergonovine

Ergonovine is used to evoke coronary artery spasm in patients with variant angina. It has been noted that some patients experience chest pain without any

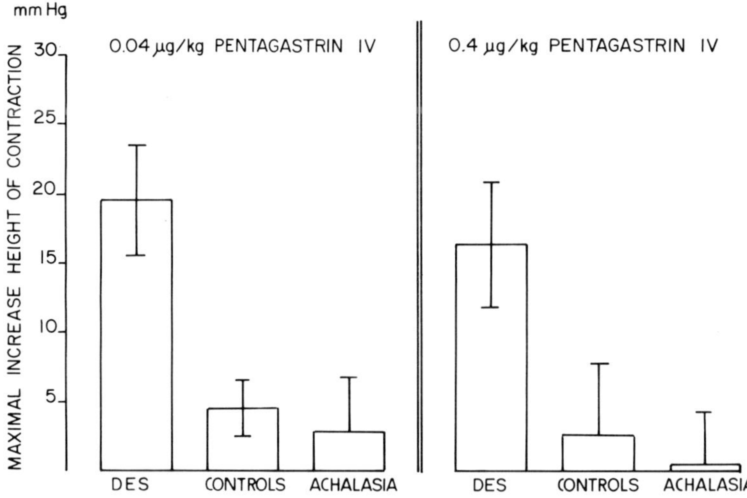

Fig. 4-11. The effect of intravenous bolus doses of pentagastrin (peptavlon), 0.04 µg/kg and 0.4 µg/kg, on the amplitude of esophageal contractions in normal subjects and in patients with diffuse esophageal spasm (DES) and with achalasia. The increase in contraction amplitude was significantly greater in patients with DES compared with the other two groups. Both dosages of pentagastrin resulted in similar responses. Reproduced by permission from McCallum RW: Diffuse esophageal spasm and gastroesophageal reflux-induced esophageal dysfunction. In: 2nd International Symposium on the Esophagus and Gastroesophageal Junction. Biomedical Information Corp., New York, 1978.

associated coronary artery spasm or ECG changes, perhaps because of esophageal spasm. Initial esophageal manometric studies performed after administration of ergonovine[53] showed an increase in peristaltic amplitude and duration in those patients who had experienced ergonovine-induced chest pain during coronary angiography but who had normal coronary angiograms. Similar results were reported in the most recent study.[54] However, there was a high incidence of side effects, some of which were potentially serious, and the investigators felt that the potential risks from ergonovine did not justify its routine use as a provocative agent.

TRANSMURAL ESOPHAGEAL POTENTIAL DIFFERENCE

An electrical potential difference (PD) exists between the mucosal and serosal surfaces of the digestive tract. It is believed to result from ionic flux.[55] Disruption of the gastric mucosal barrier is associated with a fall in this transmural PD.[56] The technique of PD measurement has been applied to the esophagus in both animals and humans.[57,58] Studies in patients with symptoms and histologic abnormalities of gastroesophageal reflux showed a reversal in polarity of the PD in 9 out of 10 subjects (and a marked fall in PD in the 10th) when compared with controls. This change in PD correlated better with symptoms than with endoscopic appearance. More recently, PD monitoring during a Bernstein test revealed a good correlation between a positive test and a fall in PD.[59]

The test is simple and appears to be sensitive. It may provide a measure of objectivity to the Bernstein test. However, more studies on both controls and patients with reflux are needed to assess reliability. In particular, it is important to know how well the PD measurement compares with histologic change and if it is altered in symptomatic patients with normal histology. The assessment of

Table 4-1. Summary of diagnostic tests for esophageal disorders

Clinical Problem	Diagnostic Test	Current Status of Test
Gastroesophageal reflux (GER)	Bernstein test	A simple reliable test to help determine if chest symptoms are due to GER.
	Standard Acid Reflux Test (SART) / Acid clearance test	More sensitive than other indicators of GER. Useful when other evidence of reflux esophagitis is lacking.
	24-hour pH monitoring	Accurate and sensitive but time-consuming. Detects GER missed by other tests and allows timing of symptoms with reflux episodes. Largely a research test.
	Gastric emptying	Applicable in patients with GER and symptoms suggestive of gastric stasis or those in whom antacid or H_2-blockers ineffective. Positive test suggests use of gastric pro-kinetic agent.
	Scintigraphy	Technically simple but not yet proven in clinical practice. Not recommended unless reliability tested in one's own laboratory.
	Potential difference	Relatively untested in clinical practice. Value yet to be determined.
Motor disorders	Scintigraphy	
	Emptying	Assessment of degree of obstruction in achalasia before and after treatment.
	Transit	Not fully established. Segmental transit studies likely to be most useful. A potential screening test. Still experimental
	Provocative stimulation	
	Bethanechol	Most helpful to diagnose achalasia. Less helpful in diffuse esophageal spasm.
	Pentagastrin	Largely a research agent. Of little clinical value.
	Ergonovine	Not recommended because of potential hazards.
Chest pain	Bernstein test	Useful to determine if chest pain is due to GER.
	24-hour pH monitoring	Useful to detect GER and to match episodes of reflux to symptom occurrence.
	Bethanechol	May add further criteria to support manometric findings of diffuse esophageal spasm or "vigorous" achalasia. Not diagnostic by itself.
	Ergonovine	Not recommended.

PD in patients with a food-sensitive esophagus[60] may also be of value. However, even if the sensitivity and accuracy of the test are confirmed, it is difficult to see, at this stage, what advantages the test offers over other tests currently available.

CONCLUSION

In summary, we have attempted to assess critically some of the more recent diagnostic tests that may be useful in evaluating esophageal disease and to discuss their accuracy and current status (Table 4-1). The applicability of an individual test is related to the presenting clinical problem. Awareness of both the limitations and the need for careful interpretation of these tests is necessary for their proper application in clinical practice.

REFERENCES

1. Kazem I: A new scintigraphic technique for the study of the esophagus. Am J Roentgenol 115:681–688, 1972.
2. Heyman S, Kirkpatrick JA, Winter HS, Treves S: An improved radionuclide method for the diagnosis of gastroesophageal reflux and aspiration in children (milk scan). Radiology 131:479–482, 1979.
3. Rudd TG, Christie DL: Demonstration of gastroesophageal reflux in children by radionuclide gastroesophagography. Radiology 131:483–486, 1979.
4. Blumhagen JD, Rudd TG, Christie DL: Gastroesophageal reflux in children: radionuclide gastroesophagography. Am J Radiol 135:1001–1004, 1980.
5. Fisher RS, Malmud LS, Roberts GS, Lobis IF: Gastroesophageal (GE) scintiscanning to detect and quantitate GE reflux. Gastroenterology 70:301–308, 1976.
6. Malmud LS, Fisher RS: Quantitation of gastroesophageal reflux before and after therapy using the gastroesophageal scintiscan. South Med J 71(Suppl 1):10–15, 1978.
7. Hoffman GC, Vansant JH: The gastroesophageal scintiscan. Comparison of methods to demonstrate gastroesophageal reflux. Arch Surg 114:727–728, 1979.
8. Menin RA, Malmud MD, Petersen RP, et al.: Gastroesophageal scintigraphy to assess the severity of gastroesophageal reflux disease. Ann Surg 191:66–71, 1980.
9. Malmud LS, Fisher RS: Gastroesophageal scintigraphy. Gastrointest Radiol 5:195–204, 1980.
10. Chernow B, Johnson LF, Janowitz WR, Castell DO: Pulmonary aspiration as a consequence of gastroesophageal reflux. A diagnostic approach. Dig Dis Sci 24:839–844, 1979.
11. McCallum RW, Berkowitz DM, Lerner E: Gastric emptying in patients with gastroesophageal reflux. Gastroenterology 80:285–291, 1981.
12. Hillemeier AC, Lange R, McCallum RW, et al.: Delayed gastric emptying in infants with gastroesophageal reflux. J Pediatr 98:190–193, 1981.
13. Gross R, Johnson LF, Kaminski RJ: Esophageal emptying in achalasia quantitated by a radioisotope technique. Dig Dis Sci 24:945–949, 1979.
14. Krosin GA, Saladino T, McCallum RW: Radionuclide quantitation of esophageal emptying of solid food in achalasia. Gastroenterology 78:1201 (abstr), 1980.
15. Tolin RD, Malmud LS, Reilley J, Fisher RS: Esophageal scintigraphy to quantitate

esophageal transit (Quantitation of esophageal transit). Gastroenterology 76:1402–1408, 1979.

16. Russell COH, Hill LD, Holmes ER III, et al.: Radionuclide transit: a sensitive screening test for esophageal dysfunction. Gastroenterology 80:887–892, 1981.

17. McCallum RW, Mensh R, Lange R: Definition of the gastric emptying abnormality present in gastroesophageal reflux patients. Gastroenterology 80:1226 (abstr), 1981.

18. Meyer JH, MacGregor IL, Gueller R, et al.: ^{99m}Tc-tagged chicken liver as a marker of solid food in the human stomach. Am J Dig Dis 21:296–304, 1976.

19. Tuttle SG, Grossman MI: Detection of gastroesophageal reflux by simultaneous measurement of intraluminal pressure and pH. Proc Soc Exp Biol Med 98:225–227, 1958.

20. Kantrowitz PH, Corson JG, Fleishli DJ, Skinner DB: Measurement of gastroesophageal reflux. Gastroenterology 56:666–673, 1969.

21. Skinner DB, Booth DJ: Assessment of distal esophageal function in patients with hiatal hernia and/or gastroesophageal reflux. Ann Surg 172:627–637, 1970.

22. Booth DJ, Kemmerer WT, Skinner DB: Acid clearing from the distal esophagus. Arch Surg 96:731–734, 1968.

23. Johnson LF, DeMeester TR: Twenty-four hour pH monitoring of the distal esophagus. A quantitative measure of gastroesophageal reflux. Am J Gastroenterol 62:325–332, 1974.

24. Benz LJ, Hootkin LA, Margulies S, et al.: A comparison of clinical measurements of gastroesophageal reflux. Gastroenterology 62:1–5, 1972.

25. Behar J, Biancani P, Sheahan DG: Evaluation of esophageal tests in the diagnosis of reflux eosphagitis. Gastroenterology 71:9–15, 1976.

26. Krejs GJ, Seefeld V, Haemmerli UP, et al.: Gastroesophageal reflux: evaluation of a diagnostic criteria. Gastroenterology 66:727 (abstr), 1974.

27. DeMeester TR, Johnson LF: The evaluation of objective measurements of gastroesophageal reflux and their contribution to patient management. Surg Clin North Am 56(1):39–53, 1976.

28. Castell DO, Harris LD: Hormonal control of gastroesophageal sphincter strength. N Engl J Med 282:886–889, 1970.

29. Siegel CI, Hendrix TR: Esophageal motor abnormalities induced by acid perfusion in patients with heartburn. J Clin Invest 42:686–695, 1963.

30. Olsen AM, Schlegel JF: Motility disturbances caused by esophagitis. J Thorac Cardiovasc Surgery 50:607–612, 1965.

31. Battle WS, Nyhus LM, Bombeck CT: Gastroesophageal reflux: diagnosis and treatment. Ann Surg 177:560–565, 1973.

32. Stanciu C, Bennett JR: Esophageal acid clearing: one factor in the production of reflux esophagitis. Gut 15:852–857, 1974.

33. DeMeester TR, Johnson LF, Guy JJ, et al.: Patterns of gastroesophageal reflux in health and disease. Ann Surg 184:459–470, 1976.

34. Johnson LF: 24-hour pH monitoring in the study of gastroesophageal reflux. J Clin Gastroenterol 2:387–399, 1980.

35. Johnson LF, DeMeester TR: Twenty-four hour distal esophageal pH monitoring (24 hour pH) and gastroesophageal reflux (GER). Gastroenterology 66:717 (abstr), 1974.

36. DeMeester TR, Wernly JA, Little AG, et al.: Technique, indications and clinical use of 24-hour esophageal pH monitoring. J Thorac Cardiovasc Surg 79:656–670, 1980.

37. Pellignini CA, DeMeester TR, Wernly JA: Alkaline gastroesophageal reflux. Am J Surg 135:177–184, 1978.

38. Wheeler HO: Water and electrolytes in bile. In Code CF (ed): Handbook of Physiology, Williams & Wilkins, Baltimore, 1968.

39. Bernstein LM, Baker LA: A clinical test for esophagitis. Gastroenterology 34:760–781, 1958.
40. Breen KJ, Whelan G: The diagnosis of reflux esophagitis: an evaluation of five investigative procedures. Aust NZ J Surg 48:156–161, 1978.
41. Fisher RS, Cohen S: Gastroesophageal reflux. Med Clin North Am 62(1):3–20, 1978.
42. Winnan GR, Meyer CT, McCallum RW: A reappraisal of criteria for the interpretation of the Bernstein test. Ann Intern Med 96:320–322, 1982.
43. Vantrappen G, Janssens J, Hellemans J, et al.: Achalasia, diffuse esophageal spasm, and related motility disorders. Gastroenterology 76:450–457, 1979.
44. Kramer P, Inglefinger FJ: Esophageal sensitivity to Mecholyl in cardiospasm. Gastroenterology 19:242–253, 1951.
45. Goyal RK, Cobb BW: Motility of the pharynx, esophagus and esophageal sphincters. In Johnson LR (ed): Physiology of the Gastrointestinal Tract, Raven Press, New York, 1981.
46. Hollis JB, Levine SM, Castell DO: Differential sensitivity of the human esophagus to pentagastrin. Am J Physiol 222:870–874, 1972.
47. Eckhardt V, Weigard H: Supersensitivity to pentagastrin in diffuse esophageal spasm. Gut 15:706–709, 1974.
48. Eckhardt V, Kruger J, Holtermuller KH, Ewe K: Alteration of esophageal peristalsis by pentagastrin in patients with diffuse esophageal spasm. Scand J Gastroenterol 10:475–479, 1975.
49. Orlando RC, Bozynski EM: The effects of pentagastrin in achalasia and diffuse esophageal spasm. Gastroenterology 77:472–477, 1979.
50. Wexler RM, Kaye MD: Pentagastrin in diffuse esophageal spasm. Gut 22:213–216, 1981.
51. McCallum RW: Diffuse esophageal spasm and gastroesophageal reflux-induced esophageal dysfunction. In: 2nd International Symposium on the Esophagus and Gastroesophageal Junction. Biomedical Information Corporation, New York, 1978.
52. Lane WH, Ippoliti AF, McCallum RW: Effect of gastrin heptadecapeptide (G-17) on esophageal contractions in patients with diffuse esophageal spasm. Gut 20:756–759, 1979.
53. Koch K, Calson G, Long A, et al.: The ergonovine stress test: a provocative test for diffuse esophageal spasm or variant angina? Clin Res 27:778 (abstr), 1979.
54. Eastwood GL, Weiner BH, Dickerson WJ, et al.: Use of ergonovine to identify esophageal spasm in patients with chest pain. Ann Intern Med 94:768–771, 1981.
55. Forte JG, Adams PH, Davies RE: Source of the gastric mucosal potential difference. Nature 197:874–876, 1963.
56. Black RB, Hole D, Rhodes J: Bile damage to the gastric mucosal barrier: the influence of pH and bile acid concentration. Gastroenterology 61:178–184, 1971.
57. Turner KS, Powell DW, Carney CN, et al.: Transmural electrical potential difference in the mammalian esophagus in vivo. Gastroenterology 75:286–291, 1978.
58. Khamis B, Kennedy C, Finucane J, Doyle JS: Transmural potential difference: diagnostic value in gastroesophageal reflux. Gut 19:396–398, 1978.
59. Herlihy KJ, Orlando RC, Bryson JC, et al.: The Bernstein test: conversion from a subjective to an objective test with potential difference (PD) measurement. Gastroenterology 80:1173 (abstr), 1981.
60. Price SF, Smithson KW, Castell DO: Food sensitivity in reflux esophagitis. Gastroenterology 75:240–243, 1978.

5 | Congenital Disorders of the Esophagus

John T. Boyle

EMBRYOLOGY OF THE NORMAL ESOPHAGUS

The esophagus develops from the embryonic foregut by the end of the first fetal month.[1,2,3] The primitive esophagus consists of the foregut, which extends from the fourth pharyngeal arch to the cephalic border of the yolk sac (Fig. 5-1). At first the stomach appears at the level of the heart, descending to its infradia-phragmatic position by the 7th week. Beginning at approximately the 3rd week, a midline cleft, called the laryngotracheal groove, forms from the ventral floor of the most caudal portion of the pharynx (Fig. 5-2). This groove rapidly elongates and gives rise to the lung buds from its caudal aspect. These buds become the mainstem bronchi and associated lung structures. The combined laryngotracheo-esophageal tube is subsequently divided in a caudal to cephalic progression by folding in and fusion of the lateral walls of the foregut. This process is completed by 33 days in such a way that the respiratory and alimentary tubes are completely separated except at the level of the larynx. The esophagus continues to elongate rapidly, and its caudal extent is delineated at the beginning of the 8th week by the developing diaphragm and stomach.

The lining of the esophagus is originally columnar epithelium. Rapid proliferation of this epithelial lining occurs between the 5th and 6th fetal weeks, converting the esophagus into an almost solid cellular cord with only a very small lumen.[4] This same phenomenon occurs in the development of the rest of the intestine. In fact, the esophagus is the only segment of the bowel where there is never complete occlusion of the lumen. As the esophagus lengthens, the cord becomes vacuolated (Fig. 5-3). Vacuolization is most marked in the 8th fetal weeks when the vacuoles begin to coalesce, so that the lumen is recanalized by approximately the 10th

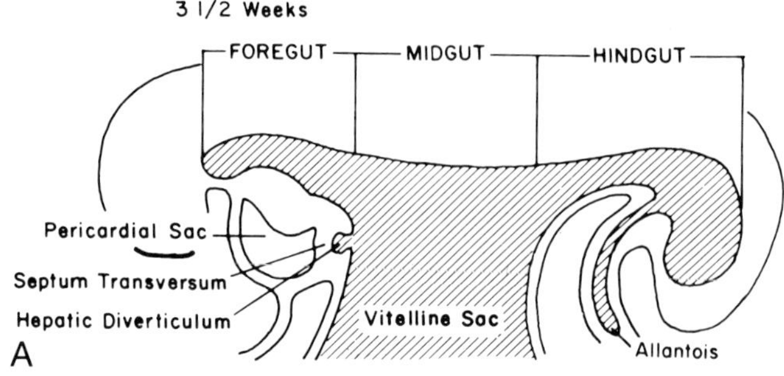

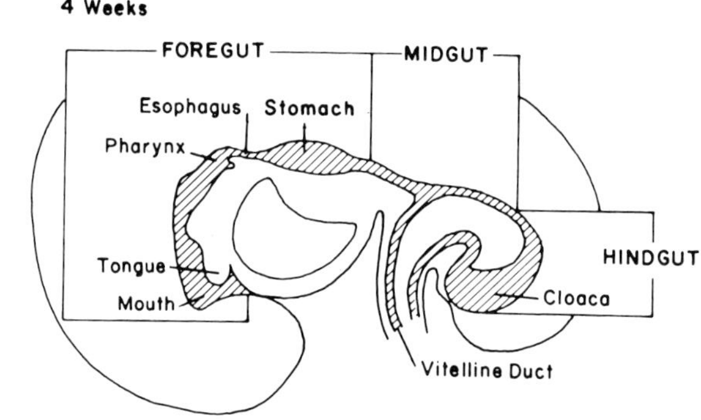

Fig. 5-1.   Segmentation of the fetal alimentary tract. From Singleton, EB et al. (eds): Radiology of the Alimentary Tract in Infants and Children, 2nd ed, WB Saunders, Philadelphia, 1977. A, 3½-week-old fetus. B, 4-week-old fetus.

week. During this same period, the inner circular layer of muscle differentiates during the 6th week, the outer longitudinal layer during the 8th week, and the muscularis mucosa is evident by the 10th fetal week. Ganglion cells appear between 8 and 10 weeks. At approximately the time that the esophageal lumen is reestablished, the columnar epithelium becomes ciliated. Stratified squamous epithelium

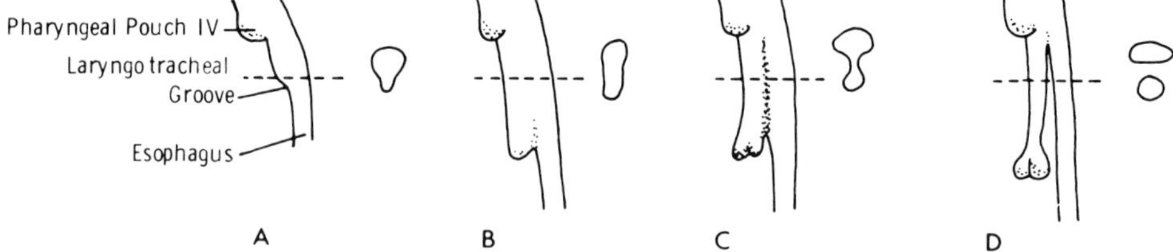

Fig. 5-2.   Separation of esophagus and tracheobronchial tree that occurs between 3rd and 5th fetal weeks. Adapted with permission from Bremer JL: Congenital Anomalies of the Viscera, Harvard University Press, Cambridge, 1957. Broken line depicts area in anatomical cross section shown to right of each longitudinal drawing.

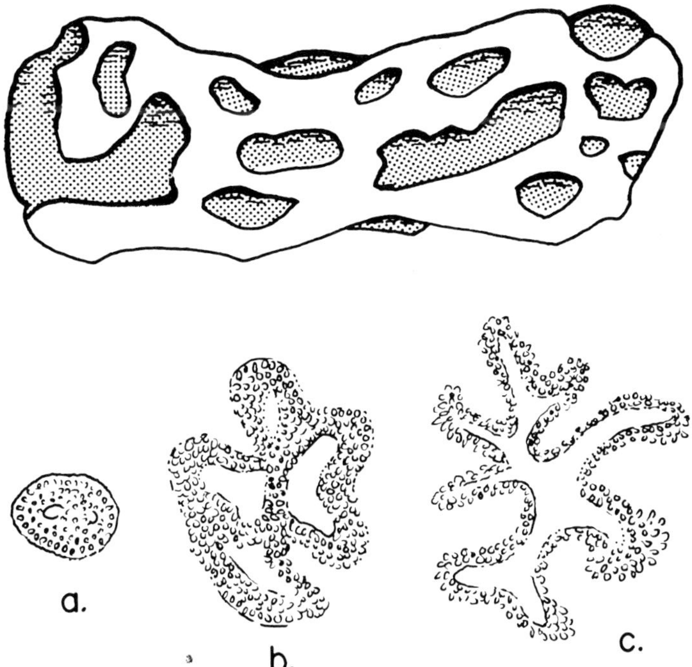

Fig. 5-3.   Longitudinal section showing development of vacuoles in esophageal lumen. A, Transverse section showing lumen almost obliterated by epithelial concrescence. B, Development of vacuoles. C, Coalescence of vacuoles with lumen reestablished. After Keibel F and Mall FP: Human Embryology, J.B. Lippincott, Philadelphia, 1912.

first appears during the 5th fetal month in the mid-esophagus and by the 7th month lines the entire esophagus. Occasional patches of columnar epithelium may remain and may still be present at birth.

At term, the esophagus is about 10 cm in length, subsequently growing approximately 0.6 to 0.7 cm/year.[5] The intra-abdominal segment of the esophagus is very short at birth. It lengthens with age and within several years measures between 0.5 and 1.5 cm. At birth, the squamous epithelium is approximately 10 cells thick, as opposed to the 20–24-cell-thick adult epithelium. Papillae are not present at birth. Since esophageal papillae are considered the equivalents of crypts in the small intestine, epithelial-cell turnover is felt to be slow at birth. The adult appearance of the mucosa is usually attained by 3 months of age.

Although the fetus can swallow at 20 weeks gestation, maturation of esophageal motor function develops postnatally.[6] Organized peristaltic activity develops in the first few postnatal weeks. During the first 2 weeks of life normal infants demonstrate decreased lower esophageal sphincter (LES) pressure as compared with adults. LES pressure subsequently increases and becomes greater than that in adults until the end of the first year of life; then values approximate adult norms.[47]

ESOPHAGEAL ATRESIA AND
TRACHEOSOPHAGEAL FISTULA

Esophageal atresia (EA) with or without tracheoesophageal fistula (TEF) is the most common congenital esophageal anomaly.

Epidemiology

The reported incidence of EA with or without TEF varies between 1:1000 and 1:4,500 live births. The figure most often cited is 1:3000. As figures for comparison, the incidence of Down's syndrome is 1:800; that of pyloric stenosis is 1:500; and for biliary atresia it is 1:10,000. There is a slight male predominance. The racial ratio (white:black) does not differ significantly from that observed in the general population. Maternal age at birth, birth rank, and season of conception are not factors. However, in one study 30% of mothers had had one or more previous abortions or stillbirths.[7]

Thirty to thirty-five per cent of affected infants are premature.[8] There is also a significant incidence of small-for-gestational-age infants, indicating intrauterine growth retardation.[7] Associated anomalies are seen in 50% of cases.[7,9] EA is also one feature of trisomy 17–18.[10]

The precise significance of genetic factors remains uncertain.[6] Familial cases are exceptional. Nevertheless, there are reports of the anomaly occuring in siblings and in two generations of a family. Both concordance and discordance in identical twins have been described.

The recurrent risk has been reported to be roughly 1.6%.[7]

Etiology

The cause of EA and TEF is unknown. Most authors consider the cause to be multifactorial, with both embryologic and environmental factors playing a major role.

The embryologic basis is poorly understood. The malformation probably develops between the 4th and 6th week of fetal life.[11] Hypotheses for the etiology of EA include (1) local disturbances in the vascular supply to the embryonic esophagus, (2) persistence of the obliterative stage of the esophageal lumen, (3) defective septation of the ventral laryngotracheal ridge, with lateral folds turning dorsally and obliterating the esophageal lumen, and (4) localized pressure on the developing esophagus by vascular anomalies. Imperfect septal development between the trachea and esophagus is considered the causative factor in TEF.

The high incidence of associated anomalies suggests a systemic insult to the fetus, possibly from an environmental teratogen, acting via the mother and placenta.[11] The same abnormalities might be produced by a number of different stimuli applied at the same period of development.

Anatomy

There have been at least 12 different anatomic classifications of EA and TEF reported. Kluth in his *Atlas of Tracheoesophageal Fistula* has described almost

100 different variations of these anomalies.[12] In practical terms, there are five basic types of EA and TEF,[8] and it is now recommended the different anomalies should be designated by simple anatomic description rather than by letters or Roman numerals (Fig. 4).[13] EA with distal TEF is by far the most common anomaly, occurring in 85–95% of cases.[6,8,14] The most common site of TEF is at or just above the tracheal bifurcation. Approximately one-half of patients with this type have a narrow gap between the upper and lower esophageal pouches; the remaining one-half having a longer atretic segment. Isolated EA, EA with proximal TEF, and EA with double TEF are all associated with long atretic gaps between the upper and lower pouches. Goodwin and associates have suggested that the incidence of EA with proximal TEF may be as high as 5%.[15] They state that many so-called postoperative recurrences of TEFs really represent original EA with proximal TEF.

Isolated TEF or so-called "H-type fistula" arises in the anterior wall of the esophagus and extends cephalad to enter the membranous posterior wall of the trachea. Seventy per cent of these fistulae occur at the level of the second thoracic vertebrae or above and thus are above the thoracic inlet.

Because of communication between the trachea and esophagus in EA with distal TEF, EA with double TEF, and isolated TEF, air is present in the abdomen. In isolated EA, and EA with proximal TEF, no air can enter the intra-abdominal gastrointestinal tract.

Associated Anomalies

Associated congenital anomalies occur in approximately 50% of the patients with EA and TEF.[6,8] The presence of these anomalies is felt to be one of the primary factors affecting ultimate prognosis in these patients. In 50% of patients with associated anomalies, there are multiple defects and in 25% the anomalies are sufficiently severe to be considered life-threatening. Associated anomalies are most common in isolated EA and least common in isolated TEF.[6] The most frequently seen of these associated lesions are congenital heart disease and gastrointestinal abnormalities.

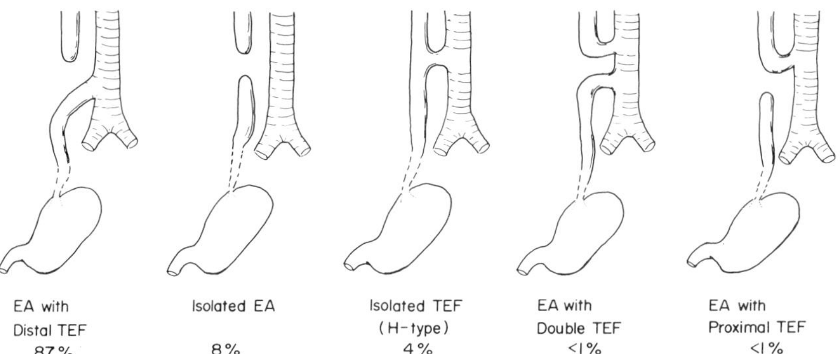

Fig. 5-4. Diagrammatic representation of the types of esophageal atresia (EA) and tracheo-esophageal fistula (TEF) malformations along with their relative incidence.[9]

Cardiovascular lesions occur in 15–25% of patients and are more likely to be seen in premature infants.[16] Vetriculoseptal defect, patent ductus arteriosis, and atrial septal defects are most common, but coarctation, vascular rings, and tetrology of Fallot have all been reported. Mortality of EA and TEF with associated cardiovascular anomalies is reported to be three times greater than that for infants without heart disease.

Gastrointestinal anomalies are also seen in 20–25% of patients.[8,17] Anorectal anomalies are the most common, occurring in 10%.[8,17] Because of the high incidence of imperforate anus associated with EA and TEF, any newborn with imperforate anus should have radiographic studies of the esophagus. Other gastrointestinal anomalies, in decreasing order of frequency, include intestinal atresia, Meckel's diverticulum, malrotation, pyloric stenosis, congenital esophageal stenosis distal to site of atresia, diaphragmatic hernia, and annular pancreas. Hiatal hernia is a relatively frequent occurrence but is thought to be an acquired defect that results from postsurgical traction.

Other less common associated lesions include genitourinary, musculoskeletal, facial, and central-nervous-system defects.

A recognizable, definite, nonrandom association of anomalies is now called the VATER syndrome[18,19] (or VACTERL syndrome).[20] Patients with this syndrome have multiple congenital defects that are associated with normal karyotypes; these include vertebral (hemivertabrae), vascular (single umbilical artery), and renal defects, anal atresia, EA with TEF, and radial dysplasia and other limb anomalies. The majority of the lesions seem to involve error of septation of developing mesoderm. The cause is unknown, but teratogenic exposure to either maternal hormones or to radiation has been implicated.

Clinical Presentation

Antepartum polyhydramnios is seen in 15–35% of mothers who give birth to infants with EA and TEF.[21] The fetus normally makes a significant contribution to the circulation of amniotic fluid. The fluid is swallowed, absorbed in the gastrointestinal tract, and transferred to the maternal circulation via the placenta. This mechanism is estimated to account for up to 50% of water transfer from the amniotic fluid to the mother. Polyhydramnios is most likely to be seen in isolated EA (85% of cases). The chance that EA and TEF will be associated with polyhydramnios is 1:12.

At birth, infants appear normal. All types of EA and TEF present shortly after birth except isolated TEF, which may be asymptomatic or may result in mild symptoms for up to several months. The triad of excessive mucus, regurgitation of feeds, and respiratory distress indicates esophageal atresia until proven otherwise. The most frequent alerting symptom is excess mucus seen soon after birth. Rarely, the secretions may be bilious if regurgitation occurs through a distal fistula to the trachea and the pharynx. In most cases, the diagnosis is not suspected until the first feeding, whereupon the infant develops choking, cough, and cyanosis associated with regurgitation or projectile vomiting of feed. Clinical signs of aspiration pneumonia are noted, primarily in the right upper lobe. Interestingly, severe pulmonary symptoms are more common in EA with distal TEF, suggesting that regurgitation of gastric contents into the lungs is a more potent cause of pulmonary complications than inhalation of saliva or milk. Abdominal distention is often seen in EA with distal TEF and may lead to worse respiratory symptoms secondary to elevation of the diaphragm.

Isolated TEF usually presents in early infancy, but symptoms may not become significant for several months or even years.[22] Rarely, cases have first been diagnosed in adults. Average age at diagnosis is 2 months. Primary symptoms involve the respiratory tract and include repeated bouts of cough and/or choking with feeding, and recurrent pneumonia. The pneumonia tends to be bilateral in contrast to the predilection for the right upper lobe that is seen in the more common aspiration syndromes. Respiratory symptoms may be episodic, thus confusing the clinician. Swallowing difficulties are uncommon. Patients often develop abdominal distention or bloating associated with crying.

The differential diagnosis in EA and TEF include laryngotracheoesophageal cleft, congenital esophageal stenosis, congenital diaphragmatic hernia, and pseudoesophageal diverticula. In cases of suspected isolated TEF, the differential also includes gastroesophageal reflux, allergic and inflammatory pulmonary disease, immunodeficiency disorder, and cystic fibrosis.

Diagnostic Evaluation

There is definite prognostic advantage in making the diagnosis of EA and TEF before significant respiratory symptoms develop. Therefore, any infant with excessive mucus, choking or vomiting with feeds, or respiratory distress should have a #10F radiopaque nasogastric tube passed as soon as possible. In EA, obstruction is usually encountered 9–13 cm from the nares. One must beware of curling of the catheter in the upper esophageal pouch, this occurrence gives the impression that the tube has passed into the stomach. Ingestion of air and auscultation over the stomach may give false-positive results because sounds are easily transmitted in the small neonate. It is therefore recommended that posterior–anterior and lateral neck and chest x-rays are obtained to document the tube position. The lateral chest x-ray may also show a dilated blind upper esophageal pouch and anterior displacement of the trachea. In addition, the chest x-ray confirms the presence or absence of pneumonia. An abdominal flat plate is obtained to evaluate the intestinal gas pattern. Air in the abdomen indicates a distal fistula whereas absence of air points toward atresia without fistula or to proximal TEF. It is important to remember that occasionally (1%) in EA with distal TEF no air enters the abdomen, presumably because of an extremely narrow or mucus-blocked fistula lumen.

There is controversy regarding the need for barium x-ray evaluation in EA and TEF. It is generally accepted that appropriate clinical symptoms, the failure of a nasogastric tube to pass into stomach, and the presence of air in abdomen are diagnostic of EA with distal TEF and that no further evaluation is needed prior to surgery.[7,14] Some authors consider that barium studies are contraindicated because of the increased risk of aspiration. Pneumonia has been reported to be three times more common in infants after a barium study.[23] Other authors advocate the contrast study of all patients for three reasons.[24] First, a definitive diagnosis is possible, since such conditions as congenital esophageal stenosis or web, pharyngeal perforation with pseudodiverticulum, and laryngotracheoesophageal cleft can be ruled out. Second, the length of the proximal atretic pouch and its relationship to the tracheal carina can be obtained; the relationship of the upper pouch to the carina is of prognostic significance for the possibility of primary closure. Last, the presence or absence of a proximal TEF can be determined. The technique involves passage of a soft red rubber catheter filled with barium sulfate fluoroscopically. The catheter tip is deflected anteriorly at the site of atresia and no more than 0.5–2.0 cc of barium injected. After anterior–posterior and lateral films are obtained, the barium is suctioned out of the pouch. Water-soluble agents are not used because they are more toxic to the bronchi and lung if aspirated.

Isolated TEF is a difficult diagnosis to make because of the small size and intermittant patency of the fistula and its oblique position in the upper esophagus. If the diagnosis is suspected, rapid infusion of dilute barium sulfate through a catheter whose tip is placed just below the mid-esophagus will usually result in enough reverse filling to show the fistula.[24] Because of the oblique nature of the fistula, the injection may have to be tried with the catheter in a number of different positions. One must be careful, because aspiration may lead to barium in the trachea and false-positive results. When the trachea fills from a fistula, there is seldom any contrast in the pharynx; the reverse is true when aspiration is present. Many authors think that when there is strong suspicion of an isolated TEF, three separate negative barium studies are needed to rule out the diagnosis. Two other x-ray findings that suggest isolated TEF include an air-filled esophagus on plain film and the presence of abnormal esophageal motility on the esophagram. Endoscopy has also been reported to be of value in confirming the diagnosis and delineating the level of the fistula. Both tracheobroncoscopy and esophagoscopy have been used.[22] Esophagoscopy is most rewarding if done under general anesthesia. During tracheobronchoscopy, one needs to remind the anesthesiologist not to insert the endotracheal tube too far down the trachea, thereby occluding the fistula. Occasionally one can see the fistula opening into the esophagus as positive pressure is applied endotracheally. Another recently described test for isolated TEF is the measurement of intragastric oxygen concentration while the patient breaths either room air or 100% O_2.[25,26] Intragastric oxygen concentrations increase or decline in response to breathing 100% O_2 or room air, respectively. The test gives best results when the patient is intubated.

Management of EA and TEF

EA with or without TEF was a uniformly fatal anomaly until 1939. In 1939, Ladd[27] and Leven[28] independently performed gastrostomy in two patients with EA and TEF, who subsequently survived. In 1941, Haight and Towsley performed primary esophagoesophagostomy in a 13-day-old infant, the first patient to survive therapy for EA and TEF because of formation of an anatomic esophagus.[29] Survival, which at that time was practically zero, has now increased to approximately 85%.[6,14,30]

There are two basic operative approaches to EA and TEF: primary anastomosis and staged operative management. Prior to the 1970s only full-term infants without significant anomalies or respiratory distress underwent primary anastomosis. Staging was the management of choice in high-risk patients, i.e., those who (1) were premature, (2) had associated anomalies, (3) had pulmonary involvement, (4) had a long gap between esophageal segments, or (5) showed deterioration during initial operative procedure. Staging involved initial gastrostomy and extrapleural division of TEF, followed at a later date by anastamosis of esophageal segments. Thus, two major thoracotomies were needed in a staging management. Because of major advances in the past 10–15 years, including increased physician awareness of the clinical presentation of EA and TEF, markedly improved neonatal care, and improved techniques of respiratory management and anesthesia, most infants today are treated by division of the TEF and primary esophageal anastomosis.[7,14,30,31,32] Prematurity and respiratory complications are rarely reasons for staging management. Staging management is still employed for desperately ill patients with severe respiratory problems and life-threatening anomalies. A long gap between the two esophageal pouches as seen in isolated EA, EA with priximal TEF, and occasionally in EA with distal TEF, together with clinical deterioration during initial surgery, are now the most important reason for staging. Staging, however, no longer requires two major thoracotomies. The necessity of having to undergo a thoracotomy with esophageal fistula division without primary repair may now be obviated by using gastrostomy decompression as a means of preventing further pulmonary complications coupled with parenteral alimentation for nutrition.[33]

Preoperative Management. Maximal stabilization of the patient prior to surgery decreases both morbidity and mortality during surgery and in the postoperative period. Thermal stability is provided by keeping the infant in an isolette. The head and thorax are elevated 30°. Continuous suction of the upper pouch is begun as soon as the diagnosis is suspected, and oxygen is provided as needed. Elective endotracheal intubation is performed early if respiratory symptoms are severe. Most surgeons employ broad-spectrum antibiotics prior to surgery. Peripheral hyperalimentation is begun, particularly if surgery is to be delayed.

1. Surgical Correction of EA with Distal TEF. Correction of this anomaly is considered an elective emergency and in most instances is performed within 12–18 hours after birth. The surgical procedure involves (1) a right thoracotomy, (2) division of TEF, (3) anastomosis of the two esophageal segments, (4) gastrostomy for postoperative gastric decompression, and (5) placement of a jejunal feeding tube to permit early postoperative feedings.

Two surgical approaches may be employed: transpleural or extrapleural.[15] The transpleural approach is technically easier, gives better exposure, and reduces operation time. However, the major disadvantage is that if postoperative anastomotic leaks occur, empyema will develop. Since such leaks occur in 10–20% of the cases,[8] most surgeons prefer the extrapleural approach; in this procedure leaks that occur drain through the thoracotomy wound.[34]

The first goal at operation is division of the TEF. (Ligation of the TEF is contraindicated as it may lead to recanalization.) Following division of the TEF, approximation of the two esophageal pouches is obtained by mobilizing the upper pouch and applying traction. It is important to rule out proximal fistulas when mobilizing proximal pouch.

End-to-end anastomosis is the standard procedure. There is some controversy over the type of anastomosis to be performed. One-layer anastomosis has been associated with fewer postoperative strictures but a higher incidence of anastomotic leaks.[7,14] Two-layer anastomosis has been reported to reduce such leaks significantly but is associated with a significantly increased incidence of stricture.[7,8,14] In one recent report no significant difference in leak rates between one- and two-layer anastomosis was found.[35] An extrapleural approach was used in these patients. Two-layer anastomosis, however, was associated with significantly increased incidence of postoperative strictures. Some surgeons performed end-to-side anastomosis and reported that the complication of postoperative stricture occurred less frequently. Advantages of the end-to-side anastomosis include[14] (1) better stability, (2) increased size of anastomosis, (3) preservation of blood supply to lower esophageal segment, and (4) diminished postoperative disturbance of motility.[14] However, there has been a report that the rate of recurrent TEF is higher with this technique.[7] Since the extrapleural approach minimizes the early postoperative morbidity of anastomotic leaks and because postoperative stricture is associated with 18–36% of the long-term operative mortality,[8,31,36] the procedure of choice would now seem to be a one-layer end-to-end anastomosis through an extrapleural approach.

Postoperative management of EA with distal TEF. The gastrostomy tube is left open to drain for 24–48 hours. The upper esophagus is suctioned through a nasal catheter placed just proximal to the esophagus at the time of surgery. Nasojejunal feedings are begun at 48–72 hours. On the 4th or 5th day after surgery, a barium swallow is performed to check the patency of the anastomosis and to rule out anastomotic leaks. A tiny crevice of barium extending from the esophagus at this time does not necessarily mean persistent leak, and if the patient is stable, a follow-up study is done in 1 to 2 weeks. Edema still causes narrowing at the anastomosis at this time so that it is impossible to evaluate it for stricture. Oral feedings are usually put off until 10–12 days after surgery. The nasojejunal tube is removed as soon as the patient is tolerating sufficient calories by oral feedings.

2. Surgical Correction of Long Gap Between Esophageal Pouches—isolated EA, EA with proximal TEF, EA with proximal and distal TEF, and occasional EA with distal TEF. A long gap is suspected if the abdomen is scaphoid and no air is present on plain x-ray, or if esophageal segments cannot be approximated at the time of thoracotomy. In this case, a staging management is employed. The initial procedure includes a gastrostomy together with extrapleural division of any TEF. Cervical esophagostomy (externalizing the upper esophagus in the neck) should be performed so that small oral feedings can be offered to maintain sucking and swallowing functions. Following the initial operation, the length of the distal esophageal pouch can be shown by barium study through the gastrostomy. Reconstruction of alimentary continuity is usually postponed until the infant weighs 15–20 lbs.[14] There are three methods of reconstructing an esophagus.[7,14]

(a) *Colon interposition.* This method is still the most popular procedure.[37] The right, transverse, or left colon may be utilized together with its blood supply.

The colon transplant can be placed retrosternally or within the thoracic cavity. It is preferable to anastomose the lower end of the colon graft to the lower esophageal pouch to maintain LES function. This procedure requires using left or transverse colon through a thoracic approach. Once again, anastomotic leaks may lead to the disastrous complication of empyema. The retrosternal approach using the right colon is easier with and involves a lower incidence of postoperative morbidity; however, the patient is left without a LES, increasing the risk of long-term acid reflux and peptic colitis.

Manometric studies have shown that there is no intrinsic muscular activity in the colon. The colon empties into the stomach simply by gravity. Whether the transplant is placed in an iso- or an antiperistaltic manner does not appear to make a difference in emptying. Because vagal fibers are disrupted during colon interposition, it is customary also to do a pyloroplasty in order to facilitate postoperative gastric emptying.

(b) *Gastric tube.* Some surgeons have advocated the use of a tube fashioned from the gastric fundus which is swung up and anastomosed to the proximal esophageal pouch.[37] The advantage of this procedure is that there is only one anastomosis, lessening the likelihood of a leak. Also, the gastric tube will not elongate and dilate like the colon. The major disadvantages are loss of the LES and decreased stomach size, which lead to significant postoperative reflux.

(c) *Mechanical elongation.* More recently, surgeons have taken advantage of the fact that the upper and lower esophageal segments seem to grow at a faster rate than the thorax, thus, with time, the gap between the segments is reduced. With substantial distal esophagus, Howard and Myers[38] and others[30,39] have recommended elongation of the upper pouch by daily passage of a Hegar dilator under fluoroscopic control. Others have also stretched the lower pouch by passing a dilator through the gastrostomy.[30] In many cases, this technique has allowed primary anastomosis of esophageal segments although there is a high rate of postoperative anastomotic leaks and stricture.

3. Surgical Correction of an Isolated TEF. Since most of these lesions are at or above the level of the second thoracic vertebrae, surgical division is almost always done by a right supraclavicular approach to avoid injuring the thoracic duct.[14] Occasionally, a transthoracic approach is necessary to reach isolated fistulae lower in the esophagus. Because of the low incidence of postoperative leaks a transpleural approach is considered safest in this case. Some surgeons advocate placing a flap of mediastinal tissue or pleura between the trachea and esophagus after division of the fistula to prevent recurrence.[14,22]

Postoperative Complications

The majority of early postoperative deaths are attributed to pulmonary complications, i.e., aspiration pneumonia, empyema and pneumothorax secondary to anastomotic leak, pulmonary edema, respiratory distress syndrome, laryngeal obstruction from edema, and accululated secretions.[7,14]

Anastomotic leaks develop in 5–10% of cases and cause 20% of early postoperative mortality.[8] Leaks are caused by undue tension, ischemia, or local infection at the site of anastomosis. They usually develop between the 2nd and 7th postoperative days, but may be delayed until 10–14 days. Anastomotic leaks are generally small and close spontaneously. Medical management includes no oral feedings, administration of broad-spectrum antibiotics, gastric decompression through gastrostomy, and continuous nasojejunal feedings. Associated mortality is negligible if an extrapleural approach has been used, since a leak results in fistulous drainage through the incision. Following the transpleural approach mortality may be as high as 50%, since the leak gives rise to empyema and pneumothorax. Management in such cases includes cervical esophagostomy and closure of the distal esophagus in addition to drainage via a chest tube.

Recurrent TEFs are rare and may be caused by anastomotic leaks or recanalization of a TEF that was only ligated; they may also represent a missed proximal TEF. Symptoms include recurrence of choking and coughing during feedings and also abdominal distention. Recurrent TEF from anastomotic leaks may close spontaneously or may require re-operation.

The incidence of esophageal stricture after anastomosis is up to 80%.[7,8,14,31,36] However, only 30–50% are severe enough to require dilitation. Clinical symptoms from stricture usually develop 3–4 weeks after surgery. Patients develop dysphagia, aerophagia, vomiting, increased secretions, and occasionally stridor secondary to distention of the upper esophagus. The cause of stricture is related to the type of anastomosis and is significantly greater following two-layer closure. Other causes include tension at the suture line, anastomotic leak, local infection, and tissue reaction to the suture material. Diagnosis is made by barium swallow. Usually only a few dilitations are required to relieve symptoms, and rarely is resection and re-anastomosis of the esophagus required. Troublesome strictures warrant careful investigation for gastroesophageal reflux.

Chronic pulmonary problems are common after repair of EA and TEF. Milligan studied lung function and bronchial reactivity in 24 patients 7–18 years after repair of EA and distal TEF.[40] Only one patient showed no abnormalities in the variables that were tested. Thirteen patients had obstructive airway disease, five had a restrictive defect, and fifteen had positive methacholine-challenge test results, indicating increased bronchial muscle responsiveness/sensitivity. Subclinical aspiration secondary to esophageal stricture, motor disorder, or gastroesophageal reflux is postulated to be the cause of these lung abnormalities. Other postulated causes include deficient ciliary activity in the trachea and bronchi with resultant retention of pulmonary secretions,[14] and milk allergy secondary to sensitization from aspiration in the neonatal period.[42] There have been reports that removing milk products from the diet has resulted in improved pulmonary function in a number of patients.

Other less common complications include hiatal hernia. There is controversy about whether this is a congenital abnormality or the result of surgical traction on the lower esophagus. Chronic diarrhea secondary to both mono- and disaccharide intolerance has been reported following TEF repair; the cause is not known.[43] Damage to the recurrent laryngeal nerve, phrenic nerve paralysis, and tracheal stenosis have all been reported.[14] These children often have a cat-like cry and barking cough, both of which seem to be self-limiting.[7] Shoulder-girdle deformity characterized by elevation of the shoulder, nipple asymmetry, disparity of size of the scapnea, and limitation of shoulder movement have been reported as a complication following thoracotomy and presumably occur secondary to nerve injury at the time of surgery.[44]

Colon interposition is associated with a high incidence of complications. Anastomotic leaks, ischemia in the colon segment, and anastomotic obstruction are early problems. Long-term complications include reflux with peptic colitis or stricture of the proximal anastomotis if the LES has not been preserved and redundant colon with associated stasis and malabsorption.[45] Gastric retention may be a problem if pyloropasty has not been performed.

Motility Disorder in EA and TEF

Motility disorder of the esophagus does not appear to be a complication of repair of EA and TEF. Peristaltic disturbances are present in 90% of patients with EA and TEF.[36,46,47] The derangement in normal motility is primarily seen in the distal half of the esophagus although in 20% of cases, the entire esophagus is involved. In the usual case the primary peristaltic wave is lost a short distance below the anastomosis. Below this level secondary and tertiary contractions occur that often result in retrograde flow of esophageal contents. The cause of the motor defect is not known. It is not thought to be secondary to EA because (1) peristaltic disturbances are not observed in dogs following esophageal transection[48,49] and (2) the motor abnormality is also present in isolated TEF without EA.[7,22] These findings suggest that there may be a congenital defect in esophageal neuromuscular coordination. Abnormal muscle mass in the esophagus may lead to abnormal nerve development. At the same time, a similar motor abnormality can be produced by local division of vagal fibers,[48,49] suggesting that surgical damage to the vagus nerve and its esophageal branches may be an important factor. Interestingly, the type of anastomosis (one-layer or two-layer, end-to-end or end-to-side) does not seem to correlate with development of motor abnormality, nor does postoperative anastomotic leak or stricture.[4,7] Clinically, disordered motility is manifested by varying degrees of dysphagia and episodes of aspiration pneumonia. Dysphagia is primarily associated with solids. The ingestion of foreign bodies is especially dangerous in patients following repair of EA and TEF. Esophageal acid clearance has been measured and is abnormal in virtually all these patients. The motility disorder has been reported to persist for 14–32 years after surgical repair; this finding leads to the belief that the condition is a permanent abnormality. Dysphagia, however, seems to decrease with time, probably reflecting the patient's adaptation to the problem.[36,50,51]

Of the esophageal sphincters, the upper is usually normal, but the lower may show increased tone with incomplete relaxation after swallowing, normal pressure and normal function, and low resting pressure with normal function.[50-55] One study reported that 40% of patients had decreased LES pressure.[53] Gastroesophageal reflux has been reported in two-thirds of the patients with EA and TEF.[55] The higher incidence of gastroesophageal reflux is also felt to be related to the increased incidence of hiatal hernia. In addition, these patients have been shown to have impaired gastric emptying.[55] Interestingly, they seem to respond well to the medical management of reflux, including upright positioning and frequent, small, thickened feedings. Studies have shown that upright positioning is associated with improved esophageal acid clearance. Bethanecol has also been reported to be useful in managing reflux.[54] Approximately 15–30% of patients with gastroesophageal reflux require antireflux surgery.[36,53,55] Indications for surgery include poor growth, pulmonary complications, and esophagitis. Experience has also shown that despite the motor disorder, the patients improve symptomatically after surgery.[53,55]

Prognosis of EA and TEF

Because so many factors influence the survival of a child with EA and TEF malformation, it is difficult to assess prognosis for any given patient. In 1964, overall survival was 60%.[8] Today the overall rate is approximately 85–90%.[6,30] This improvement in survival can be directly traced to better awareness of the anomaly and better pre- and postoperative general supportive and respiratory care.[31,32,56] Anticipation of survival and mortality is possible using the Waterston risk classification.[57] Group A consists of infants whose birthweight is greater than 2,500 g and who have no significant anomalies or pulmonary complications. Group B is comprised of infants with weight between 1800–2500 g and no significant anomalies or pulmonary complications or those with weight greater than 2,500 g and either non-life-threatening anomalies or only mild-to-moderate respiratory symptoms. Group C includes infants of less than 1800 g and any infants with life-threatening anomalies or severe pulmonary complications. Survival approximates 100% for Group A, 90% for Group B, and 40–70% for Group C.[6,41,30,31] Surprisingly survival of the VATER syndrome patients approximates 80%. Staging operation is now felt to have little influence on survival of poor-risk patients.[58]

In regard to long-term morbidity, Laks was able to obtain 15–25-year follow-up in 42 of 120 survivors who underwent surgery for EA and TEF between 1945 and 1955.[36] Of these, 90% were either asymptomatic or had mild symptoms related to swallowing, and 33% complained of respiratory difficulty that correlated with the occurrence of peri-operative pulmonary complications and/or that of early stricture of the esophagus. Today, with improved survival and aggressive management of postoperative complications and gastroesophageal reflux, the long-term prognosis for patients with this complex anomaly should be quite good.

LARYNGOTRACHEOESOPHAGEAL CLEFT

Laryngotracheoesophageal cleft is a rare and often fatal anomaly whose clinical presentation is identical with that of EA and TEF.[59-62] Approximately 40 cases have been described in the literature. The defect involves a failure of the trachea to separate from the esophagus; the extent of failure varies. The larynx is always involved. In the mildest form, the cleft is in the posterior wall of the larynx and allow communication of the airway and upper esophagus. In the most severe type, the posterior wall of the trachea and anterior wall of the esophagus are absent, and there is a common lumen for the entire length of the trachea. The cause of the anomaly is unknown. It is felt to result because the lung bud fails to separate completely from the foregut lumen and cephalic migration and posterior fusion of the lateral folds of the foregut are incomplete. The arrest in advancement of the tracheoesophageal septum is followed by a failure of the cricoid cartilages to fuse dorsally, a process that takes place in the 3rd month of gestation. In one-fifth of the cases, laryngotracheoesophageal cleft is associated with EA. Associated vertebral defects are also common. The defect is not generally associated with other anomalies.

The condition presents at birth or soon after with choking, cyanosis, massive aspiration, and abdominal distention. Associated aphonia or hoarse, feeble cry should make one suspicious of the diagnosis. Often digital examination of the pharynx will suggest the diagnosis, since the epiglottis is malformed in this anomaly. The condition is differentiated from EA and TEF by passage of a nasogastric tube into the stomach. Plain x-ray reveals persistent air in the esophagus, severe aspiration pneumonia, and gas-filled abdomen. Diagnosis is confirmed by barium cineradiography or bronchoscopy. Treatment is emergency surgical closure of the cleft. Survival figures are unknown. All patients require long-term tracheostomy.

Laryngotracheoesophageal cleft was reported in one identical twin whereas the other had tracheal stenosis; this finding indicates that one unknown teratogen is capable of causing a variety of congenital abnormalities at a given stage of embryonic development.[63]

CONGENITAL ESOPHAGEAL STENOSIS AND WEB

Both congenital esophageal stenosis and web are forms of incomplete esophageal obstruction.[64-67] They have symptoms and derivation in common and are therefore discussed together. It is now generally accepted that these anomalies are extremely rare and that the vast majority of cases of esophageal stenosis that present in infancy are acquired secondary to gastroesophageal reflux.[67]

Congenital stenosis is located in the middle third of the esophagus in 50% of cases, the lower third in 33%, and the upper third in 15%. There are basically six types of congenital stenosis.

1.   Independent esophageal web. The web is a well-defined thin structure with either a central or eccentric apperture that may be circular or crescent shaped. Webs are usually located in the cervical esophagus or at the junction of the middle and lower thirds.

2.   Segmented esophageal stenosis. The stenoses vary from 1–10 cm in length, with the majority 1–2 cm.

3.   Esophageal web within a segmental stenosis.

4.   Segmental stenosis composed of tracheobronchial elements including intra-

mural cartilagenous rings and respiratory tract glands. This defect usually occurs in the lower esophagus.[68]

5. Segmental stricture associated with proximal EA and TEF.

6. Esophageal muscular ring. In this extremely rare defect, histologically proven muscle hypertrophy causes esophageal obstruction.[69]

Pathologically, esophageal stenosis consists of a constricted lumen with normal mucosal and muscular layers. A web is comprised of thin-fold or normal squamous epithelium without muscularis that is at right angles to the esophageal lumen. The etiology of both defects is unknown but is felt to be either secondary to segmental defective recanalization of the esophageal lumen during the 7th–10th fetal weeks or to vascular insufficiency secondary to intrauterine anoxia or stress.

Clinically, the onset of symptoms depends on the degree of deformity. In most cases, symptoms begin early in infancy with regurgitation of formula that is not curdled or bile stained. Symptoms can be intermittent. It is not uncommon, however, for symptoms of vomiting and regurgitation to become manifested first when solid foods are introduced. Rarely, cases present following lodgment of a swallowed foreign body. Respiratory symptoms including stridor and wheezing may develop secondary to a dilated proximal esophagus. Recurrent aspiration pneumonia has also been reported. It is important to realize that all of the above symptoms may be secondary to stricture caused by gastroesophageal reflux. In general, the earlier the lesion presents and the higher its location in the esophagus, the more likely the lesion is to be congenital in origin. Differential diagnosis includes vascular ring, peptic stricture secondary to gastroesophageal reflux or ectopic gastric mucosa, or caustic stricture.

Diagnosis of congenital stricture requires plain chest x-ray; barium swallow; esophageal manometrics, pH monitoring and scintiscan to rule out reflux; and esophagoscopy with biopsy above and below the stricture to rule out esophagitis. Plain x-ray may show a dilated esophagus proximal to the stricture. Barium study reveals smooth tapering of the esophageal lumen at the margin of the stricture. In stricture composed of tracheobranchial elements, the contrast medium may also fill tiny crevices that are the ducts of the intramural tracheobronchial glands. On barium swallow, a web appears as a radiolucent intraluminal shelf or band of only several millimeters in width. Webs are also often difficult to delineate and are often visualized only visualized only in lateral or oblique views.

Treatment consists of esophageal dilatation. Webs are fractioned at esophagoscopy thus relieving symptoms.[70] In cases of severe stricture, feeding gastrostomy is required. The stricture may then be dilated retrograde through the gastrostomy, a safer technique than dilatation from above, which has a higher chance of perforation. The prognosis for congenital stenosis and web is excellent. Webs do not recur. A sustained good response to continued dilatation firms up the diagnosis of congenital stricture, since strictures associated with gastroesophageal reflux are rarely permanently cured by dilatation. Recurrence of congenital stenosis is very unusual. Strictures composed of tracheobronchial elements and esophageal muscular rings do not respond to dilatation and require surgical excision.

ESOPHAGEAL DUPLICATION

Several types of mediastinal cysts with overlapping histologic characteristics have been described, with the common term for all of these being foregut duplication cysts.[71-74] The esophagus is the second most common site of duplication in the alimentary tract, the most common being the ileum. Characteristics of duplication cysts of the esophagus include (1) attachment to the esophagus, (2) epithelium representing some level of the gastrointestinal tract, and (3) the presence of two layers of muscularis complete with myenteric plexus. Cysts are usually spherical or tubular, and although they may be intramural, the majority are partially or completely separated from the esophagus. They do not necessarily have muscular coat in common with the esophagus, in contrast to duplication cysts that occur elsewhere in the gastrointestinal tract. Two-thirds of the cysts are to the right of the esophagus, whereas one-third are to the left. In rare instances, the cyst may communicate with the esophageal lumen or even with the spinal canal. The lining epithelium of the cyst may be columnar, pseudostratified, ciliated, or squamous. In fact, the histology of a duplication is more frequently gastrogenic or enterogenic than esophageal. Secreting gastric mucosa may lead to rapid expansion of the cyst or peptic digestion of the wall and rupture into the esophagus.

Foregut duplication cysts also represent a developmental error in the 5th to 8th weeks of fetal life. Most authors consider that they occur secondary to incomplete recanalization of the esophagus. Another theory, put forth by Veeneklaas, hypothesizes abnormal adherence of the primative foregut to the notochord.[75] As the esophagus grows caudad, the point of adherence leads to anamolous development of future vertebrae from the notochord, and the corresponding adherent portion of the foregut becomes pinched off, forming a duplication. Vertebral anomalies such as spinabifida and hemivertebrae are commonly associated with esophageal duplication and would be explained by the above hypothesis.[73]

Esophageal duplications present most commonly as expanding mediastinal masses. The majority present in later infancy with primarily respiratory symptoms that include dyspnea, cyanosis, recurrent pneumonia, and laryngeal strider secondary to pressure in the trachea or lung. Vomiting and dysphagia may also be present secondary to pressure on the esophagus. Other presenting symptoms include (1) hemoptysis, hematemesis, or melana secondary to peptic ulceration into the lung, a pulmonary vessel, or the esophagus; (2) chest pain secondary to peptic secretions and ulcerations within the cyst; and (3) an expanding cervical mass. Patients may also be asymptomatic and present with an abnormal chest x-ray obtained for a variety of reasons.

The diagnosis is suspected on the basis of a chest x-ray finding of a posterior mediastinal mass that encroaches on the adjacent lung and displaces mediastinal structures to the opposite side. The mass usually has a smooth border. Associated vertebral anomalies are seen superior to the mass. Often it is difficult to distinguish where in the mediastium the mass arises. Barium swallow shows anterior displacement of the esophagus. Communication between the esophageal lumen and the cyst can also be ruled out by contrast study.

Table 5-1. Differential diagnosis of mediastinal masses

	Location		
	Anterosuperior	Middle	Posterior
Common	Teraloma	Lymphoma	Neurogenic tumors
	Thymus	Lymph nodes	Duplication
	Hyperplasia	Granuloma	
	Cyst	Bronchogenic	
	Lympho- sarcoma	cyst	
	Lymphangioma		
	Hemangioma		
Rare	Substernal	Pericardial	Pheochromocytoma
	thyroid	cyst	Anterior
	Thymic tumor		meningocele

Modified from Bower RJ, Kieswetter WB: Mediastinal masses in infants and children. Arch Surg 112:1003–1009, 1977. Copyright 1977, American Medical Association.

The differential diagnosis includes all causes for mediastinal masses (Table 5-1).[76] Foregut cysts are second only to neurogenic tumors as the cause of posterior mediastinal masses in infants and children.

Arteriography, myelography, or bronchoscopy may narrow the differential, but a definitive diagnosis is usually made at surgery. Treatment involves surgical excision. It is important to evaluate the entire gastrointestinal tract prior to surgery, since there is an increased incidence of duplication at other sites in the alimentary tract.

ESOPHAGEAL DIVERTICULUM

Isolated esophageal diverticula are the rarest of all esophageal anomalies.[77,78] The diverticula usually occur in the upper third of the esophagus and are squamous-epithelium lined sacs that involve all layers of the muscular wall. The vast majority of esophageal diverticula are probably acquired secondary to traumatic injury of the hypopharynx and upper esophageal mucosa and are caused by routine oropharyngeal suctioning of secretions at birth, endotracheal intubation, or passage of a nasogastric tube. Acquired diverticula are also called pseudodiverticula.[79] The clinical presentation of diverticulum may mimic that of EA and TEF, including the inability to pass a nasogastric tube, which curls in the diverticulum. Diagnosis may be suspected by the finding of blood-tinged secretions after oral suctioning and a lateral neck x-ray film showing a soft-tissue mass in the retropharyngeal area that displaces the trachea and larynx anteriorly. Diagnosis is confirmed by a barium contrast study, since barium fills the diverticulum when the patient is supine. Treatment is surgical excision.

VASCULAR RINGS

Although these are not true anomalies of the esophagus, vascular rings are the most common cause of esophageal compression and as such deserve consideration in a chapter on congenital disorders of the esophagus.[24,80] The embryologic basis for an understanding of vascular rings consists of a double aortic arch and a right and left ductus (Fig. 5-5). Normally, the right aortic arch and right ductus regress. Clinical symptoms are for the most part seen in the following variations of development, the causes of which are unknown:

1.   A double aortic arch that consists of an anterior and a posterior arch encircling the trachea and esophagus,
2.   Right aortic arch with patent left ductus or left ligamentum arteriorum to left pulmonary vein,
3.   Anomalous right subclavian artery that arises from the left side of the aortic arch and passes behind the esophagus.

In the first two anomalies, tracheal compression is more severe than esophageal compression. The conditions present with primarily respiratory symptoms including wheezing and stridor, which may be made worse by eating. Anomalous right subclavian artery produces primarily esophageal symptoms of dysphagia, vomiting, or regurgitation.

Symptoms of vascular ring usually present anywhere from birth to 6 months.

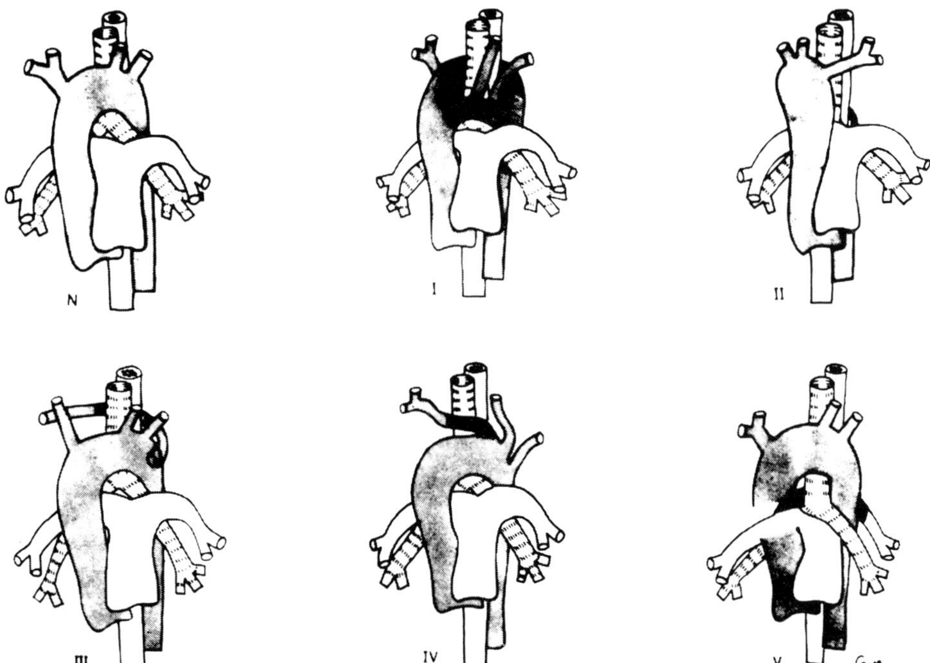

Fig. 5-5 Schematic drawings showing the various vascular anomalies. Black areas show the compressing part of the vessels. From Eklof O, Erstrom G, Eriksson BO, et al: Arterial anomalies causing compression of the trachea and/or the oesophagus. Acta Pediatr Scand 60:81–89, 1971.

These anomalies should be considered whenever both respiratory and esophageal symptoms are present in the same patient. The diagnosis is suspected from the chest x-ray and barium-swallow findings and is confirmed by arteriography.

In the double aortic-arch anomaly, usually only one component of the double arch can be visualized on P–A chest x-ray. Rarely are both right and left aortic knobs seen. Lateral chest x-ray may show anterior compression of the trachea. The barium study shows posterior compression of the esophagus at the level of the third and fourth vertebrae. This defect is formed by the posterior arch—usually the larger of the two—as it passes behind the esophagus.

In the right-aortic-arch variation, chest x-ray reveals soft-tissue prominence in the right superior mediastinum, with displacement of the trachea to the left. On barium swallow, the right arch is shown to indent on the right lateral wall of the esophagus whereas the left ligamentum anterium indents on the arteriolateral wall of the esophagus.

In an aberrant right subclavian artery, the barium study reveals an oblique filling defect on the posterior esophagus that extends from left to right. The barium x-ray appearance of an aberrant right subclavian artery can be less apparent in early infancy, and therefore repeated examination may be necessary before the diagnosis is made.

Conservative management is required on vascular rings because surgery is associated with a significant operative mortality and respiratory symptoms may persist postoperatively. This occurs because abnormalities of tracheal cartilages are frequently present at the site of compression by vascular rings. The double-aortic-arch anomaly is most likely to require surgery, usually because of recurrent pulmonary infection. Surgery is seldom needed with the anomalous subclavian artery type except in cases of significant anorexia and vomiting and failure to thrive. Symptoms associated with this anomaly tend to improve with age.

CONGENITAL SHORT ESOPHAGUS

True congenital short esophagus is an extremely rare defect, since most often short esophagus is the late result of stricture, fibrosis, and contraction secondary to peptic esophagitis caused by gastrointestinal reflux. Failure of the esophagus to elongate following septation from the trachea is considered to be the etiology. The complex of congenital short esophagus encompasses inclusion of a portion of the stomach in the thorax. The intrathoracic stomach originates above the diaphragm and derives its blood supply from the aorta, not from the celiac axis as a hiatal hernia would. There is no diaphragmatic defect. The short esophagus is lined by squamous epithelium and contains two muscle layers. The thoracic stomach is lined by functioning gastric mucosa and contains three muscle layers. There is no protective functioning LES, and reflux of gastric contents leads to severe esophagitis and stricture. Clinical symptoms are identical with complicated gastroesophageal reflux: vomiting and regurgitation, dysphagia, and recurrent bouts of pneumonia or aspiration. Barium swallow shows gastric rugae above the diaphragm and free reflux. Treatment involves fundoplication in the chest, esophageal resection with high esophagogastrostomy, or colon interposition.

SUMMARY

Congenital disorders of the esophagus are a rare spectrum of anomalies that develop following intrauterine insults in the 2nd month of fetal life. Advances in neonatal and respiratory care over the last decade have led to improved survival particularly for EA and TEF. At the same time, a greater knowledge of the spectrum of complications associated with gastroesophageal reflux has determined that many disorders previously thought to be congenital are acquired.

REFERENCES

1. Hopkins WA: The esophagus: In Gray SW, Skandalakis JE, (eds): Embryology for Surgeons, WB Saunders, Philadelphia, 1972.
2. Bremer JL: Congenital Anomalies of the Viscera, Harvard University Press, Cambridge, 1957.
3. Allan FD: Essentials of Human Embryology, Oxford University Press, New York, 1957.
4. Keibel F, Mall FP: Human Embryology, JB Lippincott, Philadelphia, 1912.
5. Bustamante S, Koldovsky O: Synopsis of development of the main morphological structures of the human gastrointestinal tract. In Lebenthal EE (ed): Gastrointestinal Development and Infant Nutrition, Raven Press, New York, 1980.
6. Herbst JJ: Development of sucking and swallowing. In Leventhall EE (ed): Gastrointestinal Development and Infant Nutrition, Raven Press, New York, 1980.
7. Chen H, Goei GS, Hertzler JH: Family studies on congenital esophageal atresia with or without tracheoesophageal fistula. Birth Defects 15,5c:117–144, 1979.
8. Ashcraff KW, Holder TM: Esophageal Atresia and tracheoesophageal fistula malformations. Surg Clin North Am 56:299–315, 1976.
9. Holder TM, Cloud OT, Lewis JE, Pilling GP: Esophageal atresia and tracheoesophageal fistula, a survey of its members by the surgical section of the American Academy of Pediatrics. Pediatrics 34:542–549, 1964.
10. Rabinowitz JG, Moseley JE, Mitty HA, Hirschorn K: Trisomy 18, esophageal atresia anomalies of the radius, and congenital hypoplastic thrombocytopenia. Radiology 89:488–491, 1967.
11. Ingalls TH, Pringle RA: Esophageal atresia with tracheoesophageal fistula. Epidemiologic and teratologic implications. N Eng J Med 240:987–994, 1949.
12. Kluth D: Atlas of esophageal atresia. J Pediatr Surg 11:901–919, 1976.
13. El Shafie M, Kippel CH, Blakemore WS: Congenital esophageal anomalies: A plea for using anatomic descriptions rather than classifications. J Pediatr Surg 13:355, 1978.
14. Myers NA, Aberdeen E: The esophagus: congenital esophageal atresia and tracheoesophageal fistula. In Ravitch MM, Welch KJ, Benson CD, et al. (eds): Pediatric Surgery, Yearbook Med Pub, Chicago, 1979.
15. Goodwin CD, Ashcraft KW, Holder TM, et al.: Esophageal atresia with double eeff. J Pediatr Surg 13:269–273, 1978.
16. Greenwood RO, Rosenthal A: Cardiovascular malformations associated with tracheoesophageal fistula and esophageal atresia. Pediatrics 57:87–90, 1976.
17. Andrassy RJ, Mahour GH: Gastrointestinal anomalies associated with esophageal atresia and tracheoesophageal fistula. Arch Surg 114:1125–1128, 1979.
18. Say B, Gerald PS: A new polydactyly, imperforate anus, vertebral anomalies syndrome. Lancet 2:688, 1968.

19. Quan L, Smith DW: The VATER association. J Pediatr 82:104–107, 1973.
20. Baumann W. Greinacherr I, Emmrich P: VATER-order VACTERL-syndrome. Klin Paediatr 188:328, 1976.
21. Scott JS, Wilson JK: Hydramnio as an early sign of esophageal atresia. Lancet 2:569–572, 1957.
22. Andrassy RJ, Ko P, Handson RA, et al.: Congenital tracheoesophageal fistula without esophageal atresia. A 22 year experience. Am J Surg 140:731–733, 1980.
23. Koop CE, Hamilton JP: Atresia of the esophagus: Factors affecting survival in 249 cases. Z. Kinderchir 5:319–325, 1968.
24. Franken EA: Gastrointestinal Radiology in Pediatrics, Harper & Row, Hagerstown, Md, 1975.
25. Korones SB, Evans LJ: Measurement of intragastric oxygen concentration for diagnosis of H-type tracheoesophageal fistula. Pediatrics 60:450–452, 1977.
26. Powers WF: Further experience with intragastric oxygen measurement to diagnose H-type tracheoesophageal fistula. Pediatrics 63:668–669, 1979.
27. Ladd WE: The surgical treatment of esophageal atresia and tracheoesophageal fistula. N Engl J Med 230:625–637, 1944.
28. Leven NL: Congenital atresia of the esophagus with tracheoesophageal fistula: report of successful extrapleural ligation of fistulous communication and cervical esophagostomy. J Thorac Surg 10:648–657, 1941.
29. Haight C, Towsley HA: Congenital atresia of the esophagus with tracheoesophageal fistula: extrapleural ligation fistula and end to end anastomosis of esophageal segments. Surg Gynecol Obstet 76:672–688, 1943.
30. Woolley MM: Esophageal atresia and tracheoesophageal fistula: 1939 to 1979. Am J Surg 139:771–774, 1980.
31. Koop CE: Recent advances in the surgery of esophageal atresia. Prog Pediatr Surg 2:41–54, 1971.
32. Louchimo I, Sulamaa M, Suutarinen T: Post-operative intensive care of esophageal atresia patients. J Pediatr Surg 5:633–640, 1970.
33. Holder TM, Leape LL, Mann CM: Esophageal atresia, tracheoesophageal fistula, and associated anomalies: hyperalimentation as an aid in treatment. J Thorac Cardiovasc Surg 63:838–840, 1972.
34. Holder TM: Transpleural versus retropleural approach in repair of tracheoesophageal fistula. Surg Clin N Am 44:1433–1439, 1964.
35. Hrabousry E, Boles ET: Long term results following esophageal anastomosis in the neonate. Surg Gynecol Obstet 147:30–32, 1978.
36. Laxs H, Wilkinson RH, Schuster SR: Long term results following correction of esophageal atresia with tracheoesophageal fistula: a clinical and cine fluorographic study. J Pediatr Surg 7:591–597, 1972.
37. Randolph JG, Anderson KD: The esophagus: replacement of the esophagus. In Ravitch MM (ed): Pediatric Surgery, Yearbook Med Pub, Chicago, 1979.
38. Howard R, Myers NA: Esophageal atresia: a technique for elongating the upper pouch. Surgery 58:725–727, 1965.
39. Gwinn JL, Lee FA: Esophageal elongation in esophageal atresia. Ann Radiol 14:279–283, 1971.
40. Milligan DWA, Levison H: Lung function in children following repair of tracheoesophageal fistula. J Pediatr 95:24–27, 1979.
41. Haddadin AJ, Emery JL: Pulmonary retention simulating pneumonia as a cause of death in children with tracheoesophageal fistula. Surgery 70:311–315, 1971.
42. Handelmann N, Nelson T: Association of milk precipitators with esophageal lesions causing aspiration. Pediatrics 34:699–703, 1964.

43. Howat JM, Aaronson I: Sugar intolerance in neonatal surgery. J Pediatr Surg 6:719–723, 1971.

44. Freeman NV, Walkden J: Previously unreported shoulder deformity following right lateral thoracotomy for esophageal atresia. J Pediatr Surg 4:627–636, 1969.

45. Louhima I, Pasila M, Visakorpi JK: Late gastrointestinal complications in patients with colonic replacement of the esophagus. J Pediatr Surg 4:663–673, 1969.

46. Burgess JN, Carlson HC, Ellis FH: Esophageal function after successful repair of esophageal atresia and tracheoesophageal fistula: a manometric and cine fluorographic study. J Thorac Cardiovasc Surg 56:667–673, 1968.

47. Moroz SP, Espinoza J, Cumming WA, Diamant NE: Lower esophageal sphincter function in children with and without gastroesophageal reflux. Gastroenterology 71:236–241, 1976.

48. Carveth SW, Schlegel JF, Code CF, Ellis FH: Esophageal motility after vagotomy, phrenicotomy, myotomy, and myomectomy in dogs. Surg Gynecol Obstet 114:31–42, 1962.

49. Haller JA, Brooker AF, Talbert JL, et al.: Esophageal function following resection. Studies in newborn puppies. Ann Thorac Surg 2:180–187, 1966.

50. Orringer MB, Kirsh MM, Sloan H: Long term esophageal function following repair of esophageal atresia. Ann Surg 186:436–443, 1977.

51. Duranceau A, Fisher SR, Flye MW, et al.: Motor function of the esophagus after repair of esophageal fistula and tracheoesophageal fistula. Surgery 82:116–123, 1977.

52. Lind JF, Blanchard RJ, Guyda H: EEE motility in tracheoesophageal fistula and esophageal atresia. Surg Gynecol Obstet 123:557–564, 1966.

53. Parker AF, Christie DL, Cahill JL: Incidence and significance of gastroesophageal reflux following repair of esophageal atresia and tracheoesophageal fistula and the need for anti-reflux procedures. J Pediatr Surg 14:5–8, 1979.

54. Whitington PF, Shermeta DW, Seto DSY, et al.: Role of lower esophageal sphincter incompetence in recurrent pneumonia after repair of esophageal atresia. J Pediatr 91:550–554, 1977.

55. Jolly SG, Johnson DG, Roberts CC, et al.: Patterns of gastroesophageal reflux in children following repair of esophageal atresia and distal tracheoesophageal fistula. J Pediatr Surg 15:857–862, 1980.

56. Brereton RJ, Zachary RB, Spitz L: Preventable death in esophageal atresia. Arch Dis Child 53:276–283, 1978.

57. Waterston DJ, Bonham-Carter RE, Aberdeen E: Oesophageal atresia: tracheoesophageal fistula: a study of survival of 218 infants. Lancet 1:819–822, 1962.

58. Weber TR, Smith W, Grosfeld JL: Surgical experiences in infants with VATER association. J Pediatr Surg 15:849–854, 1980.

59. Burroughs N, Leape LL: Laryngotracheoesophageal cleft: Report of a case successfully treated and review of the literature. Pediatrics 53:516–522, 1974.

60. Blumberg JB, Stevenson JK, Lemire RJ: Laryngotracheoesophageal cleft, the embryologic implications: review of the literature. Surgery 57:559, 1965.

61. Novaselac M, Fish U, Dangel P. Laryngotracheoesophageal cleft. J Pediatr Surg 8:963–964, 1976.

62. Fuzesi K, Young OG: Congenital laryngotracheoesophageal cleft. J Pediatr Surg 11:933–937, 1976.

63. Novak RW: Laryngotracheoesophageal cleft and unilateral pulmonary hypoplasia in twins. Pediatrics 67:732–734, 1981.

64. Greenough WG: Congenital esophageal stricture. Am J Roentgenol 92:994–999, 1964.

65. Myers NA, Aberdeen E: The esophagus: congenital esophageal stenosis and esophageal

diaphragm. In Ravitch MM, Welch KJ, Benson CD, et al. (eds): Pediatric Surgery, Yearbook Med Pub, Chicago, 1979.

66. Valerio D, Jones PF, Stewart AM: Congenital esophageal stenosis. Arch Dis Child 52:414–416, 1977.

67. Aprigliano F. Esophageal stenosis in children. Ann Otol 89:391–395, 1980.

68. Nishina T, Tsuchida Y, Scuto S: Congenital esophageal stenosis due to tracheobronchial remnants and its associated anomalies. J Pediatr Surg 16:1900–1913, 1980.

69. Heymann MB, Berquist WE, Fonkalsurd EW, et al.: Esophageal muscular ring and the VACTERL association: a case report. J Pediatr 67:683–686, 1981.

70. Huchzermeyer H, Burdelski M, Hruby M: Endoscopic therapy of a congenital oesophageal stricture. Endoscopy 4:259–262, 1979.

71. Spock A, Schneider S, Baylin GJ: Mediastinal gastric cysts: A case report and review of English literature. Am Rev Respir Dis 94:97–103, 1966.

72. Whitaker JA, Deffenbaugh LD, Cooke AR: Esophageal duplication cyst. Am J Gastroenterol 73:329–332, 1980.

73. Ravitch MM: Mediastinal infections, cysts and tumors. In Ravitch MM, Welch KJ, Benson CD, et al. (eds): Pediatric Surgery Yearbook Med Pub, Chicago, 1979.

74. Nehme AE, Rabiah R: Ciliated epithelial esophageal cyst: Case report and review of the literature. Am Surg 43:114–118, 1977.

75. Veeneklaas GM: Pathogenesis of intrathoracic cysts. Am J Dis Child 83:500–507, 1952.

76. Bower RJ, Kieswetter WB: Mediastinal masses in infant and children. Arch Surg 112:1003–1009, 1977.

77. Ravitch MM: The esophagus: Diverticulum of the esophagus. In Ravitch MM, Welch KJ, Benson CD, et al. (eds): Pediatric Surgery, Yearbook Med Pub, Chicago, 1979.

78. Borrie J, Wilson RLK: Oesophageal diverticula: Principles of management and approval of classification. Thorax 35:759–767, 1980.

79. Urrutia J, Antonmattei S: Pseudodiverticulum of the esophagus in the newborn infant. Am J Dis Child 134:417–418, 1980.

80. Eklof O, Erstrom G, Erriksson BO, et al.: Arterial anomalies causing compression of the trachea and/or the oesophagus. Acta Pediatr Scand 60:81–89, 1971.

81. Brown RE, Madge GE, Howell TR: Congenital short esophagus in the newborn. Am J Dig Dis 15:863–865, 1970.

82. Grybowski J: Gastrointestinal Problems in the Infant, WB Saunders, Philadelphia, 1975.

6 | Cricopharyngeal Disorders

Donald Gerhardt
Daniel Winship

INTRODUCTION

Anatomy

The upper esophageal sphincter (UES) is thought to consist primarily of the cricopharyngeus muscle and possibly a small portion of the circular muscle fibers of the esophagus that are immediately distal to it and/or of the inferior pharyngeal constrictor that is proximal to it.[1-7] The cricopharyngeus muscle traverses the posterior wall of the esophagus like a sling and connects anteriorly to the two lateral borders of the cricoid cartilage (Fig. 6-1). Thus, anteriorly the sphincter wall is the semirigid cricoid cartilage, and when the sphincter is closed, the esophageal lumen is a somewhat curved tranverse slit longer in the tranverse diameter than in the anterior–posterior dimension.

Examination of fresh pharynges reveals that the cricopharyngeus is located and shaped somewhat differently from that in the cadaver.[8] The muscle forms an inferior curved constriction of the posterior aspect of the hypopharynx, thus forming a floor as well as a back wall. Thus the cricopharyngeus is situated in part inferior to the cricoid cartilage rather than just posterior to it. The cricopharyngeus muscle has no central raphe as does the inferior pharyngeal constrictor superior to it. The muscle is 1–1.2 cm wide in cadaver specimens and 1.4–1.6 cm wide in fresh specimens.[8] It is most commonly located at a level between C5 and C7 vertebrae. The cricopharyngeus is bordered superiorly by the oblique fibers of the inferior pharyngeal constrictor muscle (Fig. 6-1). Its fibers pass posterior and upward from the thyroid cartilage to insert into a median raphe.[4]

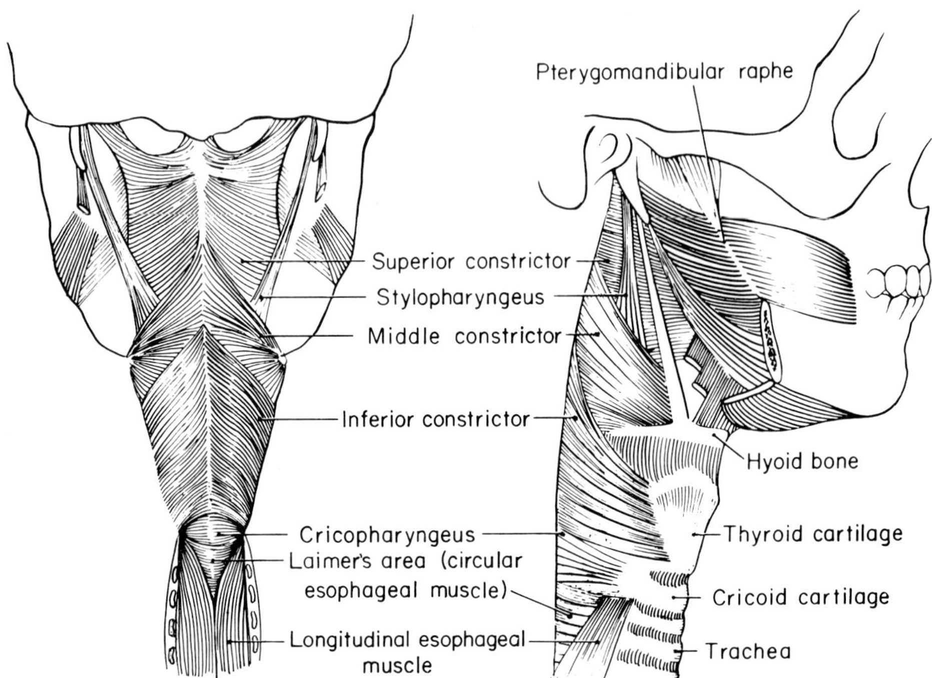

Fig. 6-1.   The muscular anatomy of the esophagus and distal pharynx; posterior and lateral views. From Payne WS, Olson AM: The Esophagus. Lea & Febiger, Philadelphia, 1974. Reprinted by permission.

Inferiorly, the cricopharyngeus muscle blends into the circular and longitudinal muscle fibers of the upper esophagus.[4] The most inferior oblique fibers of the inferior pharyngeal constrictor overlap the horizontal fibers of the cricopharyngeus and pass with it over the cricothyroid joint to insert onto the inferior border of the cricoid cartilage.[8]

The nerve supply to the UES appears to be through the pharyngeal plexus, principally from pharyngeal branches of the vagus nerve.[1,4] The IX and XI cranial nerves may supply a lesser part of the innervation.[1] There is very little information available concerning the neuropharmacology of the cricopharyngeus. The neuromuscular transmission in this muscle appears to be cholinergic and nicotinic rather than muscarinic.[9]

Physiology

The means of investigating the physiology of the UES are limited. They include radiographic, manometric, and electromyographic studies.[1,5,10] This review will focus on manometric studies. An obstacle to manometric investigation of the UES has been the marked variation and apparent lack of reproducibility of recorded intraluminal pressures. The pressures recorded from the UES were recently shown to depend on the directional orientation of the recording orifice (Fig. 6-2).[3,11] Thus,

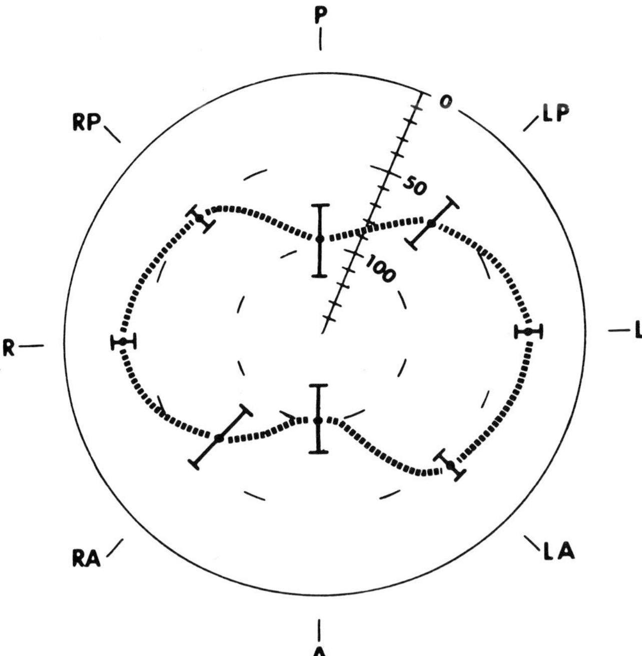

Fig. 6-2.   Spatial pressure orientation in the upper esophageal sphincter. Pressures were measured in each of eight directions in 18 subjects. Each pressure designation represents the mean maximal pressure within the pharyngoesophageal high-pressure zone for each of the eight orifices. P, posterior; LP, left posterior; L, left; LA, left anterior; A, anterior; RA, right anterior; R, right, RP, right posterior. Reprinted by permission of the publisher from The pharyngoesophageal closure mechanism: a manometric study, by Winans C: Gastroenterology 63:775. Copyright 1972 by the American Gastroenterological Association.

any attempt to study the UES must take into account the orientation of the manometric catheter within the sphincter. When such a system is used, accurate and reproducible manometric tracings can be obtained.

The major functions of the UES appear to be to prevent esophageal distention during respiration and to protect against esophagopharyngeal reflux with subsequent tracheobronchial aspiration.[1,6,11] Several characteristic features of the UES may help to explain how it achieves these functions.

UES Resting Pressure.   The UES remains closed at rest. The resting tone of the sphincter is attributable to continuous active muscle contraction.[5] It relaxes for only a short time during swallowing but then regains its resting tone.[1,2] It also opens during vomiting, regurgitation, belching, gagging, and retching.[1] This continuous resting tone may be an important factor in the competence of the UES as a barrier to regurgitation. The closed lumen that results from this continuous tone also prevents air from freely moving into the esophagus.

Normal UES resting pressures, as measured by intraluminal manometry, vary depending on the orientation of the recording orifice.[3,11] The intraluminal sphincter pressures recorded with directionally oriented manometric recording orifices in

Table 6-1. Resting UES pressure (mm Hg)

Orientation	Mean	Range
Posterior	101	(60–142)
Anterior	84	(55–123)
Lateral	48	(30–65)

Data from 20 normal subjects.
Adapted by permission of the publisher from Gerhardt DC, Castell DO, Winship DH, Shuck TJ: Esophageal dysfunction in esophagopharyngeal regurgitation. Gastroenterology 78:895, 1980. Copyright 1980 by the American Gastroenterological Association.

posterior, anterior, and lateral orientations are referred to as posterior, anterior, or lateral pressures, respectively, in this paper. Posterior pressures are significantly higher than anterior pressures, and both pressures are substantially higher than those at the lateral orifices (Table 6-1).[3,11] This directional difference in recorded intraluminal pressures is referred to as the radial asymmetry of the UES.[3]

Major improvements recently made in intraluminal recording systems have resulted in the development of low-compliance systems that can record rapid pressure changes of greater than 400 mm Hg/sec,[12] a feature necessary for faithfully recording the dynamic events of the UES.

UES Pressure Profile. The UES high-pressure zone ranges from 2.5 to 4.0 cm in length.[2,6] The peak pressures are found within a relatively narrow band of approximately 1 cm in length.[13] Recent studies have demonstrated that the peak pressures for anterior and posterior orientations do not occur at the same level in the manometric pull-through (Fig. 6-3).[5,13,14] The peak anterior pressures occurred on the average 0.55 cm more proximally than peak posterior pressures did.[13] This difference in location may be explained by the angle of attachment of the cricopharyngeus muscle to the anterior cricoid cartilage or by the fact that the inferior border of the cricopharyngeus muscle lies up to 0.5 cm below that of the cricoid cartilage, as shown by recent studies.[8] This difference in location of peak pressures is referred to as the axial asymmetry of the UES.

UES Pressure Response to Intraesophageal Fluid or Solid Bolus. The pressures recorded from the UES are not static. UES pressures increase significantly over resting pressures in response to intraesophageal fluid infused distal to the UES, to an intraluminal fluid bolus, or to intraesophageal balloon distention.[11,15,16] At present, two different types of stimuli appear to be involved in this response, namely volume and acid. An increase in volume, whether because of fluid or a balloon distention, results in increased UES pressure.[11,15,16] When 0.9% NaCl was infused at a rate of 11 ml/min in the portion of esophagus distal to the UES, there was a significant increase in UES pressure in all orientations.[11] Posterior pressures increased from 109 ± 4 mm Hg (mean ± SEM) to 127 ± 5 mm Hg after saline infusion. A bolus of fluid injected into the esophagus also causes an increase in UES pressure.[11] With intraesophageal balloon distention, the closer to the UES the distention was carried out, the greater was the UES response.[16]

Infusion of 0.1N HCL at 11 ml/min resulted in an an even more stimulatory effect upon UES pressures than did saline alone, from 109 to 138 mm Hg.[11] The

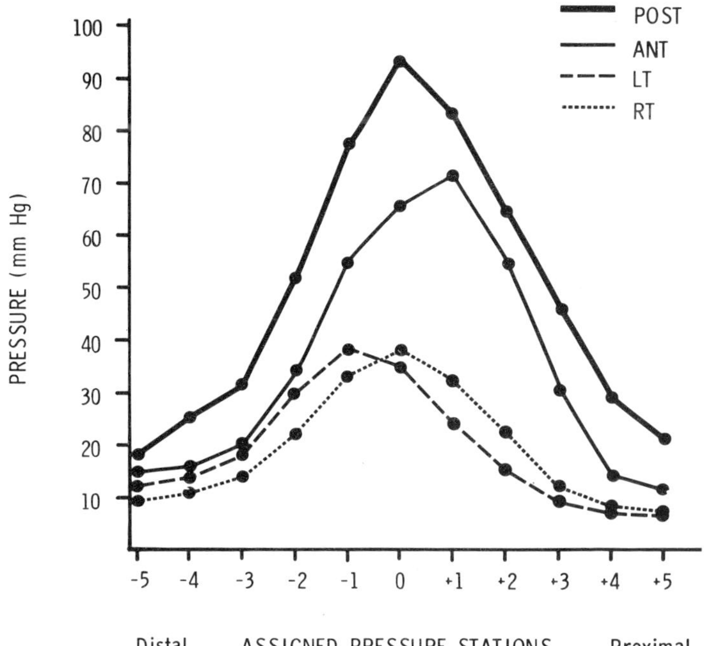

Fig. 6-3. Upper esophageal sphincter-pressure profiles for anterior, posterior, and right- and left-lateral pressure orientations. Pressure stations refer to each 0.5 cm increment at which pressure was recorded over the 6-cm pull-through. Data represented here are translated such that peak posterior pressure was designated station O and all other stations in all orientations were adjusted accordingly. Points: mean values for nine subjects. Reprinted by permission from Gerhardt D, Hewett J, Moeschberger M, et al: Human upper esophageal sphincter pressure profile. Am J Physiol 239:G51, 1980.

closer the fluid was perfused to the UES the greater was the response. This same acid response has also been observed in recent animal studies.[17] These studies suggest a protective role for the UES in preventing regurgitation of esophageal contents into the pharynx with possible resultant aspiration. This UES response of increased pressures to intraesophageal fluid infusion or bolus distention may further add to the competence of this sphincter as a barrier to regurgitation.

UES Relaxation. UES relaxation occurs early in the sequence of swallowing. In normal relaxation of the UES the resting pressure drops to pharyngeal or ambient baseline pressure. The normal sphincter always relaxes prior to the arrival of the pharyngeal peristaltic contraction. The UES resting pressure drops abruptly within 0.2–0.3 sec of a swallow, and the sphincter remains relaxed for 0.5–1.2 sec.[1,2] The timing and duration of relaxation normally vary depending on the recording position within the sphincter zone (Table 6-2).[18] The relaxation is followed by a peristaltic wave that, after propelling the bolus through the pharynx, continues to propel it through the UES on down the esophagus.

UES relaxation is attributable to inhibition of tonic contraction of the cricopharyngeus muscle, and possibly of the inferior pharyngeal constrictor as well.[5]

Table 6-2. UES relaxation intervals

Station	Duration of UES Relaxation (seconds, mean ± SD)
+1	0.55 ± 0.20
0	0.80 ± 0.21
−1	0.93 ± 0.21

Data from 7 subjects. Station 0 represents peak UES pressure; station +1 is 1 cm proximal; and station −1 is 1 cm distal to peak UES pressure.

Adapted from Fulbeck C, Gerhardt D, Henson B, Winship D: Pharyngo-cricopharyngeal coordination during swallowing in man. Clin Res 28:885A, 1980.

Forward displacement of the larynx by the geniohyoid muscle may also play a role in the relaxation.[5]

Pharyngeal Activity. Pharyngeal activity has been difficult to assess in the past partly because the manometric systems utilizing infused catheters for pressure recording markedly underestimate the pressure events. In a study using an intraluminal strain gauge recording system, peristaltic pressures in the hypopharynx averaged approximately 200 mm Hg with an average of 100 mm Hg in the oropharynx.[19] The duration of contraction (0.37–0.48 sec) is much briefer and the velocity of peristaltic waves (9–25 cm/sec) is much greater than that observed in the body of the esophagus.[19] During the act of swallowing the pharynx vigorously ejects a bolus into the esophagus. The mean velocity of the bolus front varied from 10 to 70 cm/sec.[20]

SYMPTOMS OF DISEASES OF THE PHARYNX AND THE UES

A number of symptoms correlate well with the presence of esophageal or pharyngeal disease. They include the following:

Oropharyngeal Dysphagia

Oropharyngeal dysphagia is defined as difficulty in initiating a swallow. The major problem involves the transfer of the bolus from the oropharynx to the upper esophagus. The symptom reflects a disease process that involves the pharynx, UES, or both. Patients with oropharyngeal dysphagia give a characteristic history of

1. Repeated attempts to initiate swallowing
2. Coughing spells while eating
3. Food sticking in the throat
4. Occasional nasal regurgitation of liquids while trying to swallow

Odynophagia

Odynophagia, pain on swallowing, often accompanies inflammation of the esophageal or oropharyngeal mucosa. It may be seen with severe pharyngeal or esophageal ulceration, such as may occur in peptic acid disease or with mucosal involvement by candida or by herpes virus.

Regurgitation

Regurgitation refers to the spontaneous flow of gastroesophageal contents into the pharynx. The term implies that reflux from the stomach into the esophagus occurs first, followed by regurgitation into the pharynx. The fluid may be "bitter" or "sour" tasting and yellow to green in color.

Globus Sensation

Globus sensation refers to a feeling of something always "stuck in the throat" without dysphagia.

Halitosis

Halitosis, or bad breath, usually does not indicate esophageal disease except on rare occasions when it may be associated with retention and decay of food, such as in a Zenker's diverticulum or in achalasia.

Belching

Belching and rumination do not correlate well with the presence of esophageal disease.

DISORDERS OF THE CRICOPHARYNGEUS

A number of symptoms appear to be attributable to disorders of the cricopharyngeus. As mentioned above, these include oropharyngeal dysphagia, globus sensation, and regurgitation into the pharynx. These apparent disorders of UES function may be related to changes in resting tone and/or abnormalities in sphincter relaxation.[21,22]

Abnormalities of Resting Tension

Hypertensive Sphincter. Above-normal UES pressures have been described in so-called spasm of the cricopharyngeus and in globus sensation. Some authors believe that cricopharyngeal spasm is a clinical entity, either by itself, with the Plummer–Vinson syndrome,[23] or secondary to lesions in the pharynx or nervous system. These entities have not been studied with currently available manometric systems.

Hunt et al. reported that UES resting pressures in patients with reflux esophagitis were higher than those in normal persons.[24] They suggested that this increase in resting pressure was a response to the presence of irritant material in the lower esophagus and served as a protective mechanism to prevent regurgitation of the refluxant into the pharynx. Stanciu and Bennett, however, found no difference in UES pressures between normal persons and patients with gastroesophageal reflux.[25] A recent study has demonstrated that UES pressures increase significantly when acid is perfused into the esophagus in normal volunteers.[11] In our experience some but not all patients with reflux may have elevated UES pressures. High UES resting pressures have been observed in patients with globus sensation.[26] In one study nine subjects with globus sensation had recorded UES pressures of 140–220 mm Hg (mean 176 mm Hg), compared with those of 70–140 mm Hg (mean 96 mm Hg) in control subjects.[26] It has been suggested that UES hypertension may be the cause of the globus sensation.[26]

Hypotensive UES.   UES resting pressure is attributable to continuous tonic contraction of the cricopharyngeus muscle.[5] A variety of neuromuscular diseases may result in cricopharyngeal hypotension.[21] Most such diseases also are reported to be associated with weak pharyngeal contractions.

UES hypotension usually occurs after cricopharyngeal myotomy and has been reported after laryngectomy.[8] Both the axial and the radial asymmetry of the UES disappear after laryngectomy.[8,14] Some patients with mixed connective tissue disease (MCTD) and some with scleroderma have hypotensive UES pressures.[27] Although scleroderma classically is said to involve only the distal two-thirds of the esophagus, which contains smooth muscle in its muscular coat, in our experience it is not uncommon to have involvement of the UES, which is composed of striated muscle.

UES hypotension has also been observed in some patients with chronic reflux esophagitis who experience spontaneous regurgitation of fluid into the pharynx.[28] In addition to the diminished UES resting pressures, a less than normal UES response to the presence of intraesophageal fluid was seen in some of these patients.[28] Thus, it appears that resting pressure in the UES and its response to fluid within the esophagus may be important in the competence of the sphincter to prevent regurgitation and possible subsequent aspiration.

Abnormalities of UES Relaxation

Three types of abnormalities in UES relaxation have been described: (1) incomplete relaxation, (2) premature closure, and (3) delayed relaxation.[21] The term cricopharyngeal achalasia has sometimes been used to refer to all these abnormalities, but it might be better to reserve that term specific for the disorder of incomplete relaxation of the UES.[29] Oropharyngeal dysphagia is a frequent problem associated with all of the disorders of UES relaxation.[30] Most of these disorders have been studied extensively with radiographic techniques, but few have been well studied using the manometric catheters and low-compliance recording systems that are now available.

Incomplete UES Relaxation. Upon deglutition the UES resting pressure normally drops to baseline pharyngeal pressure (atmospheric pressure) to allow a bolus to pass from the pharynx into the esophagus without its having to cross a pressure gradient. In one study UES relaxation to baseline pressure occurred 95% of the time in normal subjects.[31] In our own studies using a low-compliance manometric system, the UES relaxed to baseline pharyngeal pressure 100% of the time in normal subjects.[18]

As mentioned above, cricopharyngeal achalasia refers to incomplete relaxation of the UES. Asherson defined it as partial or complete failure of, as well as a delay in, the relaxation of the cricopharyngeus.[29] This entity was diagnosed mainly by a profile x-ray of the hypopharynx that revealed a hold-up of the bolus above the cricopharyngeus.[29] This condition has been described as an isolated phenomenon[32] or as secondary to other underlying diseases or conditions such as poliomyelitis, thyrotoxic myopathy, post-partial pharyngectomy, bilateral recurrent laryngeal nerve paralysis, and bulbar paralysis.[29] In one study of a group of patients with oropharyngeal dysphagia of various etiologies the UES relaxed to baseline pressure less than 50% of the time.[31]

Premature Closure of the UES. It has been suggested that premature closure of the UES plays a major role in the pathogenesis of Zenker's diverticulum.[33] In one study of 11 patients with Zenker's diverticulum, UES relaxation was complete, but all of the patients appeared to have an abnormal temporal relationship between pharyngeal contraction and UES relaxation.[33] Other investigators have not observed the discoordination in pharyngeal contractions and UES relaxation in patients with this entity.[34] A recent study using a low-compliance pneumohydraulic infusion system found no incoordination in patients with Zenker's diverticulum, and UES resting pressures were actually lower than in the control group.[35] In a study using an electronic pressure transducer for pharyngeal recordings and a pneumohydraulic infusion system for UES recordings, it was shown that the duration of relaxation (Table 6-2) and the temporal relationship with pharyngeal contraction varies with the location in the UES.[18] Peak pharyngeal contraction recorded with an electronic transducer that was located 3 cm above the UES occurred before the onset of UES closure and in the proximal part of the UES in only 84% of swallows in normal volunteers.[18] Thus, the abnormality leading to formation of a Zenker's diverticulum is still unclear, although clinical experience has shown that cricopharyngeal myotomy often produces favorable results.[36]

Delayed UES Relaxation. In radiographic studies, patients with familial dysautonomia were shown to have delayed opening of the UES with swallowing.[37] This abnormality has not been well studied with manometric techniques. With the older high-compliance infusion systems, even normal volunteers appeared to have delayed relaxation.

Cricopharyngeal Bar. There is no general agreement as to the significance of a cricopharyngeal bar seen on barium swallow. This posterior indentation of the barium bolus may occur in patients without swallow-related symptoms. Some investigators believe that the appearance of the cricopharyngeal bar in these studies is reliable evidence of the presence of some neuromuscular dysfunction of the cricopharyngeus.[38] Patients with a cricopharyngeal bar seen on a barium swallow have yet to be studied carefully and systematicly using good manometric techniques.

DISEASES OF THE PHARYNX AND UES

Structural lesions and neuromuscular disorders are the two major categories of diseases involving this area of the gastrointestinal tract. The structural lesions include both intrinsic and extrinsic lesions (Table 6-3). This review will focus on what is known about some of the more common neuromuscular diseases.

Disorders of Striated Muscle

Polymyositis–Dermatomyositis. Roentgenographic studies have revealed a number of swallowing abnormalities with these disorders.[39,40] They include retention of barium in the valleculae, nasal reflux of barium during swallowing, and diminished peristaltic activity in the pharynx.[40] Dysphagia is a common complaint in these disorders.[40] There are reports of cricopharyngeal dysfunction in patients with dermatomyositis[41] and polymyositis.[42] There have been few patients with polymyositis–dermatomyositis who have been studied manometrically with currently available high-fidelity manometric techniques. The few reported have decreased pharyngeal contractions, decreased UES pressures, and decreased contractions in the upper one-third of the esophagus.[21] Abnormalities of UES relaxation have been reported in a few cases.[31,43]

Table 6-3. Diseases of the pharynx and UES with
oropharyngeal dysphagia

Structural Lesions
Intrinsic
Oropharyngeal tumors
Inflammatory disorders (pharyngitis)
Esophageal web
Extrinsic
Vertebral spur
Thyromegaly
Cervical tumors
Neuromuscular Disorders
Disorders of striated muscle
Polymyositis–dermatomyositis
Other connective tissue diseases
Myotonic dystrophy
Oculopharyngeal dystrophy
Disorder of Endplate
Myasthenia gravis
Disorders of the nervous system
CVA (with brain stem involvement)
Multiple sclerosis (MS)
Parkinson's disease
Amyotrophic lateral sclerosis (ALS)
Poliomyelitis

Other Connective Tissue Diseases. Scleroderma and mixed connective tissue disease have classically been described as involving the smooth-muscle portion of the esophagus. Pharyngeal and UES pressures were not reported, however, in many of the studies. We studied 12 patients with scleroderma or mixed connective tissue disease and found UES pressures to be diminished compared with that in controls.[27] There were no observed abnormalities of relaxation. Some of these patients have disease features that overlap with those of polymyositis, and it remains to be defined if certain of these patients with scleroderma or mixed connective tissue disease are more likely to have involvement of the striated muscle portion of the esophagus.

Myotonia Dystrophica. Dysphagia is often seen in myotonia dystrophica.[44,45] Aspiration pneumonia is the most common cause of death in this disease.[45] The pharynx, UES and upper one-third of the esophagus were involved in all the patients studied in one series, and in one-half of the patients abnormalities of the smooth-muscle portion of the esophagus were present as well.[44] The patients in this study presented with characteristic clinical findings of cataracts, frontal baldness, muscle wasting, and myotonia. Although the manometric system used in the study tended to underestimate pressure events in the UES and pharynx, the mean amplitude of pharyngeal peristaltic contraction was diminished; the mean duration of pharyngeal contraction was prolonged; mean UES pressures were decreased; and duration of relaxation was prolonged as compared with controls. In a radiographic study four out of four patients studied had abnormal pharyngeal motility.[43]

Oculopharyngeal Dystrophy. The cardinal features of oculopharyngeal dystrophy are dysphagia and ptosis. Dysphagia commonly precedes ptosis in this syndrome.[46] In an esophageal manometric study of three patients, the abnormalities found were low pharyngeal pressures, problems of UES relaxation, and diminished UES pressures, with the distal esophagus being relatively normal.[46] In a recent report using a low-compliance pneumohydraulic infusion system UES pressures were found to be markedly elevated in one patient.[47] In another report UES relaxation was usually normal, but diminished pharyngeal and UES pressures were observed.[31]

Myasthenia Gravis. Dysphagia and aspiration are frequent clinical problems in myasthenia gravis. These symptoms may be the initial manifestation of the disease in a few patients. The patient with myasthenia gravis is able to swallow normally at the start of a meal but has progressive difficulty as the meal continues.[21] In a radiographic study, the four patients investigated all had abnormal pharyngeal motility, but UES relaxation appeared normal.[43] The diminished pharyngeal activity tends to recover with rest or the administration of anticholinesterase drugs.[21] These may be administered during the manometric study to quantitate changes in pharyngeal peristaltic contractions.

Disorders of the Nervous System

Cerebrovascular Accidents. Dysphagia is not an infrequent problem in patients with cerebrovascular accidents, particularly those involving the vertebrobasilar arteries or the posteroinferior cerebellar artery.[21] In one series, 19 of 25 patients with posteroinferior cerebellar artery syndrome had abnormal pharyngeal motility, and 9 of the 25 had apparent UES dysfunction.[43] In a manometric study that included 13 patients with cerebral vascular disease only one of the nine with unilateral central nervous system involvement had dysphagia.[48] Dysphagia and abnormal peristalsis were seen in all four patients with bilateral pyramidal tract signs compatible with pseudobulbar palsy.[48] No systematic study using currently available manometric techniques has been reported.

Multiple Sclerosis. Disturbances of swallowing are not unusual in multiple sclerosis. In one report of 29 patients, 16 had experienced some dysphagia.[49] Disordered swallowing may occur either early or late in the course of this disease. Four of the patients had oropharyngeal dysphagia, but UES relaxation was observed to be abnormal in only one case. Eleven patients had abnormalities in motility in the body of the esophagus.

Parkinson's Disease. Disordered swallowing may be observed in Parkinson's disease. All seven patients reported in one radiographic study had abnormal pharyngeal motility.[43] Five of the seven had stasis of barium in the hypopharynx, and four had UES dysfunction. There may be some improvement in swallowing with treatment of the underlying disease.[50]

Amyotrophic Lateral Sclerosis (ALS). The disorders of deglutition in ALS are similar to those seen in some of the other neurologic diseases reported above. In one report four of five patients studied had abnormal pharyngeal motility, and three were reported to have UES dysfunction.[43] Three patients out of the four studied by manometry had abnormal peristalsis.[48] Incomplete UES relaxation has also been reported.[31]

Poliomyelitis. Difficulty in swallowing is not uncommon in acute epidemic bulbar-type poliomyelitis.[51] It occurred in 87 of 123 patients in one center.[51] In all but five patients it resolved within 3 weeks. Although most patients with this problem improve, a number of those who survive the illness are left with residual problems in deglutition.[52] The pharynx appears to be the most frequent site of involvement.

Other Conditions. There are numerous other neuromuscular diseases that present with oropharyngeal dysphagia as part of the clinical picture. These are covered in some recent references.[6,21,31,43,48] None have been well studied with present-day manometric systems.

MANAGEMENT

There is very little available information concerning the treatment of the pharyngeal and UES disorders associated with many of the diseases described above. If the underlying disease is treatable—e.g., as polymyositis is with steroids or myasthenia gravis with anticholinesterase drugs—the disordered deglutition may improve with the treatment of the underlying disease. Very little is known about the pharmacology of this area of the GI tract.[9] In the absence of a specific treatment for the underlying disease, cricopharyngeal myotomy has been helpful in a number of patients who have severe problems with swallowing.[4,30,36,53] In one manometric study of patients who underwent cricopharyngeal myotomy, the postoperative UES Pressure was decreased as compared with that measured before surgery—as one would expect.[54] Unfortunately, directional orientation of the recording orifices was not controlled in that study, and therefore the information provided may not be totally accurate.

REFERENCES

1. Ingelfinger FJ: Esophageal motility. Physiol Rev 38:533–584, 1958.
2. Code CF, Schlegel JF: Motor action of the esophagus and its sphincters. In Code CF (ed): Handbook of Physiology, Sec 6, Alimentary Canal; Vol 4 Motility; American Physiological Society, Washington, D.C., 1968, pp 1821–1839.
3. Winans CS: The pharyngoesophageal closure mechanism: a manometric study. Gastroenterology 63:768–777, 1972.
4. Ellis, FH: Upper esophageal sphincter in health and disease. Surg Clin North Am 51:553–565, 1971.
5. Asoh R, Goyal R: Manometry and electromyography of the upper esophageal sphincter in the opossum. Gastroenterology 74:514–520, 1978.
6. Palmer ED: Disorders of the cricopharyngeus muscle: a review. Gastroenterology 71:510–519, 1976.
7. Zaino C, Jacobson HG, Lepow H, Ozturk C: The pharyngoesophageal sphincter. Radiology 89:639–645, 1967.
8. Gates GA: Upper esophageal sphincter: pre- and post-laryngectomy—a normative study. Laryngoscope 90:454–464, 1980.
9. Christensen J: Pharmacology of the esophageal motor function. Ann Rev Pharmacol 15:243–258, 1975.
10. Sokol EM, Heitmann P, Wolf BS, Cohen BR: Simultaneous cineradiographic and manometric study of the pharynx, hypopharynx, and cervical esophagus. Gastroenterology 51:960–974, 1966.
11. Gerhardt DC, Shuck TJ, Bordeaux RA, Winship DH: Human upper esophageal sphincter: response to volume, osmotic and acid stimuli. Gastroenterology 75:268–274, 1978.
12. Arndorfer RC, Stef JJ, Dodds WF, et al.: Improved infusion system for intraluminal esophageal manometry. Gastroenterology 73:23–27, 1977.
13. Gerhardt D, Hewett J, Moeschberger M, et al.: Human upper esophageal sphincter pressure profile. Am J Physiol 239:G49–G52, 1980.
14. Welch RW, Luckmann K, Ricks PM, et al.: Manometry of the normal upper esophageal sphincter and its alterations in laryngectomy. J Clin Invest 63:1036–1041, 1979.
15. Creamer B, Schlegel J: Motor responses of the esophagus to distention. J Appl Physiol 10:498–504, 1957.
16. Gray JE, Lockard O, Shuck TJ, Winship DH: Response of the upper esophageal sphincter and upper esophagus to intraluminal esophageal balloon distention. Gastroenterology 76:A1143, 1979.
17. Freiman JM, El-Sharkawy TY, Diamant NE: Effect of bilateral vagosympathetic nerve blockade on response of the dog upper esophageal sphincter (UES) to intraesophageal distention and acid. Gastroenterology 81:78–84, 1981.
18. Fulbeck C, Gerhardt D, Henson B, Winship D: Pharyngo-cricopharyngeal coordination during swallowing in man. Clin Res 28:885A, 1980.
19. Dodds WJ, Hogan WJ, Lydon SB, et al.: Quantitation of pharyngeal motor function in normal human subjects. J Appl Physiol 39:692–696, 1975.

20. Fisher MA, Hendrix TR, Hunt JN, Murrills AJ: Relation between volume swallowed and velocity of the bolus ejected from the pharynx into the esophagus. Gastroenterology 74:1238–1240, 1978.
21. Kilman WJ, Goyal RL: Disorders of pharyngeal and upper esophageal sphincter motor function. Arch Intern Med 136:592–601, 1976.
22. Roed-Petersen K: The pharyngooesophageal sphincter. Dan Med Bull 26:275–281, 1979.
23. Hurst A: Nervous disorders of swallowing. J Laryngol Otol 58:60–71, 1943.
24. Hunt PS, Connell AM, Smiley TB: The cricopharyngeal sphincter in gastric reflux. Gut 11:303–306, 1970.
25. Stanciu C, Bennett JR: Upper esophageal sphincter yield pressure in normal subjects and in patients with gastroesophageal reflux. Thorax 29:459–462, 1974.
26. Watson WC, Sullivan SN: Hypertonicity of cricopharyngeal sphincter: cause of globus sensation. Lancet 2:1417–1418, 1974.
27. Gerhardt D, Shuck T, Winship D: Upper esophageal sphincter resting pressures in patients with esophago-pharyngeal regurgitation and connective tissue disease. Clin Res 25:50A, 1977.
28. Gerhardt DC, Castell DO, Winship DH, Shuck TJ: Esophageal dysfunction in esophago-pharyngeal regurgitation. Gastroenterology 78:893–897, 1980.
29. Asherson N: Achalasia of the cricopharyngeal sphincter. J Laryngol Otol 64:747–758, 1950.
30. Hurwitz AL, Duranceau A: Upper esophageal sphincter dysfunction: pathogenesis and treatment. Dig Dis 23:275–281, 1978.
31. Hurwitz AL, Nelson JA, Haddad JK: Oropharyngeal dysphagia: manometric and cine esophagraphic findings. Dig Dis 20:313–324, 1975.
32. Reichert TJ, Bluestone CD, Stool SE, et al.: Congenital cricopharyngeal achalasia. Ann Otol 86:603–610, 1977.
33. Ellis FH, Schlegel JF, Lynch VP, Payne WS: Cricopharyngeal myotomy for pharyngo-esophageal diverticulum. Ann Surg, 170:340–349, 1969.
34. Kodicek J, Creamer B: A study of pharyngeal pouches. J Laryngol Otol 75:406–411, 1961.
35. Knuff TE, Benjamin SB, Castell DO: Zenkers diverticulum: a reappraisal. Gastroenterology 78:A1196, 1980.
36. Ellis, FH: Surgical management of esophageal motility disturbances. Ann J Surgery 139:752–759, 1980.
37. Margulies SI, Brunt PW, Donner MW, Silbiger ML: Familial dysautonomia: a cineradiographic study of the swallowing mechanism. Radiology 90:107–112, 1968.
38. Seaman WB: Cineroentgenographic observations of the cricopharyngeus. Am J Roentgenol 96:922–931, 1966.
39. O'Hara JM, Szemes G, Lowman RM: The esophageal lesions in dermatomyositis: a correlation of radiologic and pathologic findings. Radiology 89:27–31, 1967.
40. Feldman F, Marshak RH: Dermatomyositis with significant involvement of the gastrointestinal tract. Am J Roentgenol 90:746–752, 1963.
41. Porubsky ES, Murray JP, Pratt LL: Cricopharyngeal achalasia in dermatomyositis. Arch Otolaryngol 98:428–429, 1973.
42. Dietz F, Logeman JA, Sahgal V, Schmid F: Cricopharyngeal muscle dysfunction in the differential diagnosis of dysphagia in polymyositis. Arthritis Rheum 23:491–495, 1980.
43. Silbiger MI, Pikielney R, Donner MW: Neuromuscular disorders affecting the pharynx: cineradiographic analysis. Invest. Radiology, 2:442–448, 1967.

44. Siegel CI, Hendrix TR, Harvey JC: The swallowing disorder in myotonia dystrophica. Gastroenterology 50:541–550, 1966.
45. Garrett JM, DuBose TD, Jackson JE, Norman JR: Esophageal and pulmonary disturbances in myotonia dystrophica. Arch Intern Med 123:26–32, 1969.
46. Bender MD: Esophageal manometry in oculopharyngeal dystrophy. Am J Gastroenterol 65:215–221, 1976.
47. O'Laughlin JC, Bredfeldt JE, Gray JE: Hypertonic upper esophageal sphincter in the oculo-pharyngeal syndrome. J Clin Gastroenterol 2:93–98, 1980.
48. Fischer RA, Ellison GW, Thayer WR, et al.: Esophageal motility in neuromuscular disorders. Ann Intern Med 63:229–248, 1965.
49. Daly DD, Code CF, Anderson HA: Disturbances of swallowing and esophageal motility in patients with multiple sclerosis. Neurology 12:250–256, 1962.
50. Nowack WJ, Hatelid JM, Sohn RS: Dysphagia in parkinsonism. Arch Neurol 34:320, 1977.
51. Brahdy MB, Lenarsky M: Difficulty in swallowing in acute epidemic poliomyelitis. JAMA, 103:229–234, 1934.
52. Bosma JF: Residual disability of pharyngeal area resulting from poliomyelitis. JAMA 165:216–221, 1957.
53. West EM, Baker HW: Esophageal dysphagia treated by cricopharyngeal myotomy. Ann Surg 43:703–708, 1977.
54. Henderson RD, Marryatt G: Cricopharyngeal myotomy as a method of treating cricopharyngeal dysphagia secondary to gastroesophageal reflux. J Thorac Cardiovasc Surg 74:721–725, 1977.

7 | Chest Pain of Esophageal Origin

Douglas L. Brand

Chest pain is taken seriously by all who deal with it. Its cardiac connotations place it among the most frightening of symptoms to the patient and convey diagnostic urgency to the physician. Its frequency and multiple causes make it highly pertinent to the primary care physician and a wide range of specialists, including the cardiologist, pulmonary physician, gastroenterologist, and rheumatologist; the neurologist and psychiatrist; and surgeons of general, cardiac, thoracic, orthopedic, and neurologic persuasion. The role of the gastroenterologist has been enlarged in recent years as the esophagus has gained notoriety as a frequent noncardiac cause of chest pain; in the two esophageal manometry laboratories with which I have been associated, chest pain has replaced reflux symptoms as the leading reason for referral. This chapter, in addressing the problem of chest pain and the esophagus, will delineate the types and causes of esophageal pain and place it in the broader perspective of all the major causes of chest pain.

NEUROANATOMIC CONSIDERATIONS

The esophagus contains afferent fibers, some travelling centrally in the vagus and others in the sympathetic nerves. It is presumed but not completely established that the former participate largely in reflex pathways and the latter serve as sensory afferents.[1,2] The sensory afferents are thought to terminate largely in the submucosa, where specialized endings in the form of Ruffini's corpuscles (a type often associated with the sensation of warmth) have been seen in the rabbit.[3,4] However, there is a thin web of fibers in the lamina propria, with fibrils penetrating into the lower layers of the squamous epithelium; these functionally undefined nerves might well participate in transmitting mucosal stimuli.

137

The sensory afferents of the esophagus, along with all other sensory pain fibers, enter the spinal cord through the dorsal roots, reaching their cell bodies in the dorsal root ganglia. Synapse of the neurones occurs in the dorsal horn of the cord, where they join the spinothalamic tract. Esophageal and other visceral pain is felt at the level or levels where the overlying skin and body wall structures are supplied by sensory *somatic* fibers of the same dermatome segments. A listing of these segments for various organs explains the overlap in location of esophageal pain with that from other thoracic and abdominal organs: esophagus C8–T10; heart T1–T4; stomach, liver, and gall bladder T6–T9; and pancreas T6–T11. The overlap with pain from cervical spine arthritis and thoracic outlet syndromes is dependent on the fact that the cervical nerves C5–8 and thoracic nerve T1 all participate in the formation of the brachial plexus; injury to the plexus or to its roots produces arm pain as well as neck or chest pain.

TYPES OF PAINFUL STIMULI

The sketchiness of the defined sensory neuroanatomy makes impossible any precision in describing mechanisms of esophageal pain production. However, it can be postulated that the disorders known to produce pain in the esophagus all cause one or more of the following phenomena: direct noxious stimulation, inflammation, abnormal muscular contractions, and esophageal distention.

Noxious Stimuli; Inflammation

Noxious stimuli, such as acid or extremes of temperature, may act directly to irritate and stimulate sensory nerve endings. Demonstration of damage to the very small, unmyelinated nerve fibers present in the esophageal mucosa is a difficult and as yet unaccomplished histologic feat, but there is electron microscopic evidence of changes in the epithelial cell walls, organelles, and basement membrane in patients who have gastroesophageal reflux,[3] suggesting that the acid may have access to the nerve endings in the epithelium and lamina propria. It is likely that extremely cold beverages also produce chest pain by directly stimulating nerve endings, in light of recent evidence that the pain is accompanied by failure of contraction rather than spasm of the esophageal body.[5] If a noxious substance also produces inflammation, at least one other mechanism could be brought into play, e.g., the stretching of nerve fibers by the cellular infiltrate and tissue edema. As I shall discuss in more detail below, noxious stimuli and inflammation may trigger abnormal motor events known to produce pain in turn. These events may also serve as sensitizers, resulting in the perception of normal contractions as unpleasant or even painful, as is exemplified by the occasional patient with reflux who can feel normal peristaltic contractions as they move down the length of the esophagus.

Abnormal Muscular Contractions; Esophageal Distention

Such contractions, with diffuse spasm as the prototype, have long been recognized as a possible cause of esophageal pain.[6] More recent developments, which are discussed below, are the recognition of other contraction abnormalities associated with pain and the discovery that painful motor abnormalities can be secondary phenomena, induced by reflux. The pain associated with these motor abnormalities is similar to pain from esophageal balloon distention; both can be angina-like.[7] However, the mechanisms may well differ, since pain from distention does not seem dependent on contraction of esophageal muscle, either in balloon distention experiments[8] or in the dilated gullet of achalasia. Resolution of this issue will depend on an animal model for hypercontractility that will make possible better definition of the nerve-receptor types and pathways stimulated by distention and hypercontraction.

TYPES OF PAIN

Discomfort from the esophagus is usually categorized into heartburn (pyrosis), odynophagia (pain on swallowing), and central or angina-like pain.[2,9] However, the three are not strictly comparable terms, since the first is descriptive of the quality, the second primarily of the circumstance, and the third of the location of the discomfort. Nonetheless, they retain their dominant usage, probably because in each case the term reflects that aspect of the sensation that is most striking to the patient.

Heartburn

Heartburn is regarded as the bellwether of gastroesophageal reflux in excess of the occasional episodes seen in the posturally upright, asymptomatic person.[10] The reflux that produces heartburn tends to occur with the patient supine and is cleared less rapidly than that in asymptomatic people.[11] Heartburn can also be an expression of sensitivity to alkali.[12] With respect to the mechanisms of discomfort mentioned above, heartburn's close association with direct contact of acid (or alkali) and the esophageal mucosa points toward direct irritation and stimulation of sensory nerve endings; its association with histologic damage and polymorphonuclear leukocyte infiltration and its rarity in volunteers with normal mucosa[13,14] suggest that mucosal disruption is necessary to provide access of the acid to the nerve endings and that inflammation itself may have a role in causing the painful stimulus.

Odynophagia

Odynophagia, which can range from sharp pain to a pressure sensation, occurs commonly in diseases that cause severe mucosal damage, such as ulceration, severe esophagitis from any of the recognized causes, and carcinoma. Although the pain (by definition) occurs with swallowing, hypercontraction need not be and usually is not present, leading to my conjecture that the mechanisms involved, solely or in combination, may be direct nerve stimulation, inflammation, or sensitization to normal contractile activity. Odynophagia also occurs occasionally in motility disorders such as diffuse spasm; there the most likely pathway is that of abnormal contraction.

Central or Angina-like Pain

Pain of this type is less obviously tied to the esophagus, is possessed of a larger and more alarming differential diagnosis, and has been studied most avidly in recent years. The confusion of central chest pain that originates in the esophagus with angina pectoris of cardiac origin arises from several similarities. Often, both are aches or pressure sensations; both spread into the upper chest, neck, jaws, or arms; and both are relieved by nitroglycerin. There are contrasting points that are helpful when present. Esophageal pain may be tied to swallowing, recumbency, regurgitation, or heartburn and is usually not related to physical exertion; it also more commonly radiates through to the back than does cardiac pain. Angina pectoris tends to be exertional, relenting promptly on rest, and its link with meals, if any, tends to be distinctly postprandial. Unfortunately, the points in common often outweigh the differences.

It is likely that all the mechanisms involved in producing heartburn and odynophagia are involved, separately or in concert, in producing central chest pain of esophageal origin; thus, nonspecificity reigns within the organ as well as among the organs. The remainder of this chapter will deal with the current information on the esophageal causes of central chest pain; the main points of differential diagnosis that arise; the diagnostic approach to such patients; and the modes of therapy available for the esophageal causes.

ESOPHAGEAL DISORDERS CAUSING CENTRAL CHEST PAIN (Table 7-1)

Motility Disorders

Diffuse Spasm. The production of pain by muscular spasm of the esophagus was postulated by Greco-Roman writers, perhaps the first being Soranus in the 2nd century A.D.[6] The association with swallowing of solids or liquids is also

Table 7-1. Esophageal disorders associated with central chest pain

Motility Disorders
Diffuse spasm
High-amplitude peristaltic contractions
Long-duration peristaltic contractions (?)
Achalasia
Esophageal Reflux
Acid
Alkaline
Nonreflux Esophagitis
Monilial infection
Herpetic infection
Caustic esophagitis
Carcinoma
Esophageal Perforation

long-established; it was described by Osgood in 1889 as "simple oesophagismus."[15] With the advent of esophageal manometrics, the quantitation of esophageal pressures became possible, and considerable jousting in quest of the correct pathophysiologic definition ensued. Most investigators accept a definition similar to that proposed by DiMarino and Cohen: diffuse spasm is present when the patient has chest pain, dysphagia, and tertiary contractions that are evidenced by x-ray and correspond to repetitive simultaneous contractions shown by manometry; the patient usually displays some peristaltic contractions as well.[16]

The pain of diffuse spasm is variable in location, character, and duration. Often, however, it is substernal and radiates through to the back. It may occur following a swallow, is sometimes triggered by very hot or very cold liquids, and often awakens the patient from sleep. The intensity ranges from mild to excruciating, and the quality is more often a pressure sensation than a sharp pain. As Castell has stated, "the real (diagnostic) challenge is the patient who, after a meal, suddenly develops severe substernal pain that is squeezing in quality, radiates through to the back and down both arms, and is relieved by sublingually administered nitroglycerin. This symptom complex—and a number of variations on it—is encountered relatively frequently, and could equally well be caused by diffuse spasm or angina pectoris."[17]

Although this graphic symptomatic and manometric display characterizes the well-developed case of diffuse spasm and represents the prototype of esophageal chest pain, it is nonetheless relatively uncommon, even among chest-pain patients suspected of having an esophageal disorder. In a study of 43 patients with central chest pain who were proven to be free of coronary artery disease, Brand, Martin, and Pope found that 14 patients had abnormal manometric patterns, only three of which were that of diffuse spasm.[18] This scarcity of patients with diffuse spasm was confirmed in a recently published extension of the series, in which 62 of 160 patients with chest pain had abnormal manometric findings but only 10 of the 62 had diffuse spasm.[19]

What do all the other patients have? Two new motility disorders—one probable and one possible—have emerged from the sea of manometric squiggles; they are, respectively, high-amplitude peristaltic contractions and long-duration peristaltic contractions, which occur either concurrently or in isolation. The chest pain associated with these manometric findings cannot be distinguished from that seen with diffuse spasm, so the manometric patterns are currently the sole defining factor.

High-amplitude Peristaltic Contractions. The study from Pope's laboratory that originally proposed high-amplitude peristaltic contractions as a manometric abnormality associated with chest pain defined them as being of a mean amplitude greater than two standard deviations above that of asymptomatic control subjects (Fig. 7-1).[18] This corresponded to a value of at least 125 mm Hg (normal value, 60–80 mm Hg), and often the amplitude reached 250–300 mm Hg,[19] (leading to the somewhat facetious description of these patients as "super-squeezers"). The abnormality characteristicly occurred in the distal esophagus and was present in 29 of the 63 patients with abnormal manometry findings (three times the frequency of diffuse spasm). Benjamin and coworkers published a study of similar patients, describing seven individuals—five with chest pain and five with dysphagia—with

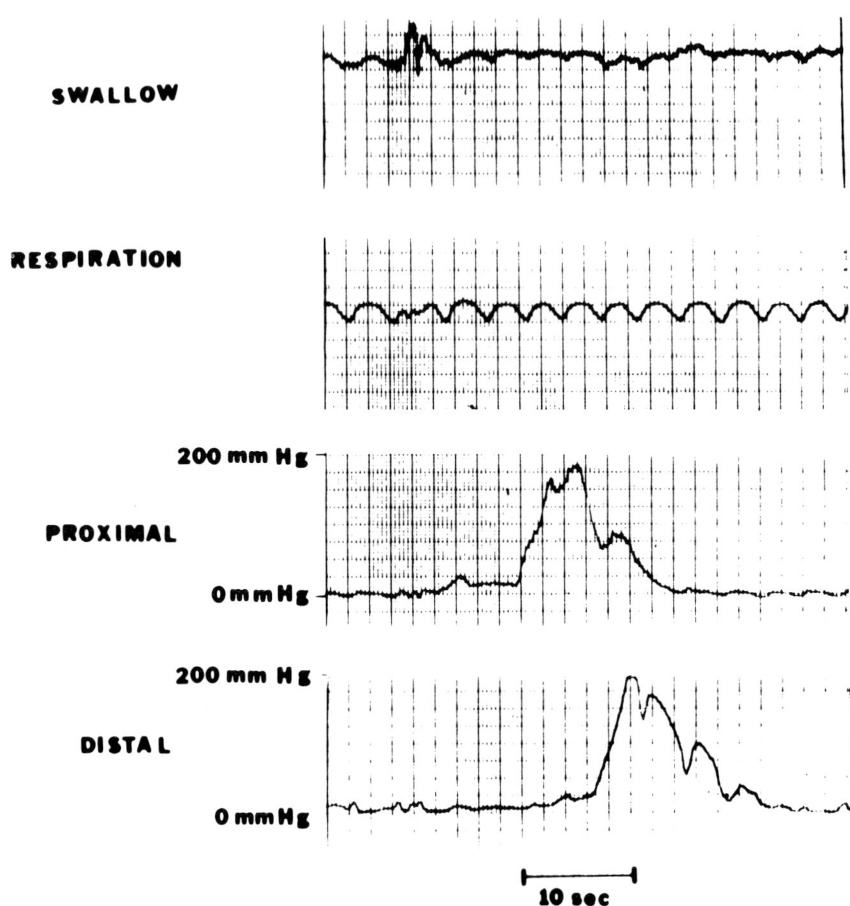

Fig. 7-1. High-amplitude peristaltic contraction occurring in conjunction with chest pain. From Brand DL, Martin D, Pope CE II: Esophageal manometrics in patients with angina-like chest pain. Am J Dig Dis 22:300–304, 1977. With permission.

mean contraction amplitudes ranging from 100 to 200 mm Hg and maximum amplitudes from 225 to 430 mm Hg.[20]

Does this manometric finding have anything to do with chest pain? Two points speak to this question; one is the indirect evidence of the presence of dysphagia, a symptom specific to the gullet, in over half of these patients.[18,20] More convincing, perhaps, is that almost half of the 29 patients with high-amplitude peristaltic contractions experienced their typical chest pain *during* the manometric demonstration of the abnormality, with the onset, duration, and intensity of the pain correlating with those parameters of the contractions.[19]

Long-duration Peristaltic Contractions and Simultaneous Contractions. The link between long-duration contractions (in which a given segment of the distal esophagus remains in the contracted state longer than normal) and chest pain is more tenuous. Although the high-amplitude contractions discussed above are often of long duration, only three patients of the 63 with abnormal manometry findings had prolonged contractions as their sole abnormality, and none of the three experienced chest pain during the manometric study.[19] It may well be that at the times when these patients actually experience such pain, they are having contractions of high amplitude as well as long duration.

A better case can be made for long-duration contractions producing dysphagia. Herrington and coworkers studied 22 patients with long-duration, normal-amplitude contractions; 82% of them had dysphagia.[21]

Simultaneous (nonperistaltic) contractions warrant brief mention. Although such contractions are the second most frequently occurring isolated abnormality in patients with chest pain, they, like prolonged contractions, were not associated with chest pain during manometric study.[19] For the time being, they should probably be regarded either as a sign of spasm or high-amplitude contractions occurring at other times, or alternatively, of no significance with regard to the source of chest pain.

Achalasia.   Achalasia is the final motor disorder pertinent to a discussion of esophageal chest pain. Although dysphagia is the hallmark of achalasia, substernal chest pain not related to swallowing is reported in 60% of a series of 133 patients.[22] The characteristic motility phenomenon in the esophageal body—low-amplitude, simultaneous (nonperistaltic) contractions—seems unlikely to produce pain. A better clue may be in the characteristic dilation of the organ, calling to mind distention as a more likely mechanism. A few achalasia patients step outside these bounds, having strong contractions as well as chest pain; this variant has been dubbed "vigorous achalasia."[23]

The motility disorders that produce chest pain usually appear as primary or idiopathic conditions, with no recognizable underlying cause. Kaye[24] and Debas et al.[25] have pointed out that these disorders, while producing their symptoms of chest pain and dysphagia, can probably also produce the anatomic changes of mid- or distal-esophageal diverticula. Thus, it would seem that diverticula should not be considered as the cause of chest pain or dysphagia; they are rather a result of an underlying motility disorder, usually diffuse spasm or achalasia, which is also responsible for the symptoms.

Similarly, severe, nonpleuritic chest pain and dysphagia have been described in two patients with systemic lupus erythematosus.[26] Pericarditis could not be demonstrated and manometry studies revealed painful episodes of diffuse spasm. Since the chest pain was limited to periods of activity of the systemic lupus erythematosus, the authors speculate that the spasm may have resulted from the underlying disease. Whether or not this is the case, it seems reasonable to conclude that the spasm produced the chest pain.

Esophageal Reflux

The possibility that reflux or acid perfusion can induce central (or angina-like) chest pain was clearly articulated by Bernstein, Fruin, and Pacini in their description of four patients with exertional substernal chest pain and no evidence of cardiac disease whose pain (not heartburn) was induced by acid perfusion of the esophagus.[27] The authors reasonably suggest that in these patients exertion induced reflux; they do not offer an explanation for the nonburning, pressure-sensation quality of the discomfort. Bennet and Atkinson subsequently confirmed these findings, describing "tight, gripping, or vise-like" pain in 8 of 35 (23%) patients with esophagitis and no heart disease, as well as exertional pain in 24% of the esophagitis patients.[28] Henderson et al. also found that exertional pain was common (55%) in patients with atypical pain and esophageal reflux and noted radiation of the pain to the arm in the same percentage; all of these patients had negative cardiac stress tests and/or coronary angiograms.[29] Looking at the converse situation, we found that reflux was commonly found among patients with central chest pain; it was present in 17 of 28 patients tested with a pH probe.[18] Also, our series of 163 chest-pain patients yielded 14 who experienced their pain during spontaneous reflux or acid infusion.[19] Thus, it is well documented that reflux can be associated with pain characteristics that are considered typical for ischemic heart disease. Much less clear is the explanation for this phenomenon: is the direct effect of acid on the esophageal mucosa simply expressed as a different sensation in these patients, or is something additional occurring? There is reason to entertain the hypothesis that reflux can induce motility abnormalities that in turn produce central chest pain.

Reflux and the Motility Disorders. The first systematic attempt at recording motor abnormalities during an acid-perfusion (Bernstein) test was reported by Siegel and Hendrix.[30] In 25 patients with heartburn reproduced by acid infusion, these authors described three manometric abnormalities; each was present in nearly all of the patients during acid perfusion and was absent during saline perfusion. These were a modest increase in contraction amplitude and duration; the appearance of spontaneous (no swallows involved), simultaneous contractions; and a gradual rise in resting esophageal pressure. A possible interpretation of the findings, pertinent to this discussion, is that these abnormalities represent the *forma fruste* of more severe contraction abnormalities that are now linked with angina-like pain; thus, the contractions of modestly increased amplitude would become distinctly high-amplitude contractions in the patient with chest pain, and the spontaneous, simultaneous contractions and elevated resting pressure would turn into full-blown diffuse spasm.

Unfortunately, most manometrists have not routinely recorded esophageal motility during acid-perfusion tests, so there are few data to confirm or disprove the study by Siegel and Hendrix. However, there are some convincing reports that acid—either infused or spontaneously refluxed—produces angina-like pain together with diffuse spasm or high-amplitude peristaltic contractions. Henderson et al. report one such individual with acid-induced pain and spasm.[29] Benjamin et al. report on acid-perfusion tests in six patients with high-amplitude contractions; five had positive results. Four of the five experienced heartburn; of these, two had no change in their manometric pattern during the infusion; one developed repetitive simultaneous contractions (diffuse spasm?); and one showed increases in the (already high) amplitude of her peristaltic contractions.[20] The fifth—and most intriguing patient—felt severe central chest pain during the acid infusion simultaneous with changes in her manometry pattern from high-amplitude contraction to diffuse spasm. Just as interesting as this patient's flagrant response to acid infusion is the fact that all but one patient tested were in some way symptomatically sensitive.

The final line of evidence connecting reflux with motility disorders is the frequency of dysphagia—a symptom more specific for esophageal dysfunction than is chest pain—and central chest pain among patients with reflux. In a study of the effects of antireflux surgery, 15 of 25 reflux patients (with no strictures) had dysphagia prior to surgery and only seven had it afterwards. Among the nine patients who had chest pain (distinct from heartburn) preoperatively, five were free of it after surgery.[31] These changes, the former reaching and the latter just short of statistical significance, suggest that correction of the reflux problem improved motility.

Thus, there is considerable support for an association between reflux, motility disorders, and chest pain. What is unclear is the nature of the relationship. It remains a possibility that abnormal contractions, such as those seen in diffuse spasm or those of high-amplitude peristalsis, result from a neuromuscular lesion of unknown cause and are, by dint of their extensiveness or force, experienced as painful; reflux, although often present, may not be at all important in production of the symptom. Secondly, the reflux of acid may cause damage to the nerve or muscle of the esophageal body, leading to the motility disorders in question; these abnormal contractions may then produce the pain. A third possibility is that the reflux may directly produce sensory nerve irritation or damage, provoking the experience of pain during contractions; these contractions, although they are abnormal (in the sense that they occur infrequently in asymptomatic individuals), would not be painful in the absence of the sensory pathway damage. Lastly, the sensory nerve damage may itself be sufficient to produce pain, and the abnormal contractions, whether or not they result from acid damage, have nothing to do with the pain.

Descriptions of symptoms from specific patients have been used to lend support to each of these possibilities. To choose among them requires much more anatomic and physiologic knowledge of the afferent and efferent neurologic pathways and the muscular function of the esophageal body, in the normal state and in the presence of reflux or the motility disorders. Animal models of reflux and motility dysfunction will be helpful in this regard but are, of course, at a distinct disadvantage in eliciting the specific conditions necessary for the production of pain. Careful prospective evaluation of a large series of patients with the complaints of chest pain and/or dysphagia is required, a study that not only looks at patients' motility patterns and symptoms but also searches for the occurrence of reflux and defines its histologic, electron-microscopic, and motility imprints. Similar study of a series of reflux patients, with and without chest pain and dysphagia, will separate those motility events that are simply epiphenomena of reflux from those with symptomatic consequences. These studies may benefit from new techniques, such as the radio-isotopic methods of assessing reflux and motility, which are noninvasive and, in the case of motility testing perhaps even more sensitive than the traditional catheter methods.[32-34] Finally, therapeutic investigations should be carried out, studies that examine the effect on chest pain and dysphagia of eliminating reflux, on the one hand, and of eliminating abnormal contractions, on the other. Our therapeutic tools for accomplishing these feats are reasonable and improving; urecholine, cimetidine, metoclopramide, and antireflux surgery are either established or promising in dealing with reflux, and long-acting nitrates and calcium-channel blockers may be effective in modifying abnormal contractions.

Nonreflux Esophagitis

Inflammation of the esophageal lining from causes other than acid reflux can produce central chest pain. *Moniliasis* or *herpes infection* of the esophagus, although more often characterized by odynophagia and dysphagia, can also produce substernal pain radiating into the back.[35-37] *Alkaline reflux,* carefully defined via 24-hour pH monitoring by Pellegrini et al.[12] produces endoscopically convincing esophagitis and heartburn indistinguishable from that of acid reflux; although central chest pain, as opposed to heartburn, was not sought in the symptom survey, it probably occurs just as it does in some acid-reflux patients. Certainly, central chest pain occurs in the extreme instance of alkaline esophagitis, that resulting from lye ingestion.[38]

Carcinoma

Dysphagia and odynophagia, as symptoms of luminal obstruction, are the usual local symptoms of presentation for esophageal cancer. Central chest pain often denotes extension of the disease beyond the confines of the esophagus and is unusual as an isolated symptom in this disease.[39]

Perforation of the Esophagus

Esophageal perforation, called Boerhaave's syndrome when associated with vomiting after a heavy meal, produces the abrupt onset of epigastric or subxyphoid pain that may radiate through to the back. Other manifestations are dyspnea, cyanosis, diaphoresis, tachycardia, and shock.[40] The presence of subcutaneous emphysema and fluid at the left-lung base distinguishes this condition from similarly painful abdominal and thoracic catastrophes, such as a perforated ulcer, acute pancreatitis, a dissecting aortic aneurysm, or myocardial infarction.

NONESOPHAGEAL CAUSES OF CENTRAL CHEST PAIN (Table 7-2)

Cardiopulmonary Disorders

Coronary Artery Disease. Considerable reference has been made to the similarities in the pain produced by esophageal dysfunction and by coronary-artery disease with consequent myocardial ischemia. Harrison has written an excellent characterization of angina pectoris, based on 77 patients, which was first published

Table 7-2. Nonesophageal disorders associated
with central chest pain

Cardio-Pulmonary Disorders
    Coronary artery disease
    Pericarditis
    Pulmonary embolism
    Dissecting aortic aneurysm
Mediastinal Disorders
    Mediastinal emphysema
    Mediastinal tumors
Gastrointestinal Disorders
    Peptic ulcer disease
    Biliary colic
    Acute cholecystitis
    Pancreatitis, acute and chronic
    Pancreatic pseudocysts
Musculo-Skeletal Disorders
    Cervical and thoracic osteoarthritis
    Costochondral, costosternal inflammation
    Thoracic outlet syndromes
Functional Chest Pain Disorders
    Psychogenic
    Psychophysiologic

in 1944 and 1945 and recently reprinted.[41] He defines angina pectoris as "a condition characterized by recurrent attacks of discomfort in or near the chest, commonly induced by conditions which impose an additional burden on the heart, ordinarily dependent on disturbance of the oxidative processes in the myocardium and always attended by the likelihood of sudden death." It is useful to review his main points in depicting the nature of this chest pain. Localization to the substernal region was present in 55% of the patients, to the precordium in 39%, to the left arm, shoulder, and hand in 30%, and to the front of the neck in 18%. Rarely (5%) was the pain epigastric, and never was it solely so. The duration of the pain was 1–30 min in 90% of the patients. Intensity was variable, being mild or minimal in about 50%. The pain was characterized as constrictive in 40%, aching in 20%, and burning in 5%. More reliable than these parameters was induction of pain by general exertion (as opposed to specific local muscular activity) seen in 91%; in patients without this feature there were extenuating circumstances such as extreme inactivity. With respect to factors suggestive of esophageal disorders in these patients with coronary artery disease, pain was felt immediately after meals in 8% and was induced by recumbency in 15% and by acute emotional stress in 18%. Table 7-3 summarizes the features that Harrison considered most helpful in diagnosing angina pectoris.

A relatively uncommon variant of angina pectoris is confusing to all doctors concerned with the heart and gullet. Characterized by onset without exertion and often awakening the patient from sleep, it was described by Prinzmetal and his group in 1959[42] and is now considered an associate of coronary artery spasm with ST-segment elevation.[43] The pain and electrocardiographic and angiographic changes can be reproduced in these patients by injection of ergonovine.[44]

There have been several efforts to delineate esophageal pain. Bennet and Atkin-

Table 7-3. Summary of the most important clinical features in the diagnosis of angina pectoris[a]

Features of Positive Value (present in over 90% of patients)	Features of Negative Value (tend to exclude angina pectoris)
1. History of relation of pain to effort	1. Location limited to periapical, axillary, or abdominal regions
2. Substernal or precordial location	2. Duration of less than 1 min
3. Duration of 1–30 min	3. Lancinating or throbbing pain
4. Demonstration that nitroglycerine increases the amount of effort required to induce pain	4. Aggravated by breathing, coughing, swallowing, sitting or standing

[a] From Harrison TR: Clinical aspects of pain in the chest. Am J Med Sci 269:74–110, 1975. Reprinted with permission.

son, in comparing esophagitis and ischemic chest pain, found that esophageal pain was brought on by stooping or lying in 43% of patients and immediately after eating in 30%; the figures for cardiac patients were 7% in both situations.[28] Davies and Rhodes, in studying patients with diffuse spasm or coronary artery disease, found the two most discriminating points in the patients' histories to be persistence of pain as a dull ache for hours at a time (esophageal spasm, 82%; coronary artery disease, 33%) and radiation of the pain from the chest to the stomach area (esophageal spasm, 32%; coronary artery disease, 0%).[45]

Thus, the features most helpful for defining coronary artery-disease pain seem to be its relation to generalized exertion and its duration of a few minutes, whereas for esophageal pain, symptoms that suggest reflux (pain occurring right after meals or with recumbency) or spasm (pain associated with swallowing) or pain that radiates into the epigastrium are helpful. The critical point, or course, is the frequency of overlap of the two symptom complexes. This was graphically demonstrated by Henderson et al., who compared two large groups of patients, one with "atypical" esophageal disease and the other with reflux esophagitis.[29] The former had a much more frequent occurrence of pain that radiated to the arm and occurred with general exercise and much less frequent relief from antacids, traits commonly ascribed to cardiac pain. At best, the symptom differences can serve merely as a guide toward the initial selection of specific diagnostic tests.

Pericarditis, Pulmonary Embolism, Dissecting Aortic Aneurysm. The discomfort from pericarditis usually falls into three categories, one of which mimics esophageal pain. Fortunately, the most commonly occurring type is pleuritic pain, usually left-sided. The least common one is synchronous with the heartbeat and is also left-sided. The third diagnostically confusing category encompasses pain that is substernal, steady, and crushing and—in the absence of either of the other two types of pain—resembles that of myocardial infarction or protracted diffuse esophageal spasm.[46]

Pulmonary embolism, when massive, can also produce central crushing pain. Dyspnea is very commonly present in this setting and is uncommon in esophageal spasm.

A *dissecting aortic aneurysm* causes severe anterior chest pain, which radiates to the back. It is maximal at its onset and persists longer than that of myocardial infarction; usually it remains severe for hours, which diffuse spasm rarely does.

Mediastinal Conditions

Mediastinal emphysema, occurring "spontaneously" as a result of the rupture of peripheral alveoli and entry of the air along perivascular channels, is announced by the abrupt onset of severe substernal pain, which may radiate to the shoulders and is often exacerbated with breathing. The pain is frequently preceded by coughing, vomiting, sneezing (activities that presumably produce the alveolar rupture). Diagnosis is made by the physical findings of subcutaneous emphysema and a clicking sound accompanying the heartbeat together with radiographic evidence of air in the mediastinum and in the soft tissues. Treatment is rarely required. A secondary form, following rupture or perforation of the esophagus or tracheo-bronchial tree, is less common; it is often accompanied by acute mediastinitis and fever.

Mediastinal masses such as lymphomas, thymomas, bronchogenic cysts, teratodermoid tumors, and neurogenic tumors sometimes produce chest pain described as a vague sensation of heaviness.[47]

Other Gastrointestinal Conditions

The gastrointestinal disorders associated with chest pain have recently been reviewed by Long and Cohen, who point out that aside from esophageal causes, the pertinent gastrointestinal conditions nearly always have additional features that distinguish them from other causes of central chest pain.[9] Thus, a *peptic ulcer* can cause lower-chest pain, but the usual epigastric component, the burning nature of the pain, and the relief obtained with food or antacids point toward its true origin. *Biliary colic* can be felt high in the epigastrium but often radiates to the right upper quadrant or right scapular area and is associated with nausea and vomiting. *Acute cholecystitis* also can cause pain in the high epigastrium; usually right upper-quadrant pain and tenderness and systemic signs of inflammation are also present. The pain of *pancreatitis,* acute or chronic, spreads through to the back from the epigastrium; abdominal tenderness is the rule. *Pancreatic pseudocysts* can produce central chest pain when they dissect into the mediastinum or pleural space; here, a history of previous pancreatic disease must be sought to elicit a diagnostic clue.

Musculo-Skeletal Disorders

Osteoarthritis of the cervical or thoracic spine can produce neck, shoulder, arm, and chest pain, generally of a radicular nature corresponding to the involved segment. Actual arthritic changes may not be necessary for symptoms from the thoracic spine area, which have been described in association with decreased mobility, of uncertain cause, of one vertebral body on the next; in this situation, direct tenderness over the spinous process is a useful sign.[48] Anteriorly, tenderness over the costochondral or chondrosternal articulations implicates them as causes of chest pain; the uncommon presence of swelling graces the conditions with the name of Tietze's syndrome.

The *thoracic outlet syndromes* have in common the compression of the neuro-vascular bundle, as it journeys toward the arm from the neck and thorax, by musculoskeletal structures; such compression commonly results in the typical nerve-compression symptoms of pain and paresthesia in the neck, shoulder, arm and hand, and at times, anterior pain in the chest on the afflicted side. Motor weakness is present in only 10% of the patients. Vascular symptoms, also relatively uncommon, consist of coldness, weakness, easy fatigability of the arm, and more diffuse pain.[49] Roos recommends that objective neural findings should be sought as follows: (1) pain on percussion over the brachial plexus supraclavicularly, infraclavicularly, or on the ipsilateral neck; (2) pain on pressure applied for 30 sec over the brachial plexus; (3) hypesthesia to touch and pinprick over the inner forearm and the ulnar side of the hand; (4) early fatigue, heaviness, and pain when the fists are opened and closed for 3 min with arms elevated and shoulders braced; and (5) weakness of the grip, the triceps, and the interosseus muscles.[50]

Roos also points out that the most common structural abnormality in these patients is the presence of an anomalous fibromuscular band, rather than that of bony abnormalities. This may explain the relative rarity of vascular compression and the frequently negative tests for diminution of the radial pulse in the neurologically symptomatic patients. Also, normal individuals sometimes have pulse changes when tested. Thus, the traditional tests for thoracic outlet syndrome, which include Adson's test (full inspiration, head turned to the side), hyperextension or hyperabduction of the arms, and the exaggerated military (or "backpack") position, are important only if they reproduce the symptoms.

Functional Causes of Chest Pain

It is useful to separate functional chest pain into two categories, psychogenic and psychophysiologic.[51] *Psychogenic* pain, the less common type, is regarded as a misperception of an emotional state, similar to classic conversion reactions or hysteria, in which an emotional conflict is converted into a functional impairment of voluntary muscles or special sensory organs. With chest pain, as in other psychogenic pain or disability, the locale of the symptom conforms to the person's lay concept of anatomy; thus, conceived of as heart pain, it is often localized over the apex rather than substernally. It tends to fluctuate in severity or frequency with emotional state or life situation.

Psychophysiologic (or psychosomatic) chest pain describes the situation in which the emotional component is mediated through hypothalamic and autonomic innervation to produce muscle or blood-vessel spasm—and consequent pain—with or without additional symptoms. Examples include the *hyperventilation syndrome,* which may produce pain as well as dyspnea, presumably from chest-wall and intercostal-muscle spasm. *Aerophagia* may produce left-sided chest pain, perhaps by displacing the left diaphragm through gastric distention. Similar discomfort, sometimes radiating to the left shoulder, may result from the *splenic flexure* syndrome, a variant of the irritable bowel syndrome, which is associated with abnormal postprandial colonic spike potentials and contractions.[52] The so-called *cardiac neurosis* (or neurocirculatory asthenia) may involve elements of all of these, with the hyperventilation syndrome most prominent.

APPROACH TO THE PATIENT WITH CHEST PAIN

From the discussion thus far, it is apparent that there are two important reasons why it is often difficult to arrive at a diagnosis of esophageal chest pain. One is the wide scope of the differential diagnosis, and the other is the necessity of relying on findings associated with esophageal chest pain, a necessity proceeding from the lack of suitable pain-provoking diagnostic tests.

If we turn first to cope with the large differential diagnosis, the usual approach to this problem—a careful history of the symptom—is the appropriate measure. Figure 7-2 is an algorithm that uses the history, physical examination, and simple screening tests to choose an initial direction for the diagnostic evaluation. As we have seen, the most helpful historic point in defining the pain of cardiac ischemia is that it correlates with generalized physical exertion. If present, this relationship demands a cardiac evaluation, starting with a resting electrocardiogram (ECG) and exercise stress testing. If the latter demonstrates the presence of pain and ECG changes, the specificity of the test is high and coronary artery disease is very likely.[53] If the pain is not reproduced but ECG changes are present or if the test is in some other way equivocal, it is recommended that exercise thallium-

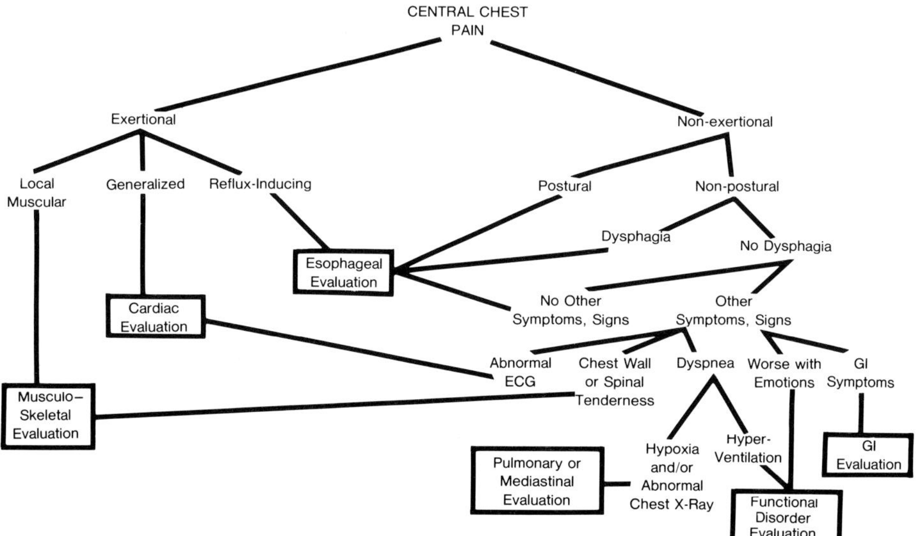

Fig. 7-2. Use of symptoms, signs, and screening tests to select initial organ or system for evaluation.

201 imaging be carried out; this procedure, which detects segmental changes in myocardial perfusion, has a sensitivity of 82% and a specificity of 95% for coronary artery disease. For the few remaining equivocal cases, exercise radionuclide angiography provides a means of evaluating regional cardiac wall-motion and ejection-fraction changes with exercise; this test has a sensitivity and specificity comparable with that of exercise thallium-201 imaging. Okada et al. have comprehensively reviewed these testing procedures and their sequential use.[54]

The importance of carefully delineating the type of exertion that produces the pain has been stressed by Tibbling; this investigator, using a questionnaire designed to elicit the presence of angina pectoris, found a positive exertional response (i.e., exertional pain) in 50% of 217 patients with positive Bernstein tests, compared with 13% in a general population.[55,56] She suggests that we separate out those types of generalized exertion that might also produce reflux (e.g. digging in the garden, scrubbing a floor) from those that are less likely to do so (e.g. brisk walking, bicycling). Similarly, chest pain that occurs only with movement or a certain position of an arm, a shoulder, or the neck suggests a musculoskeletal or thoracic-outlet problem and thus has a different significance from that of generalized exertional pain.

If the pain is not exertional, then the physician taking the history should seek other ways to tie it to the esophagus. Does it occur with the patient recumbent or bending over? If not, is there associated dysphagia? If, again, the response is negative, the patient has earned a temporary stay from an esophageal evaluation, and the physician should do a thorough review of systems, seeking additional symptoms that would point to other gastrointestinal disorders, to functional pain, or to pulmonary or mediastinal problems mentioned earlier in the chapter as causes of chest pain. Chest-wall tenderness, an abnormal electrocardiogram, or an abnormal chest x-ray can also provide an initial direction for the work-up. If, however, there are no specific clues, the esophagus should be the initial point of focus.

How do we select from what has become a large roster of esophageal tests? Figure 7-3 presents a proposed sequence of tests used to evaluate the esophagus as a cause of central or angina-like chest pain. The barium esophagogram should be followed by endoscopy if a structural defect such as a stricture, a mass, an ulcer, or diffuse or nodular mucosal changes (perhaps denoting moniliasis) are present; appropriate biopsies or brushings can be obtained. If the x-ray is normal or shows only abnormal motility, then manometry, pH-probe acid-reflux testing, and the acid-infusion (Bernstein) test should be performed, at the same session, through the same catheter assembly. This trio of tests is the "heart" of the work-up, and each test asks a separate, relevant question. Is one of the motility disorders closely associated with pain present, i.e., diffuse spasm, high-amplitude contractions, or achalasia? Is there reflux? Does acid infusion reproduce the pain?

If these tests are negative, the option of attempting to entice abnormal contractions from the esophagus is available; however, this endeavor has met with only limited success. The discovery that very cold stimuli can produce pain while diminishing contractions (rather than producing spasm)[5] has dampened the enthusiasm for ice water as a stimulant during manometry. There has been no systematic study of acid's effect on motility since the study by Siegel and Hendrix described

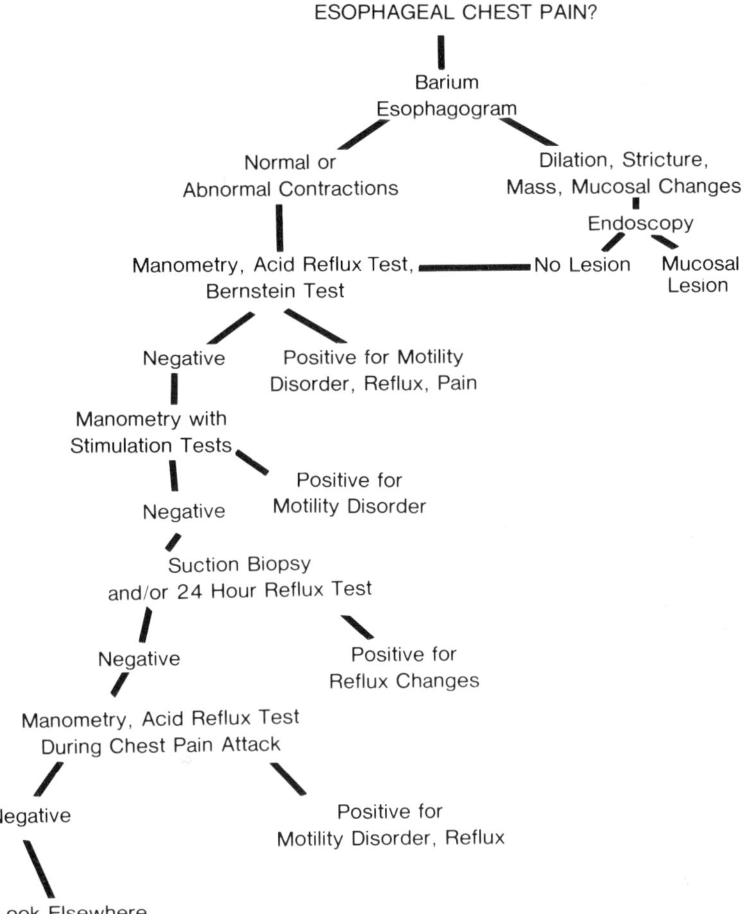

Fig. 7-3. Sequence of esophageal test selection in evaluation for chest pain of esophageal origin.

above.[30] Pentagastrin was found to increase mean contraction amplitude and lower sphincter (LES) pressure in patients with diffuse spasm and achalasia, and it produced chest pain and dysphagia in over half of the patients in both groups; normal subjects displayed only a rise in LES pressure, with no symptoms.[57] However, pentagastrin did not contribute to the diagnosis in either patient group, since the characteristic motility patterns were present without its use, nor did it bring forth abnormalities in patients with symptoms suggesting a motility disorder and normal prepentagastrin-manometry studies. Benjamin et al. recently studied 20 consecutive patients referred for evaluation of chest pain or dysphagia; central chest pain was induced in these patients as follows: acid, 0; pentagastrin, 2 (no manometry changes); edrophonium, 3 (with manometry changes); hethanechol, 2 (no manometry changes).[58]

The most successful *agent provocateur* is ergonovine. Davies and coworkers report that 13 of 22 patients experienced their chest pain with manometric changes of diffuse spasm after 500 mg of intravenous ergonovine; only 2 of the 13 had had abnormal manometric findings without medication.[59] Unfortunately, as the authors point out, this agent can also cause coronary spasm and angina pectoris in patients with or without the presence of coronary-artery disease; furthermore, it has caused deaths and myocardial infarction.[60] Therefore, its use should be limited to patients whose coronary angiographic findings, including response to ergonovine stimulation, were normal.

Proceeding down the algorithm of Fig. 9-3, we come to suction biopsy of the esophagus. This procedure provides an additional means of documenting acid-induced changes in the esophageal mucosa[13] and thus is reasonable to do when the acid-reflux test and acid-infusion test results are ambiguous or negative in the presence of reflux symptoms; it may also provide a means of separating trivial reflux from that capable of inducing chest pain, although this ability is still unproven. Another means of making this distinction may be the 24-hour reflux test, with the patient dutifully recording symptoms throughout the monitoring period.[61] With the recent development of a portable monitoring system,[62] this test may become significantly more practical and applicable during ordinary activities.

Finally, if all else has failed to implicate the esophagus, the dogged manometrist may wish to repeat the manometry study during an episode of pain if, as is usually the case, the first study was done during a pain-free period. If nothing comes of it, there is at least the rare satisfaction of having performed an emergency esophageal study.

How should this sequence be altered if the symptom is clearly heartburn or odynophagia? Very little, in my opinion, since the esophageal conditions that are associated with central chest pain are also associated with these other types of chest discomfort. One modification is suggested by Silverstein and Pope.[63] In the classic heartburn patient with no dysphagia, a trial of therapy is reasonable, following (or perhaps even prior to) a barium esophagogram; if the heartburn responds well, no further testing is required. In the patient with odynophagia, endoscopy should play a more prominent role and precede manometry because of the symptom's more frequent association with carcinoma, on the one hand, and monilial or herpetic esophagitis, on the other.

Finally, it remains to put forth a method of evaluating the positive and negative results of these tests. Although all of them may be pertinent to esophageal chest pain, the circumstances of their occurrence are critical. Figure 7-4 presents such a framework, with the most important branch point being the presence or absence of pain during the manometry testing. If pain is present, a much higher degree of certainty surrounds one's conclusions. Thus, if the patient has pain while displaying high-amplitude peristaltic contractions or diffuse spasm or while acid is bathing the esophageal mucosa, it seems clear that the esophagus is the offending organ. Similarly, if pain is present but the manometry pattern is normal and no acid reflux or pain intensification occurs during acid infusion, the esophagus, within the limits of our ability to evaluate it, is exonerated.

More often, however, pain does not occur during manometry, and our conclusions must be more tentative. If diffuse spasm or high-amplitude contractions are present, the gullet is highly suspect, for we know that these disorders are often

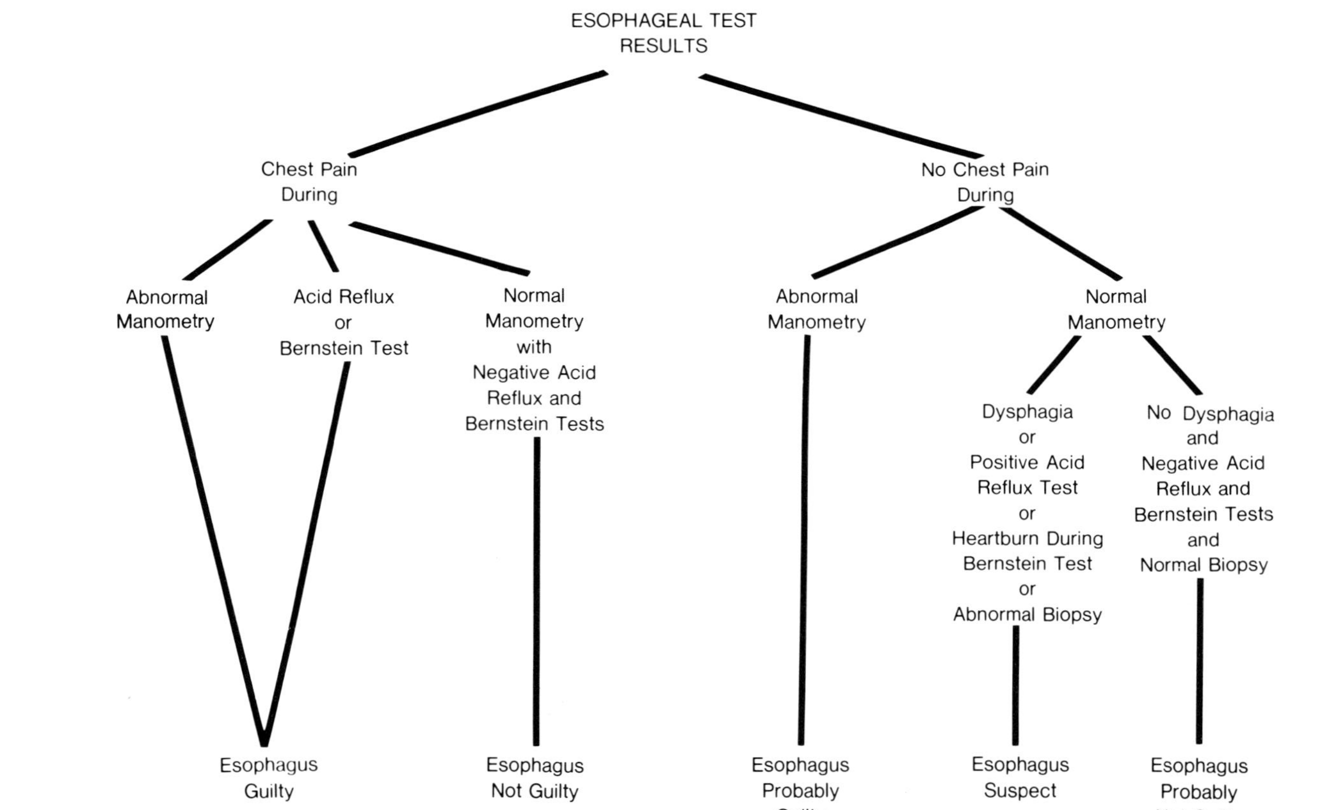

Fig. 7-4. Interpretation of esophageal test results in patients with central chest pain. Reproduced with modifications by permission from Brand DL, Martin D, Pope CE II: Esophageal manometrics in patients with angina-like chest pain. Am J Dig Dis 22:300–304, 1977.

associated with pain and are not found in the asymptomatic person. When the manometry pattern is normal during the painless study, we remain suspicious of the esophagus if our patient has dysphagia, a positive pH-probe acid-reflux test, heartburn during acid infusion, or an abnormal suction biopsy; after all, dysphagia is quite esophagus-specific, and reflux might at times produce angina-like pain. Finally, in the absence of these fellow-travelers, it is likely, but not certain, that the esophagus is not involved in the patient's chest pain.

TREATMENT OF ESOPHAGEAL CHEST PAIN

The obvious guide to treating chest pain from the esophagus is to treat the associated or underlying disorder. The treatment of all of these conditions—the motility disorders, reflux, esophagitis, and carcinoma—is thoroughly discussed elsewhere in this volume. Thus, the comments to follow deal with selected points of interest to the physician managing esophageal pain.

In regard to the motility disorders, often the major source of relief to the patient with chest pain is the knowledge that it is the esophagus, not the heart, that is the miscreant. Fortunately, such knowledge can be sufficient treatment, since the pain is often mild in severity or infrequent in occurrence. When this is not the case, therapy has been problematic in the absence of underlying reflux or achalasia. With diffuse spasm or high-amplitude peristaltic contractions, nitroglycerin and isosorbide dinitrate are inconsistently helpful.[18,64-66] Two newer agents deserve further investigation. One is hydralazine; Mellow has reported that this drug decreased both the pain and the duration of the bethanecol-induced spasmodic contractions in five patients with diffuse spasm.[66] The second is verapamil, a calcium-channel blocking agent that has been extensively evaluated for cardiovascular effects, which Richter et al. have studied in the baboon esophagus.[67] It produced a 63% decrease in contraction amplitude, a 40–50% decrease in duration, and a 74% decrease in LES pressure. These profound effects, coupled with its relative safety in cardiovascular patients, justify a trial in patients with severe pain from diffuse spasm or high-amplitude contractions.

In patients with reflux and chest pain, the reflux should be treated for a trial period of several weeks with an aggressive medical regimen that employs 300 mg of cimetidine four times daily, antacids as needed, and the usual postural precautions. Because of the safety and efficacy of this regimen,[68,69] it seems a reasonable ploy even when the reflux symptoms themselves are mild or the connection between the reflux and the chest pain is tenuous. If, however, medical therapy fails, antireflux surgery should be considered only when (1) the chest pain (not heartburn) is reliably reproduced by acid infusion, or (2) the reflux symptoms or recognized complications are severe enough to warrant the surgery, regardless of the chest pain. In the latter situation, the patient must be told that the chest pain may or may not be helped by the operation.

REFERENCES

1. Davenport HW: Chewing and swallowing. In: Physiology of The Digestive Tract. 4th Ed., Year Book Med Pub, Chicago, 1977, pp. 3–21.

2. Lorber SH: Symptom dynamics. In Van Der Reis L (ed): Fronteirs of Gastrointestinal Research, Vol. 3, S. Karger, Basel, New York, 1978, pp. 33–48.

3. Geboes K, Desmet V: Histology of the esophagus. In Van Der Reis L (ed): Frontiers of Gastrointestinal Research, Vol 3, S. Karger, Basel, New York, 1978, pp. 1–17.

4. Cecio A, Califano G, Lobello R: Further histophysiological observations on the lower esophagus of the rabbit. Cell Tissue Res 168:475–485, 1976.

5. Meyer GW, Castell DO: The "slurpee" esophagus: effects of rapid ingestion of cold liquids on human esophageal peristalsis. Dig Dis Sci 25:714 (A-1), 1980.

6. Frank PI: Some historical aspects of chest pain. Practitioner 211:96–104, 1973.

7. Kramer P, Hollander W: Comparison of experimental esophageal pain with clinical pain of angina pectoris and esophageal disease. Gastroenterology 29:719–743, 1955.

8. Flood CA, Fink S, Mathers J: Pain due to esophageal distension. Am J Dig Dis 8:632–638, 1963.

9. Long WB, Cohen S: The digestive tract as a cause of chest pain. Am Heart J 100:567–572, 1980.

10. DeMeester TR, Lawrence FJ, Joseph GJ, et al.: Patterns of gastroesophageal reflux in health and disease. Ann Surg 184:459–469, 1976.

11. Boesby S: Gastro-oesophageal acid reflux and sphincter pressure in normal human subjects. Scand J Gastroenterol 10:731–736, 1975.

12. Pellegrini CA, DeMeester TR, Wernly JA, et al.: Alkaline gastroesophageal reflux. Am J Surg 135:177–184, 1978.

13. Ismail-Beigi F, Horton PF, Pope CE II: Histological consequences of gastroesophageal reflux in man. Gastroenterology 58:163–174, 1970.

14. Hopwood D, Milne G, Logan KR: Electron microscopic changes in human oesophageal epithelium in oesophagitis. J Pathol 129:161–167, 1979.

15. Osgood H: A peculiar form of oesophagismus. Boston Surg J 120:401–405, 1889.

16. DiMarino AJ, Cohen S: Characteristics of lower esophageal sphincter function in symptomatic diffuse esophageal spasm. Gastroenterology 66:1–6, 1974.

17. Castell DO: Achalasia and diffuse esophageal spasm. Arch Intern Med 136:571–579, 1976.

18. Brand DL, Martin D, Pope CE II: Esophageal manometrics in patients with angina-like chest pain. Am J Dig. Dis 22:300–304, 1977.

19. Brand DL, Ilves R, Pope CE II: Evaluation of esophageal function in patients with central chest pain. Acta Med Scand [Suppl] 644:53–56, 1981.

20. Benjamin SB, Gerhardt DC, Castell DO: High amplitude, peristaltic esophageal contractions associated with chest pain and/or dysphagia. Gastroenterology 77:478–483, 1979.

21. Herrington JP, Burns TW, Balart LA: Dysphagia in patients with prolonged peristaltic contractile duration—a clinical and manometric analysis. Gastroenterology 80:1173 (abstr), 1981.

22. VanTrappen G, Hellemans J: Esophageal motility disorders. In Van Der Reis L (ed): Frontiers of Gastrointestinal Research, Vol 3, S. Karger, Basel, New York, 1978, pp. 49–75.

23. Sanderson DR, Ellis FH Jr, Schlegel JF, et al.: Syndrome of vigorous achalasia; clinical and physiological observations. Dis Chest 52:508–517, 1967.

24. Kaye MD: Oesophageal motor dysfunction in patients with diverticula of the mid-thoracic oesophagus. Thorax 29:666–672, 1974.

25. Debas HT, Payne WS, Cameron AJ, et al.: Physiopathology of lower esophageal diverticulum and its implications for treatment. Surg Gynecol Obstet 151:593–600, 1980.

26. Peppercorn MA, Docken WP, Rosenberg S: Esophageal motor dysfunction in systemic lupus erythematosus. JAMA 242:1895–1896, 1979.

27. Bernstein LM, Fruin RC, Pacini R: Differentiation of esophageal pain from angina pectoris: role of the esophageal acid perfusion test. Medicine 41:143–162, 1962.

28. Bennett JR, Atkinson M: The differentiation of oesophageal and cardiac pain. Lancet 2:1123–1127, 1966.

29. Henderson RD, Wigle ED, Sample K, et al.: Atypical chest pain of cardiac and esophageal origin. Chest 73:24–27, 1978.

30. Siegel CI, Hendrix TR: Esophageal motor abnormalities induced by acid perfusion in patients with heartburn. J Clin Invest 42:686–695, 1963.

31. Brand DL, Eastwood IR, Martin D, et al.: Esophageal symptoms, manometry, and histology before and after anti-reflux surgery: a long-term follow-up study. Gastroenterology 76:1393–1401, 1979.

32. Fisher RS, Malmud LS, Roberts GS, et al.: Gastroesophageal (GE) scintiscanning to detect and quantitate GE reflux. Gastroenterology 70:301–308, 1976.

33. Tolin RD, Malmud LS, Reilley E, et al.: Esophageal scintigraphy to quantitate esophageal transit (quantitation of esophageal transit). Gastroenterology 76:1402–1408, 1979.

34. Russell COH, Hill LD, Holmes ER III, et al.: Radionuclude transit: a sensitive screening test for esophageal dysfunction. Gastroenterology 80:887–892, 1981.

35. Bucke RM, Nichol WD: Painful dysphagia due to monilial oesophagitis. Br Med J 1:821–822, 1964.

36. Kodsi BE, Wickremesinghe PC, Kozinn PJ, et al.: Candida esophagitis: a prospective study. Gastroenterology 71:715–719, 1976.

37. Lightdale CJ, Wolf DJ, Marcucci RA, et al.: Herpetic esophagitis in patients with cancer: ante mortem diagnosis by brush cytology. Cancer 39:223–226, 1977.

38. Ray JF III, Myers WO, Lawton BR, et al.: The natural history of liquid lye ingestion. Arch Surg 109:436–439, 1974.

39. Pope CE II: Tumors. In Sleisenger MH and Fordtran JS (eds): Gastrointestinal Disease, 2nd Ed., WB Saunders, Philadelphia, 1978, pp. 574–586.

40. Bombeck CT, Boyd DR, Nyhus LM: Esophageal trauma. Surg Clin North Am 52:219–230, 1972.

41. Harrison TR: Clinical aspects of pain in the chest. Am J Med Sci 269:74–110, 1975.

42. Prinzmetal M, Kennamer R, Merliss R, et al.: Angina pectoris I. A variant form of angina pectoris. Preliminary report. Am J Med 27:375–388, 1959.

43. Oliva PB, Potts DE, Pluss RG: Coronary arterial spasm in Prinzmetal angina. N. Engl J Med 288:745–751, 1973.

44. Curry RC Jr, Pepine CJ, Sabom MB, et al.: Similarities of ergonovine-induced and spontaneous attacks of variant angina. Circulation 59:307–312, 1979.

45. Davies HA, Rhodes J: How often does the gut cause anginal pain? Acta Med Scand [Suppl] 644:62–65, 1981.

46. Braunwald E: Chest pain and palpitation. In Isselbacher KJ, Adams RD, Braunwald E et al. (eds): Principles of Internal Medicine, 9th Ed., McGraw-Hill, New York, 1980. pp. 28–34.

47. Duffell GM: Chest pain due to mediastinal disorders. In Hurst JW and Spiro HM (eds): Chest Pain: Problems In Differential Diagnosis, Vol. 5, No. 2, Biomedical Information Corp, New York, 1979.

48. Hamberg J, Lindahl O: Angina pectoris symptoms caused by thoracic spine disorders. Acta Med Scand [Suppl] 644:84–86, 1981.

49. Urschel HC, Razzuk MA: Management of the thoracic-outlet syndrome. N Engl J Med 286:1140–1143, 1977.

50. Roos DB: Congenital anomalies associated with thoracic outlet syndrome. Am J Surg 132:771–778, 1976.

51. Flinn DE: Functional chest pain. Aerospace Med 38: 1167–1170, 1967.
52. Sullivan MA, Cohen S, Snape WJ: Colonic myoelectric activity in irritable bowel syndrome: effect of eating and anticholinergics. N Engl J Med 298:878–883, 1978.
53. Ellestad MH, Cooke BM Jr, Greenberg PS: Stress testing: clinical application and predictive capacity. Prog Cardiovasc Dis 21:431–460, 1979.
54. Okada RD, Boucher CA, Strauss HW, et al.: Exercise radionuclide imaging approaches to coronary artery disease. Am J Cardiol 46:1188–1204, 1980.
55. Tibbling L: Angina-like chest pain in patients with oesophageal dysfunction. Acta Med Scand [Suppl] 644: 56–59, 1981.
56. Tibbling L: Oesophageal dysfunction and angina pectoris in a Swedish population selected at random. Acta Med Scand [Suppl] 644:71–74, 1981.
57. Orlando RC, Bozymski EM: The effects of pentagastrin in achalasia and diffuse esophageal spasm. Gastroenterology 77:472–477, 1979.
58. Benjamin SB, Richter JE, Cordova CC, et al.: Pharmacologic provocation in patients with chest pain and suspected esophageal motility dysfunction: a prospective evaluation. Gastroenterology 80:1109 (abstr), 1981.
59. Davies HA, Dart AM, Lowndes RH, et al.: Ergometrine provocation in the diagnosis of oesophageal spasm. Acta Med Scand [Suppl] 644:77–79, 1981.
60. Buxton A, Goldberg S, Hirshfeld JW, et al.: Refractory ergonovine-induced coronary vasospasm: importance of intracoronary nitroglycerin. Am J Cardiol 46:329–334, 1980.
61. DeMeester TR: Wang C-I, Wernley JA, et al.: Technique, indications, and clinical use of 24 hour esophageal pH monitoring. J Thorac Cardiovasc Surg 79:656–670, 1980.
62. Ravich WJ, Klein DB, Schneider W, et al.: Development of a portable pH monitor for ambulatory continuous gastroesophageal reflux studies. Gastroenterology 80:1258 (abstr), 1981.
63. Silverstein BD, Pope CE II: Role of diagnostic tests in esophageal evaluation. Am J Surg 139:744–748, 1980.
64. Orlando RC, Bozymski EM: Clinical and manometric effects of nitroglycerin in diffuse esophageal spasm. N Engl J Med 289:23–24, 1973.
65. Swamy N: Esophageal spasm: clinical and manometric response to nitroglycerine and long-acting nitrates. Gastroenterology 72:23–27, 1977.
66. Mellow MH: The effect of isosorbide and hydralazine on esophageal motility in symptomatic diffuse esophageal spasm. Gastroenterology 80:1229 (abstr), 1981.
67. Richter JE, Sinar DR, Cordova CC, et al.: Verapamil—a potent inhibitor of esophageal peristalsis. Gastroenterology 80:1261 (abstr), 1981.
68. Behar J, Brand DL, Brown FC, et al.: Cimetidine in the treatment of symptomatic gastroesophageal reflux—a double blind controlled trial. Gastroenterology 74: 441–447, 1978.
69. Wesdorp E, Bartelsman J, Pope K, et al.: Oral cimetidine in reflux esophagitis: a double blind controlled trial. Gastroenterology 74:821–824, 1978.

8 | Esophageal Motor Disorders

G. Vantrappen
J. Hellemans

INTRODUCTION

Normal esophageal motility is characterized by peristaltic contractions in the esophageal body and by sphincteric mechanisms at the proximal and distal ends of the tubular esophagus. The main role of primary and secondary peristaltic contraction (provoked by swallowing and local distention respectively) is to transport a swallowed bolus into the stomach and to clear the esophagus from refluxed material. The sphincters function as antireflux barriers that must relax to allow passage of swallowed boluses.

In cases of disordered motility, the peristaltic nature of the contraction may get lost, often resulting in simultaneous pressure waves. The contractions may be too strong or too weak. Repetitive contractions may follow a single swallow, or "spontaneous" motor activity may occur. Sphincters may be hypo- or hypertensive; they may open too easily and allow an abnormal quantity of reflux; they may fail to relax sufficiently so that stasis develops proximally. In most cases of disordered motility several of these abnormalities are combined. However, the combination is not always sufficiently typical and specific to be pathognomonic.

The esophageal motor disorders have been classified as primary or secondary. In primary motor disorders the esophagus is the site of major involvement. Achalasia, diffuse spasm, and related disorders belong to this group. In secondary motor disorders the esophageal abnormalities are due to more generalized neural, muscular, or systemic diseases, to metabolic disturbances, or to inflammatory or tumoral lesions of the esophageal wall. This review will focus on the primary motor disorders.

Achalasia

Definition. Typical achalasia may be defined as a disease of unknown etiology, characterized by absence of peristalsis in the body of the esophagus and failure of an often hypertensive sphincter to relax normally in response to swallowing. Loss of the propulsive peristaltic contractions together with the defective sphincter opening result in stasis of food in a progressively dilating gullet. This esophageal stasis brings about most of the symptoms and complications.

Symptoms. The symptoms are summarized in Fig. 8-1. Dysphagia for liquids and solids is the most prominent symptom and is present in nearly all patients. In our study, 69% of the patients had more trouble with solids than with liquids, 25% did not notice any difference, and only 7% experienced more difficulties with liquids.[1,2] The degree of swallowing difficulties varied considerably from day to day, particularly in the initial stages of the disease. However, the dysphagia tended to get worse with time. Active prandial or postprandial regurgitation (often mistaken for vomiting) occurred in 91% of these patients. Retention of large quantities of food in a dilated esophagus may lead to regurgitation when the patient is in the recumbent position (noticed by 57%) or to aspiration into the airways. Thirty percent of the patients had coughing spells at night, and 7.5% had bronchopulmonary complications. Substernal pain was experienced by 60%. Pain occurs especially in the initial stage of the disease and in cases of vigorous achalasia. The degree of weight loss is related to the severity of the dysphagia.

Manometry. The manometric criteria that must be met are aperistalsis in the body of the esophagus and defective relaxation of the lower esophageal sphincter (LES). In addition, there is an increased sensitivity to cholinergics and to gastrin.

After deglutition, simultaneous pressure waves are recorded throughout the

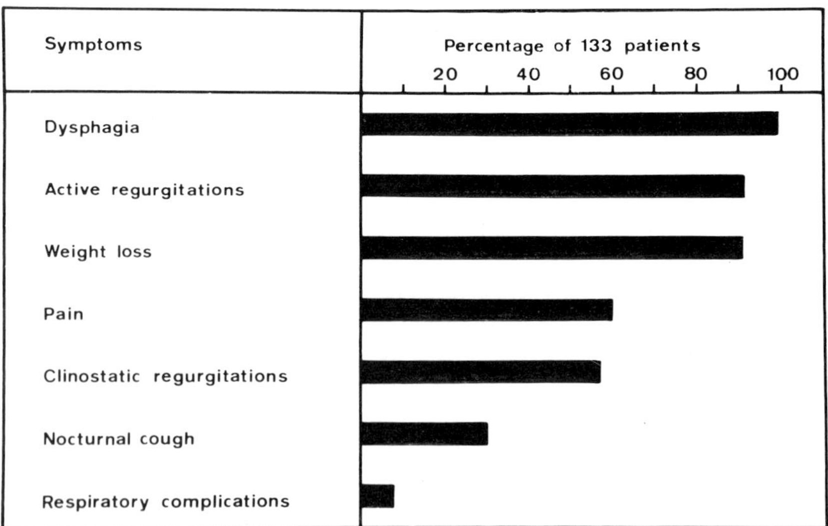

Fig. 8-1. Symptoms of achalasia. From Vantrappen G , Hellemans J , Deloof W et al., Gut 12:268–275, 1971.

esophageal body. In many cases progressive contractions may occur in the upper few centimeters, which probably correspond to the striated muscle part. According to the classic description the presence of (even occasional) normal peristaltic waves excludes the diagnosis of achalasia. However, one wonders if manometry in a dilated esophagus does not overestimate the incidence of nonperistaltic contraction. It is possible that weak peristaltic contractions produce simultaneous pressure peaks in a widely dilated gullet. After treatment the esophageal diameter decreases and (occasional) peristaltic contractions reappear in nearly one-third of the patients.[3] Perhaps this third represents patients in the initial stages of the disease.

When the esophagus becomes dilated, the amplitude of the pressure waves decreases. The pressure waves then become rather typically broad-based in shape (Fig. 8-2). Absence of any mechanical contraction may indicate muscle changes secondary to dilation or may represent advanced degeneration of intramural neurons.[4] In cases of "vigorous" achalasia,[5] the amplitude of the contractions is high, the pressure waves are repetitive, and spontaneous contractions occur. The motility of the esophageal body and some clinical features resemble the pattern of symptomatic diffuse esophageal spasm (SDES). However, peristaltic waves are not seen, and the sphincteric relaxations are defective. The vigorous character may persist, or it may disappear spontaneously. In some cases it seems to be determined by esophageal stasis, since in 19 of 32 patients the vigorous character disappeared after pneumatic dilatation whereas it did not disappear in six cases of SDES.[3]

The resting pressure of the LES is increased.[6] Pressures above 30 mm Hg have been measured in 40%[7] to 90%[6] of the patients. In achalasia patients, the sphincter relaxes incompletely ($\pm$ 30% relaxation) after swallowing, whereas a normal sphincter relaxes completely (to the level of the pressure in the gastric fundus). The residual LES pressure seems responsible for obstructing passage from the esophagus into the stomach.[6,8]

Radiology. Cineradiography may visualize the absence of peristaltic contraction waves and the disorganized and nonpropulsive nature of the contractions. Because the LES fails to open normally following deglutition, the head of the barium column takes a smoothly tapered "bird-beak" appearance, which is rather characteristic although not entirely specific.[9] The esophageal body becomes dilated and eventually elongated; the gastric air bulb disappears. In approximately 20% of cases, there is a symmetrical or asymmetrical dilation in the narrowed sphincter zone that may simulate an ulcer niche.[1]

Nonidiopathic Achalasia. Chagas' disease closely resembles idiopathic achalasia in many respects. Clinical symptoms, manometric and radiologic findings, and pharmacologic responses are similar. The main difference is the involvement of other organs, although clinical manifestation is not always apparent.

Achalasia secondary to a carcinoma has been reported in association with pancreatic, bronchogenic, and gastric cancer[10-12] and with lymphoma of the distal esophagus.[13] The manometric features are identical with those in idiopathic achalasia, but the clinical history is somewhat different. Patients are usually about 50 years of age (mean age 65 years), have a history of dysphagia of short duration (less than 1 year), and weight loss is prominent.[12] The mechanism of this achalasia

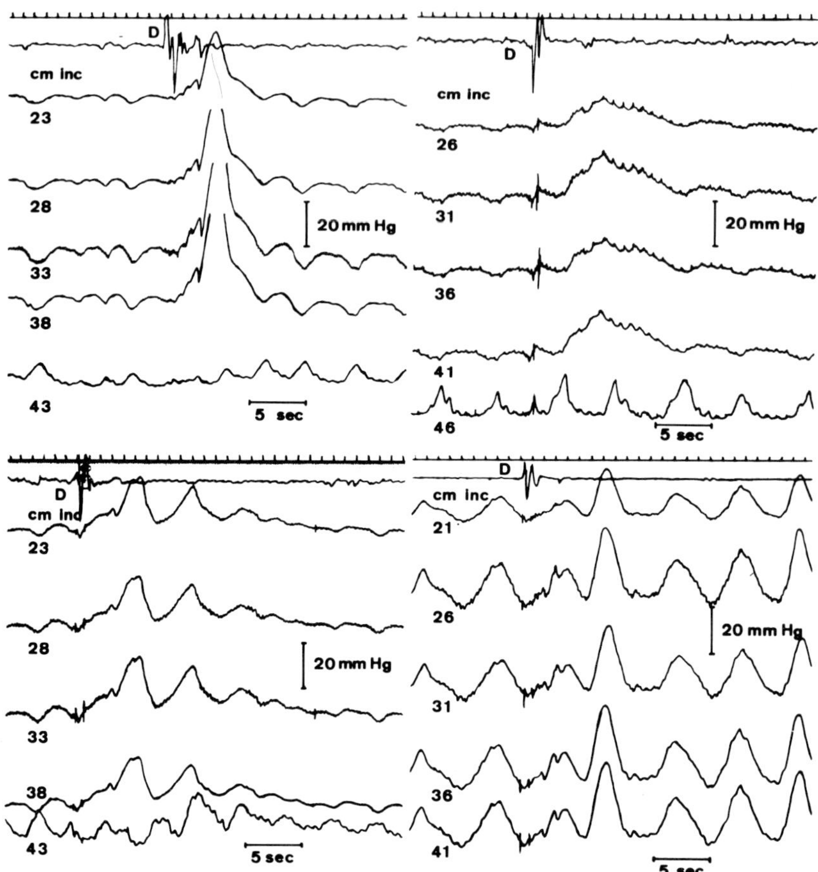

Fig. 8-2. Deglutitive pressure patterns in patients with achalasia. Upper left. Simultaneous pressure peaks after deglutition. Upper right. Pressure waves decrease in amplitude and become wider when the esophagus dilates. Lower figures. Repetitive waves. The tracing at the right is from a patient with vigorous achalasia. Cm. inc., centimeters from incisors. D, deglutition signal. Reproduced with permission from Vantrappen G, Hellemans J: Achalasia. In Vantrappen G, Hellemans J (eds): Diseases of the Esophagus, Springer-Verlag, New York, 1974, p. 877.

is not firmly established. Tumors of the esophageal wall can destroy the myenteric plexus,[14] induce a peripheral neuropathy,[13] or produce a distal obstruction with aperistalsis as a nonspecific reaction.[12] Peristalsis may return after successful treatment or removal of the tumor.[13,15]

Intermediate Achalasia-related Motility Disorders. Although achalasia and SDES have distinctive properties, a number of cases do not fit into this simple classification. In patients who would otherwise fit the criteria of achalasia, occasional peristaltic waves and/or sphincter relaxations have been reported.[5,16,17] Up to 24% of patients with motility disorders that were severe enough to justify treatment with dilatation did not fit well into the two classic entities (Fig. 8-3).[3] After dilata-

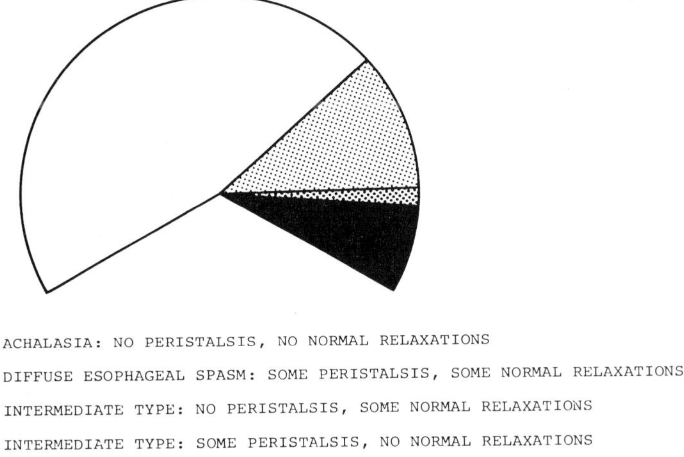

Fig. 8-3.   Spectrum of motility patterns in primary esophageal motility disorders. Reprinted by permission of the publisher from Achalasia, diffuse esophageal spasm, and related motility disorders, by Vantrappen G, Janssens, J, Hellemans, J, Coremans G, Gastroenterology, 76:450–457. Copyright 1979 by the American Gastroenterological Association.

tion, as many as 45% of the patients fell into the "intermediate" categories. These patients presented either with a complete absence of peristalsis and the presence of (at least some) normal LES relaxations or with some degree of peristalsis and complete absence of normal LES relaxation. These observations suggest that the primary esophageal motility disorders constitute a spectrum of motor disorders composed of achalasia, SDES, and intermediate types.[3] Moreover, transition from SDES to achalasia has been documented,[3,18] although most cases of SDES remain unchanged over long periods of time. There also seems to be some relation between SDES and "symptomatic esophageal peristalsis" (SEP) (see section on SEP below). On the other hand, real return of peristalsis after pneumatic dilatation[3,19] may occur.

Do these different syndromes constitute separate entities or do they result from the same degenerative lesion, and are the differences more quantitative than qualitative? The question will probably remain open as long as we do not know the precise neuromuscular defects in achalasia and SDES and as long as we are not able to perform pharmacologic tests on the lesions that are present.

Pathophysiology.   Both vagal and intramural neural pathways seem to be involved in achalasia.[4] Abnormalities have been demonstrated in the dorsal vagal nucleus,[20] in the vagal nerves,[21] in the Auerbach's plexuses, and in the esophageal wall[22,23] and muscle.[20] There is also pharmacologic evidence of denervation. Both the esophageal body[24] and the sphincter[25,26] react strongly upon direct cholinergic stimulation by methacholine (Mecholyl) or carbachol. Extremely dilated and "decompensated" esophagi may fail to react. Interestingly, edrophonium, a cholinesterase inhibitor, also increases the pressure of the LES in achalasia patients. This suggests that some acetylcholine is still released[27] and that complete postganglionic denervation is unlikely.

The sphincter[28] and the esophageal body[29] are also supersensitive to gastrin.

Serum gastrin levels are normal. The mechanism of this gastrin supersensitivity is unknown.[30]

There is some pharmacologic evidence that the nonadrenergic, noncholinergic inhibitory postganglionic nervous system is impaired in achalasia patients. This system mediates the sphincter relaxation in the opossum.[31] It probably also plays a role in the peristaltic progression of the contractions in the esophageal body.[32] Cholecystokinin (CCK) octapeptide induces relaxation in normal subjects but a paradoxical increase in LES pressure in most achalasia patients.[33] The CCK-induced relaxation in a normal sphincter is the result of an indirect effect via inhibitory nonadrenergic nerves to the sphincter that overwhelms a direct excitatory effect on LES smooth muscle.[34] In most achalatic patients, the direct excitatory effect is unmasked because the inhibitory neurons are impaired. Achalasia patients demonstrating relaxation after CCK (1 of 24)[33] may have neural impairment limited to preganglionic fibers. However, CCK also has a stimulating effect on the LES in SDES patients who exhibit complete relaxations after swallowing. This observation is difficult to explain, but it does not necessarily invalidate the interpretation given for achalasia patients.[35]

Treatment.   Current treatment of achalasia is palliative and aims at improving esophageal emptying by reducing the resistance at the cardia sufficiently to allow aboral flow but insufficiently to favor gastroesophageal reflux. Dysphagia is more readily improved than the esophageal stasis iteslf. The crampy pain attacks are more resistant.[36]

Several drugs, such as anticholinergics, short-acting nitrites and gastrointestinal hormones, have been tried but are of doubtful value. Recently interest in drug trials in achalasia patients has been revived. Anticholinergics (e.g. dicyclomine)[37] may lower the LES pressure and improve the dysphagia, but experience in current practice has been disappointing.[38] Long-acting nitrites (e.g. isosorbide) relieved or significantly improved the dysphagia in 19 of 23 patients and reduced sphincter pressures by 66% for more than 1 hour.[39] Nifedipine (30–40 mg/day) gave 70% excellent or good results in a group of 20 patients who were followed for 6–18 months.[40] This confirms previous reports.[41] In contrast, verapamil seems to have no effect on the achalatic sphincter.[42] Prostaglandins of the E-type also decrease the LES pressure in achalasia patients[43] and seem to be worth trying.[44] Most of these drug regimens lower the LES pressure only intermittently in the prandial period. Is this an advantage to prevent reflux during the night? Or does it perpetuate the dangers of esophageal stasis? The series of patients tested are rather small, the follow-up periods are short, and side effects (headache) are noted in a considerable portion of patients. Only trials in larger groups of patients and over a longer period of time will make it clear if drug therapy has its place along with the two currently accepted forms of therapy: forceful dilatation and myotomy.

The literature on dilatation and myotomy has been recently reviewed in detail.[45,46] Forceful dilatations give approximately 77% excellent or good results if recurrences are treated again. In our series 93% of the patients showed improvement. If one follows the policy of dilating only once, the success rate is approximately, 60–65%. Mortality is very low (0.2%), and perforations occur in approximately 2.6% of the patients. These perforations can be treated conservatively in most cases.[47]

Endoscopic myotomy of the lower esophageal circular muscle above the Z-line has recently been advocated. Three to 25 months after the procedure 88% of 17 patients had excellent to good results.[48] Further experience is needed. Surgical myotomy yields excellent or good results in 64–88% of the patients, with a very low mortality. The overall incidence of serious surgical complications amounts to 3–4%.[49,50] Persistent dysphagia is due to incomplete section of the circular muscle or to reflux esophagitis and peptic stricture.[51,52] The incidence of reflux esophagitis has been sufficiently high for most surgeons to combine the Heller myotomy procedure with an antireflux operation. Good to excellent results are reported in 54–100% of the patients treated by the combined procedure. The need for these combined operations and the type of procedure remain controversial. Large series with sufficiently long follow-up are very important for evaluating the results. Patients may develop a recurrence of symptoms many years after treatment. The reason for this late recurrence is unknown but may be related to slow progression of the degenerative process of nervous structures. Symptomatic reflux and stenosis may appear after a long time. In a recent study[53] the incidence of symptomatic reflux increased from 24% after 1 year to 48% after 10 years and stabilized at 52% after 13 years.

Few studies have compared the results of dilatation and myotomy. Some find equally good results for both,[54,55] but the majority suggest that surgical treatment yields better results.[38,50,56,57] In some of these studies, however, the results of dilatation are obviously less good than what can be achieved. In some such study[56] 6% of the dilated patients suffered a perforation, and 33% failed to show any degree of improvement. In the other series[38] only 46% of the patients did well 1 year after pneumatic bag dilatation versus 85% of the 24 surgically treated patients. The largest series of patients was described by the Mayo group. Okike et al.[50] found better late results in 468 myotomized patients (97% with follow-up) than Sanderson et al.[58] in 408 patients (only 76% with follow-up) treated with hydrostatic dilatation. The mean follow-up period of the surgical group (6.5 years) was considerably shorter than that of the dilated group (9.5 years). This may explain at least part of the different outcome. The 85% excellent or good results after surgery, obtained in spite of only 3% severe reflux esophagitis, have obviously not been reproduced by those surgeons who insist upon the necessity of an additional antireflux procedure.

The only prospective and randomized study compares 18 dilated and 20 myotomized patients, with a mean follow-up period of 42–43 months.[57] Excellent or good results (adverse symptoms, at most occasional mild dysphagia) were obtained in 100% of the patients who underwent surgery and in only 60% of those who underwent dilatation. Sphincter pressures were decreased by 75% after myotomy and by only 49% by dilatation. The gastroesophageal junction had a larger diameter as shown by x-ray, in the surgically treated patients. However, a test for provoked acid reflux was positive in 31% of the group who underwent surgery and in only 7% of those treated with dilatation. This carefully evaluated series of patients certainly deserve to be followed further, particularly in view of the higher incidence of reflux in patients who underwent surgery.

One factor that is largely unknown is the true incidence of pathologic reflux, reflux esophagitis, and its complications after both procedures, but the currently available evidence suggests that the problem is far more important after surgery than after dilatation. Another important parameter for evaluating the therapeutic results is the degree of esophageal stasis that remains years after treatment. Radiologic techniques for measuring this parameter are difficult to standardize, because of the great variation in size and shape of the gullet and of the apparently unpredictable variability in the emptying pattern. Recently a scintigraphic method has been proposed that allows construction of an esophageal emptying curve. This may prove to be a useful tool for quantitative analysis.[59]

Although many advocate myotomy as the primary treatment,[50,57,58] we consider that it is justified to reserve operation for those patients in whom dilatation fails or is contraindicated. In experienced hands the results of dilatation are much better and the complication rate much lower than has been quoted in some (mainly small) series, and the incidence of peptic stricture is only 0.7% in a series of 403 patients.[46] Good to excellent "palliation" is possible in 65–75% of patients with achalasia without thoracotomy.[60]

Symptomatic Diffuse Esophageal Spasm (SDES)

Definition. SDES is characterized by clinical symptoms of intermittent chest pain, dysphagia, or both in the absence of a demonstrable organic lesion and by abnormal nonperistaltic contractions on manometry or radiological examination.[8,44,61-63] To make a diagnosis of SDES, three conditions must be fulfilled: clinical symptoms should be present, organic lesions should have been excluded, and the motor disorder of the esophagus should meet certain criteria.[8,44]

In asymptomatic subjects, motor disturbances may occur that closely resemble those found in SDES.[44,64] It is not known in what respect symptomatic subjects are different and to what extent the motor disorders in both groups can be distinguished by other means than by a Methacholine test. Therefore the term "asymptomatic diffuse spasm"[65,66] should be used with caution. Some authors[67] take the view that DES is not a well-defined disease but rather a motility disorder that can be caused by several conditions.

One of the main problems is the relation between DES and acid sensitivity of the esophagus.[44,68,69] As long as the basic neuromuscular defect of SDES cannot be demonstrated, it seems wise to limit the diagnosis to patients in whom other lesions (such as reflux disease) have been excluded. Moreover the secondary motor disturbances, for example in reflux esophagitis, are not identical with those found in SDES.

Symptoms. Most patients have pain and dysphagia. Of the 46 patients with severe symptoms reported by Ellis et al.[70] 15 had pain only, 24 had pain and dysphagia, and 7 only dysphagia. The symptoms are intermittent and vary from mild and occasional to severe and daily. In approximately half of the instances, the pain is precipitated by a meal, is often associated with dysphagia, and may worsen during periods of emotional stress.[71] The pain may closely mimic angina pectoris. Both types of pain are relieved by nitroglycerin. However, dysphagia is not a symptom of angina.

Gastroesophageal reflux may also provoke pain rather than heartburn. The dysphagia is of variable severity and lacks the persistance seen in achalasia or organic stenoses. It occurs after intake of both fluids and solids. The belief that cold or carbonated fluids precipitate symptoms has not been documented very well. Food impaction,[72] syncope on swallowing,[65,73] and weight loss caused by fear of eating[61] have been described but are rather exceptional.

Manometry. SDES affects mainly the distal half or two-thirds of the esophageal body. Although some swallows produce normal peristaltic contraction waves, the typical deglutitive response in this part of the gullet consists of nonsequential pressure peaks of high amplitude and long duration, which may or may not be repetitive.[67,74,75] Two-thirds of the patients have normal LES function.[64] Recently, interrupted peristalsis and abnormally slow distal propagation have been described.[63] However, the manometric abnormalities found in different patients are variable, and there are no uniform or generally accepted criteria for manometric diagnosis of SDES.[63] The following criteria are generally considered:

Simultaneous contractions. Although the esophagus retains its capability of producing some peristaltic waves, these contractions are frequently nonperistaltic in the lower half of the gullet. However nonperistaltic waves can be seen in patients with reflux,[76] in those with neuropathies,[77,78] in the elderly,[79,80] and even in normal persons.[81] The mere presence of simultaneous contractions is not a sufficient diagnostic criterion. A minimum of 30% high-amplitude nonperistaltic contractions has been proposed as a diagnostic criterion.[64] Others propose that at least 30% of responses to swallowing should be abnormal (simultaneous and/or repetitive contractions of high amplitude and duration).[82] If all pressure waves are nonsequential and some deglutitions are followed by normal sphincter relaxations or if the sphincter relaxations are absent or incomplete and some sequential pressure waves occur in the body of the esophagus, the esophageal motor disorder is of the intermediate type.[3] If all contractions are peristaltic but of increased amplitude and duration and if they correlate with clinical symptoms, the disorder can be called "symptomatic esophageal peristalsis" (SEP, see below).

Contractions of high amplitude and duration. Peristaltic or simultaneous "giant" waves have long been recognized as typical for DES.[74] A mean esophageal contraction duration of 7.5 sec has been proposed as a criterion for SDES because this value is greater than 2 standard deviations (SD).[69,82] The high amplitude of the contractions is less well documented, since the less accurate high-compliance systems that were used in many previous studies underestimate the pressures generated in the esophagus.[83] If miniature intraesophageal pressure transducers are used, deglutitive pressure peaks in the lower two-thirds of the esophagus reach mean values of 70 mm Hg with dry swallows and of 123 mm Hg with a water bolus.[84,85] A low compliance perfusion system registers mean peristaltic amplitudes of 81 ± 15 mm Hg[69] for wet swallows and maximal peristaltic amplitudes varying between 75 and 175 mm Hg in 40 normal individuals. There are only few reports document-

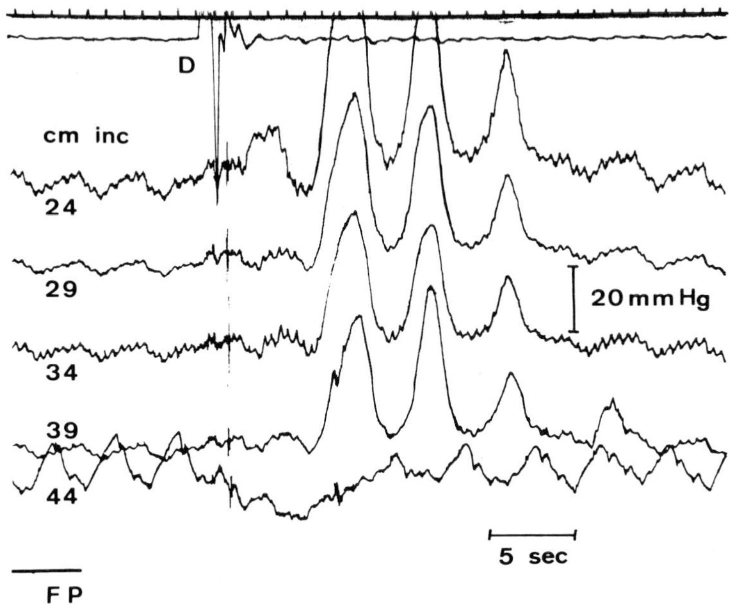

Fig. 8-4. Deglutitive pressures in patient with diffuse esophageal spasm. Reproduced with permission from Vantrappen G, Hellemans J: Diffuse esophageal spasm. In Vantrappen G and Hellemans J (eds): Diseases of the Esophagus, Springer-Verlag, New York, 1974: 361.

ing how high the "high-amplitude contractions" really are in SDES. With a low-compliance perfusion system and a water bolus, mean pressure values of 104 ± 49 mm Hg[29] and 140 ± 17 mm Hg[30] have been reported. However, the amplitude and the duration are not increased in every patient with SDES.[63] In Cohen's criteria "high-amplitude" simultaneous contractions need not to be higher than peristaltic contractions of normal subjects. The amplitude of the simultaneous contractions is higher in SDES than in gastroesophageal reflux.[8,44,82] This and the low LES pressures in reflux may help to distinguish SDES from reflux disease.

Repetitive waves.   Repetitive contractions (two or more pressure waves in response to a single swallow) occurred in nine of the 16 patients of Roth and Fleshler[65] and in all but one of the 21 reported by Gillies et al.[61] According to Castell[83] such contractions are the most typical aspect of esophageal spasm. The entire complex of repetitive waves may be simultaneous, the first wave may be peristaltic and may be followed by a series of simultaneous waves, or a distal peak may be simultaneous with the second pressure wave that is recorded on a more proximal pressure sensor (see below, "slow distal propagation"). "Spontaneous" esophageal contractions (not related to a swallow) occur in more than half of these patients.[82]

Interrupted peristalsis and abnormally slow distal propagation.   Interrupted peristalsis—defined as a simultaneous rise in pressure at two or more proximaly recording points, with a later pressure rise at a distal recording point—was observed in 7 of 12 SDES patients. In six of them and in one other patient the apparent distal propagation in the distal esophageal segment was slowed down to only 0.8–1.5 cm/sec (the minimal value in normal subjects is 2.1 cm/sec). Both abnormalities were found to occur intermittently.[63] They possibly reflect failure of normal lumen obliteration during esophageal contraction in an esophageal segment.

LES.   Most patients with SDES have a normal LES pressure and complete LES relaxation on swallowing. The relaxation was impaired in 10 of 27 patients and a hypertensive sphincter was found in 9 (33%) of them.[64] Incomplete sphincter relaxations occurred more frequently (8 of 12 patients) in another series of individuals with SDES-like disturbances.[63] Some authors even hesitate to accept the diagnosis of SDES when the LES relaxation is incomplete.[29,30,63,82] Whether the finding of a "complete" manometric relaxation means that the sphincter opens normally or merely indicates that the LES has relaxed to the point where its minimal diameter is as great as that of the recording catheter[63] is an interesting point that cannot be answered at the present time. If the hypothesis is correct that some patients with apparently normal manometric relaxations open their sphincters incompletely and that many apparently simultaneous pressure waves are to be ascribed to a common cavity phenomenon, the two main features that distinguish SDES from achalasia would become very questionable. To eliminate the other possibility, that spastic esophageal body contractions displace the sphincter and cause "pseudo-relaxations," a number of these patients should be examined with a sleeve.[86]

Sphincter disorders may occur as apparently isolated motor abnormalities in patients with clinical symptoms of substernal or high epigastric pain or dysphagia. Several abnormalities have been described: hypertensive sphincter[87-89] and hyper-reacting or hypercontracting sphincter.[90] However, the amplitude of the peristaltic esophageal contraction was increased[7] or was not measured accurately, so that some of these cases might belong to the "symptomatic esophageal peristalsis" group.

Individual patients do not necessarily have all the manometric features described above; in fact, most of them do not. Some patients have almost identical motility patterns on different manometric examination.[82] On the other hand, loss of peristalsis and of LES relaxations over a period of a few months or years has been observed, and this manometric evolution may be accompanied by corresponding changes in the radiologic picture.[3,18] Repeated manometric studies in patients with "typical" manometric tracings may fail to reproduce the typical abnormalities.[29]

Provocative Tests.   The lack of strict diagnostic criteria, the need to distinguish SDES from achalasia on the one hand and from nonspecific or asymptomatic motor disorders on the other, makes provocative tests highly desirable. A provocative test would be extremely useful in patients with chest pain, in whom no coronary disease can be demonstrated and in whom the radiologic and manometric findings do not prove a motility disorder.

Most authors perform manometric examination with a water bolus, and this seems a reasonable policy,[74] because it reduces the number of non peristaltic waves in normal individuals[91,92] and probably also in those with nonspecific motor disorders. There are no data comparing "dry" and "wet" swallows in patients with SDES. It is generally believed that in these patients the intake of cold fluids may elicit clinical symptoms and the appearance of high-amplitude, repetitive pressure waves of long duration,[8] but hard facts for this belief are lacking.[83] The esophagus of many patients with SDES is hypersensitive to cholinergics such as methacholine,[66,93] betanechol,[82] or carbachol[94]—the latter two drugs have fewer cardiovascular side effects than methacholine—and is also hypersensitive to a cholinesterase inhibitor, edrophonium chloride.[82] The methacholine test, however, is also positive in patients with primary achalasia, those with Chagas' disease, and in some patients with carcinomatous infiltration of Auerbach's plexus.[14] The test can be useful to distinguish SDES from asymptomatic similar motor disorders[66] and from reflux-related spasm.[82]

Patients with SDES have been found to respond to subcutaneously injected pentragastrin with a marked increase in amplitude and duration of esophageal contractions.[30,94] In healthy persons there is no such effect on esophageal peristalsis.[84,94] Other investigators found only an increase in amplitude but not in duration[29] or no exaggerated response at all.[95] In some patients repetitive contractions[30,94] and clinical symptoms[29,94] developed after a pentagastrin bolus. Continuous infusion of pentagastrin, in both physiologic and pharmacologic range, had only small effects on contraction amplitude and duration in SDES patients,[96] and intravenous infusion of gastrin G17 in a dose that mimicked postprandial gastrin concentrations had no significant effect at all.[30] In a group of 22 patients with clinically suspected esophageal motor disorders, the pentagastrin test was disappointing, since none of the 10 patients with a final diagnosis of SDES developed dysphagia, chest pain, repetitive waves, or increased esophageal pressure.[29] Moreover, the test is also positive in patients with achalasia[29] and in some elderly patients.[97]

There is need for a provocative test that induces SDES in patients with chest pain or dysphagia and radiologic or manometric data that do not meet the criteria of SDES. There is also a need for a pharmacologic test that gives some idea about the degree of denervation. The available data indicate that the pentagastrin test is not the diagnostic test that is needed. Ergonovine maleate, an alpha-adrenergic agonist has been used as a provocative test for coronary artery spasm[98] and for esophageal spasm.[99] However, serious side-effects may occur. In a group of 13 patients, ergonovine induced chest pain without any localized coronary artery spasm or electrocardiographic or metabolic evidence of myocardial ischemia. In these patients subsequent manometry showed that their pain was associated with esophageal spasm.[99] No evidence for a generalized sensitivity to alpha-adrenergic stimulation could be demonstrated in SDES patients.[100]

Radiology.   Roentgenographic study reveals segmental lumen-obliterating contractions. The radiologic appearances of SDES are described as "curling," "segmental spasm," "ladder spasm," "rosary bead esophagus," "spastic pseudo-diverticulosis," "corkscrew esophagus," "diffuse spasm," etc. Often the barium is trapped and pushed back and forth before entering the stomach. This is best demonstrated when the patient is in the recumbent position. A second, but less common, appearance is a tight contraction of the esophagus over a length of several centimeters or a slight diffuse narrowing of the lower half of the esophagus with a slightly dilated upper segment.[62] Marked dilation of the esophagus and prolonged stasis of food and fluids are rare in diffuse spasm. In many cases the esophageal wall is thickened[101,102] because of muscular hypertrophy.[103]

The extent and severity of radiologic abnormalities may vary widely from patient to patient and from one time to another in the same patient.[67] The severity of the radiologic changes correlates poorly with the clinical, manometric or pathologic findings.[61] Patients with SDES may appear normal on routine radiological examination,[65,74,102,103] and "typical" radiologic pictures may occur in asymptomatic, mainly elderly, patients or in patients with SDES at a symptom-free moment.[44]

Treatment. Other causes of disordered esophageal motility and of gastroesophageal reflux must be excluded first. Drug treatment of SDES is still disappointing. Anticholinergics and nitrites[102,104] have been used with moderate success. In one trial isosorbide or hydralazine did not affect amplitude or duration of esophageal contraction, but hydralazine resulted in a significant inhibition of the spastic response to betanechol and of the resulting chest pain.[105] Nifedipine led to a decrease of contraction frequency lasting for more than 60 min. Neither the amplitude nor the pattern of contraction were affected.[41]

If patients with severe symptoms fail to respond to medical therapy, pneumatic dilatations can be performed. This treatment is clearly less successful than in achalasia[45] and influences the dysphagia rather than the pain.

Severe cases can benefit from a long esophagomyotomy[61,70,103,106] extending to just above the level of involvement of the esophagus muscle (usually to the level of the aortic arch)[103] or even higher.[102,106] Here again the results obtained in achalasia patients cannot be equalled. The procedure can be completed by an antireflux procedure.[102,107] However, some caution has been exercised against the routine addition of an anti-reflux procedure, except in cases of hiatal hernia.[103] The question has been raised (but not answered) concerning whether SDES patients with a normotensive relaxing or a hypertensive sphincter with incomplete relaxations deserve a different approach.[103,108]

Symptomatic Esophageal Peristalsis (SEP)

Definition. The development of measurement systems able to pick up rapid pressure rises has enabled different investigators to identify patients with angina-like chest pain that is caused by peristaltic contractions of increased amplitude or duration. This condition ("nutcracker esophagus") was found to be more frequent than SDES or achalasia in patients with thoracic pain.[69,109,110] Brand et al.[68] examined 43 patients with chest pain but no evidence for coronary heart disease. Of the 14 patients with pain of esophageal origin one had achalasia and three met the criteria for diffuse spasm, but nine had disorders of amplitude and one a disorder of duration of peristalsis. Similar cases of SEP with increased amplitude or duration have been described by others.[69,111] Increased amplitude and duration occur together in most cases. Brand et al.[68] observed only one patient with isolated increased duration of peristalsis whereas increased duration frequently occurs in high-amplitude patients[68] and vice versa.[111]

During the test the chest pain bears a direct relationship to the amplitude of the peristaltic wave. The sequence of a completely normal manometric tracing during an asymptomatic period followed by an abnormal tracing during an episode of chest pain was seen in a few patients.[68]

Manometry. Criteria proposed for the diagnosis of SEP are a mean amplitude above 120 mm Hg in the lower third of the esophagus[69,109] or a peak pressure about 200 mm Hg.[69] A reasonable criterion for prolonged contraction seems to be a duration time that equals or exceeds the normal mean + 2 SD (i.e., 7.5 sec).[69,82] The mean value in a group of 22 patients with prolonged peristalsis was 7.8 sec.[111] The relationship of SEP to reflux and to SDES is still to be defined. Some patients improve with antacids[68] or develop a manometric tracing consistent with SDES after acid perfusion.[69]

Ergonovine, by acting via an alpha-adrenergic receptor, precipitates the pain in these patients. These pain attacks are time-related to the occurrence of high-amplitude and long-duration peristaltic waves.[110] Nitroglycerine did not change these waves.[112]

REFERENCES

1. Vantrappen G, Hellemans J, Deloof W, Vandenbroucke J: Treatment of achalasia with pneumatic dilatations. Gut 12:268–275, 1971.
2. Vantrappen G, Hellemens J: Achalasia. In Vantrappen G, Hellemans J (eds): Diseases of the Esophagus, Springer-Verlag, New York, Heidelberg, Berlin, 1974.
3. Vantrappen G, Janssens J, Hellemans J, Coremans G: Achalasia, diffuse esophageal spasm, and related motility disorders. Gastroenterology 76:450–457, 1979.
4. Goyal RK: Pathophysiology of achalasia and diffuse esophageal spasm. In American Gastroenterological Association: Postgraduate Course. The Neuromuscular Disorders of the Gastrointestinal Tract, New York, 1981.
5. Sanderson DR, Ellis FH Jr, Schlegel JF, Olsen AM: Syndrome of vigorous achalasia: clinical and physiologic observations. Dis Chest 52:508–517, 1967.
6. Cohen S, Lipshutz W: Lower esophageal sphincter dysfunction in achalasia. Gastroenterology 61:814–820, 1971.
7. Berger K, McCallum RW: The hypertensive lower esophageal sphincter: a clinical and manometric entity. Gastroenterology 80:1109, 1981.
8. Cohen S: Motor disorders of the esophagus. New Engl J Med 301:184–192, 1979.
9. Dodds WJ, Harell GS: Motility disorders. In Margulis AR, Burhenne J (eds): Alimentary Tract Roentgenology, CV Mosby, St. Louis, 1973.
10. Kolodny M, Schrader ZR, Rubin W, et al.: Esophageal achalasia probably due to gastric carcinoma. Ann Intern Med 69:569–573, 1968.
11. Shulze KS, Goresky CA, Jabbari M, Lough JO: Esophageal achalasia associated with gastric carcinoma: lack of evidence for widespread plexus destruction. Can Med Assoc J 112:857–864, 1975.
12. Tucker HJ, Snape WJ Jr, Cohen S: Achalasia secondary to carcinoma: manometric and clinical features. Ann Intern Med 89:315–318, 1978.
13. Davis JA, Kantrowitz PA, Chandler HL, Schatzki SC: Reversible achalasia due to reticulum cell sarcoma. N Engl J Med 293:130–132, 1975.
14. Herrera AF, Colon J, Valdes-Dapena A, Roth JLA: Achalasia or carcinoma? The significance of the Mecholyl test. Am J Dig Dis 15:1073–1081, 1970.

15. Kline MM: Successful treatment of vigourous achalasia associated with gastric lymphoma. Dig Dis Sci 25:311–313, 1980.
16. Moersch HJ, Code CF, Olsen AM: Dyschalasia of the esophagus. Coll Papers Mayo Clin 49:19–27, 1957.
17. Hogan WF, Caflisch CR, Winship DH: Unclassified oesophageal motor disorders simulating achalasia. Gut 10:234–240, 1969.
18. Kramer P, Harris LD, Donaldson RM Jr: Transition from symptomatic diffuse spasm to cardiospasm. Gut 8: 115–119, 1967.
19. Mellow MH: Return of esophageal peristalsis in idiopathic achalasia. Gastroenterology 70:1148–1151, 1976.
20. Cassella RR, Brown AL Jr, Sayre GP, Ellis FH Jr: Achalasia of the esophagus: pathologic and etiologic considerations. Ann Surg 160:474–486, 1964.
21. Cassella RR, Ellis FH Jr, Brown AL: Fine-structure changes in achalasia of the esophagus. I. Vagus nerves. Am J Pathol 46:279–288, 1965.
22. Trounce JR, Deuchar DC, Kauntze R, Thomas GA: Studies in achalasia of the cardia. Q J Med 26:433–443, 1957.
23. Misiewicz JJ, Waller SL, Anthony PP, Gummer JWP: Achalasia of the cardia: pharmacology and histopathology of isolated cardiac sphincteric muscle from patients with and without achalasia. Q J Med 38:17–30, 1969.
24. Kramer P, Ingelfinger FJ: Esophageal sensitivity to Mecholyl in cardiospasm. Gastroenterology 19:242–253, 1951.
25. Heitmann P, Espinoza J, Csendes A: Physiology of the distal esophagus in achalasia. Scand J Gastroenterol 4:1–11, 1969.
26. Cohen BR, Guelrud M: Cardiospasm in achalasia: demonstration of supersensitivity of the lower esophageal sphincter. Gastroenterology 60:769, 1971.
27. Cohen S, Fisher R, Tuch A: The site of denervation in achalasia. Gut 13:556–558, 1972.
28. Cohen S, Lipshutz W, Hughes W: Role of gastrin supersensitivity in the pathogenesis of lower esophageal sphincter hypertension in achalasia. J Clin Invest 50:1241–1247, 1971.
29. Orlando RC, Bozymski EM: The effects of pentagastrin in achalasia and diffuse esophageal spasm. Gastroenterology 77:472–477, 1979.
30. Lane WH, Ippoliti AF, McCallum RW: Effect of gastrin heptadecapeptide (G17) on oesophageal contractions in patients with diffuse oesophageal spasm. Gut 20:756–759, 1979.
31. Goyal RK, Rattan S: Neurohumoral, hormonal, and drug receptors for the lower esophageal sphincter. Gastroenterology 84:589–619, 1978.
32. Diamant NE, El-Sharkawy TY: Neural control of esophageal peristalsis. a conceptional analysis. Gastroenterology 72:546–556, 1977.
33. Dodds WJ, Dent J, Hogan WJ, et al.: Paradoxical lower esophageal sphincter contraction induced by cholecystokinin-octapeptide in patients with achalasia. Gastroenterology 80:327–333, 1980.
34. Behar J, Biancani P: Effect of cholecystokinin-octapeptide on lower esophageal sphincter. Gastroenterology 73:57–61, 1977.
35. Ippoliti AF, Varner AA: Does denervation of the lower esophageal sphincter occur in diffuse esophageal spasm? In Christensen J (ed): Gastrointestinal Motility, Raven Press, New York, 1980.
36. Menzies-Gow N, Gummer JWP, Edwards DAW: Results of Heller's operation for achalasia of the cardia. Br J Surg, 65:483–485, 1978.
37. Lobis IF, Fisher RS: Anticholinergic therapy for achalasia. A controlled trial. Gastroenterology 70:977, 1976.

38. Yon J, Christensen J: An uncontrolled comparison of treatments for achalasia. Ann Surg 182:672–676, 1975.
39. Gelfond M, Rozen P, Keren S, Gilat T: Effect of nitrates on LOS pressure in achalasia: a potential therapeutic acid. Gut 22:312–318, 1981.
40. Bortolotti M, Labó G: Clinical and manometric effects of nifedipine in patients with esophageal achalasia. Gastroenterology 80:39–44, 1981.
41. Weiser HF, Lepsien G, Golenhofen K, Siewert R: Clinical and experimental studies on the effect of nifedipine on smooth muscle of the esophagus and LES. In Duthie HL (ed): Gastrointestinal Motility in Health and Disease, MTP Press Limited, Lancaster, 1978.
42. Becker BS, Burskoff R: Differential effect of verapamil on LESP in normal subjects and those with achalasia. Gastroenterology 80:1107, 1981.
43. Goyal RK, Mukhopadhyay A, Rattan S: Effect of prostaglandin E on the lower esophageal sphincter in normal subjects and patients with achalasia. Clin Research 23:358A, 1974.
44. Castell DO: Achalasia and diffuse esophageal spasm. Arch Intern Med 136:571–579, 1976.
45. Vantrappen G, Hellemans J: Treatment of achalasia and related motor disorders. Gastroenterology 79:144–154, 1980.
46. Vantrappen G: Treatment of primary esophageal motility disorders. In American Gastroenterological Association: Postgraduate Course. The Neuromuscular Disorders of the Gastrointestinal Tract, New York, 1981.
47. Vantrappen G, Hellemans J, Coremans G: Perforation of the cardia by penumatic dilatations can be treated by conservative means. Gut 21:A456–A457, 1980.
48. Ortega JA, Madureri V, Perez L: Endoscopic myotomy in the treatment of achalasia. Gastrointest Endosc 26:8–10, 1980.
49. Ellis FH Jr, Olsen AM: Achalasia of the esophagus. In Dunphy E (consulting ed.): Major Problems in Clinical Surgery. WB Saunders, Philadelphia, London, Toronto, 1969.
50. Okike N, Payne WS, Neufeld DM, et al.: Esophagotomy versus forceful dilation for achalasia of the esophagus: results in 899 patients. Ann Thorac Surg 28:119–125, 1979.
51. Patrick DL, Payne WS, Olsen AM, Ellis FH Jr: Reoperation for achalasia of the esophagus. Arch Surg 103:122–128, 1971.
52. Nelems JMB, Cooper JD, Pearson FG: Treatment of achalasia: esophagotomy with antireflux procedure. Can J Surg 23:588–589, 1980.
53. Jara FM, Toledo-Pereyra LH, Lewis JW, Magilligan DJ Jr: Long-term results of esophagomyotomy for achalasia of esophagus. Arch Surg 114:935–936, 1979.
54. Bennett JR, Hendrix TR: Treatment of achalasia with pneumatic dilatation. In Bayless TM (guest ed.): Management of Esophageal Disease. Modern Treatment Vol 7, no. 6, Harper & Row, New York 1970.
55. Spitzer G, Hessler C, Sailer FX: Therapie des Kardiospasmus und ihre Spätergebnisse. Med Welt 24:1256–1259, 1973.
56. Arvanitakis C: Achalasia of the esophagus. A reappraisal of esophagomyotomy vs forceful pneumatic dilation. Dig Dis 20:841–846, 1975.
57. Csendes A, Velasco N, Braghetto I, Henriquez A: A prospective randomized study comparing forceful dilatation and esophagomyotomy in patients with achalasia of the esophagus. Gastroenterology 80:789–795, 1981.
58. Sanderson DR, Ellis FH Jr, Olsen AM: Achalasia of the esophagus: results of therapy by dilation, 1950–1967. Chest 58:116–121, 1970.

59. Tolin RD, Malmud LS, Reilley J, Fisher RS: Esophageal scintigraphy to quantitate esophageal transit. Gastroenterology 76:1402–1408, 1979.
60. Orringer MB: The treatment of achalasia: controversy resolved? Ann Thorac Surg 28:100–102, 1979.
61. Gillies M, Nicks R, Skyring A: Clinical, manometric, and pathological studies in diffuse oesophageal spasm. Br Med J 2:527–530, 1967.
62. Vantrappen G, Hellemans J: Diffuse muscle spasm of the oesophagus and the hypertensive lower oesophageal sphincter. Clin gastroenterol 5:59–72, 1976.
63. Kaye MD: Anomalies of peristalsis in idiopathic diffuse oesophageal spasm. Gut 22:217–222, 1981.
64. DiMarino AJ Jr, Cohen S: Characteristics of lower esophageal sphincter function in symptomatic diffuse esophageal spasm. Gastroenterology 66:1–6, 1974.
65. Roth HP, Fleshler B: Diffuse esophageal spasm. Ann Intern Med 61:914–923, 1964.
66. Kramer P, Fleshler B, McNally E, Harris LD: Oesophageal sensitivity to Mecholyl in symptomatic diffuse spasm. Gut 8:120–127, 1967.
67. Bennett JR, Hendrix TR: Diffuse esophageal spasm: a disorder with more than one cause. Gastroenterology 59:273–279, 1970.
68. Brand DL, Martin D, Pope CE: Esophageal manometrics in patients with angina-like chest pain. Dig Dis 22:300–304, 1977.
69. Benjamin SB, Gerhardt DC, Castell DO: High Amplitude peristaltic esophageal contractions associated with chest pain and/or dysphagia. Gastroenterology 77:478–483, 1979.
70. Ellis FH Jr, Olsen AM, Schlegel JF, Code CF: Surgical treatment of esophageal hypermotility disturbances. JAMA 188:862–866, 1964.
71. Cohen S, Snape WJ: The Role of psychophysiological factors in disorders of oesophageal function. Clin Gastroenterol 6:569–579, 1977.
72. Creamer B: Motor disturbances of the esophagus. In Code CF (ed): Handbook of physiology; Sec 6, Alimentary Canal; Vol 4, Motility, American Physiological Society, Washington DC, 1968.
73. Alstrup P, Pedersen SA: A case of syncope on swallowing secondary to diffuse oesophageal spasm. Acta Med Scand 193:365–368, 1973.
74. Creamer B, Donoghue FE, Code CF: Pattern of esophageal motility in diffuse spasm. Gastroenterology 34:782–796, 1958.
75. Fleshler B: Diffuse esophageal spasm. Gastroenterology 52:559–564, 1967.
76. Ahtaridis G, Snape WJ, Cohen S: Clinical and manometric findings in benign peptic strictures of the esophagus. Dig Dis Sci 24:858–861, 1979.
77. Winship DH, Caflisch CR, Zboralske FF, Hogan WJ: Deterioration of esophageal peristalsis in patients with alcoholic neuropathy. Gastroenterology 55:173–178, 1968.
78. Mandelstam P, Siegel CI, Lieber A, Siegel M: The swallowing disorder in patients with diabetic neuropathy–gastroenteropathy. Gastroenterology 56:1–12, 1969.
79. Soergel KH, Zboralske FF, Amberg JR: Presbyesophagus: esophageal motility in nonagenarians. J Clin Invest 43:1472–1479, 1964.
80. Khan TA, Shragge BW, Crispin JS, Lind JF: Esophageal motility in the elderly. Am J Dig Dis 22:1049–1054, 1977.
81. Nagler R, Spiro HM: Serial esophageal motility studies in asymptomatic young subjects. Gastroenterology 41:371–379, 1961.
82. Mellow M: Symptomatic diffuse esophageal spasm. Manometric follow-up and response to cholinergic stimulation and cholinesterase inhibition. Gastroenterology 73:237–240, 1977.
83. Castell OD: Motor disorders of the esophagus. N Engl J Med 301:1124, 1979.

84. Hollis JB, Levine SM, Castell DO: Differential sensitivity of the human esophagus to pentagastrin. Am J Physiol 222:870–874, 1972.

85. Humphries TJ, Castell DO: Pressure profile of esophageal peristalsis in normal humans as measured by direct intraesophageal transducers. Dig Dis 22:641–645, 1977.

86. Dent J: What's new in the esophagus. Dig Dis Sci 26:161–173, 1981.

87. Code CF, Schlegel JF, Kelley ML Jr, et al.: Hypertensive gastroesophageal sphincter. Proceed Staff Meet Mayo Clin 35:391–399, 1960.

88. Vantrappen G, Van Derstappen G, Vandenbroucke J: The syndrome of the hypertonic gastroesophageal sphincter. In: Proceedings of the International Congress of Gastroenterology, Excerpta Medica, Leiden. Amsterdam, 1960.

89. Graham DY: Hypertensive lower esophageal sphincter: a reappraisal. South Med J 71 (Suppl 1):31–37, 1978.

90. Garrett JM, Godwin DH: Gastroesophageal hypercontracting sphincter. JAMA 208:992–998, 1969.

91. Dodds WJ, Hogan WJ, Reid DR, et al.: A comparison between esophageal peristalsis following wet and dry swallows. J Appl Physiol 35:851–857, 1973.

92. Hollis JB, Castell DO: Effect of dry swallows and wet swallows of different volumes on esophageal peristalsis. J Appl Physiol 38:1161–1164, 1975.

93. Kaye MD: Dysfunction of the lower esophageal sphincter in disorders other than achalasia. Am J Dig Dis 18:734–745, 1973.

94. Eckardt VF, Krüger J, Holtermüller K-H, Ewe K: Alteration of esophageal peristalsis by pentagastrin in patients with diffuse esophageal spasm. Scand J Gastroenterol 10:475–479, 1975.

95. Morris SJ, Perez C, Rogers AI: Sensitivity of esophageal peristalsis to pentagastrin (PG) in patients with symptomatic esophageal spasm (SDES). Gastroenterology 74:1137, 1978.

96. Wexler RM, Kaye MD: Pentagastrin in diffuse oesophageal spasm. Gut 22:213–216, 1981.

97. Guelrud M, Simon C, Gomez G, Villalta B: Pentagastrin supersensitivity of the lower esophageal sphincter (LES) in the elderly. Gastroenterology 80:1165, 1981.

98. Heupler FA Jr, Proudfit WL, Razavi M, et al.: Ergonovine maleate provocative test for coronary arterial spasm. Am J Cardiol 41:631–640, 1978.

99. Dart AM, Davies H, Lowndes R, et al.: Oesophageal spasm and "angina": diagnostic value of ergometrine provocation. Eur Heart J 1:91–95, 1980.

100. Dalal JJ, Dart AM, Davies HA, et al.: Coronary and peripheral arterial responses to ergometrine in patients susceptible to coronary and oesophageal spasm. Br Heart J 45:181–185, 1981.

101. Johnstone AS: Diffuse spasm and diffuse muscle hypertrophy of lower esophagus. Br J Radiol 33:723–735, 1960.

102. Henderson RD, Pearson FC: Reflux control following extended myotomy in primary disordered motor activity (diffuse spasm) of the esophagus. Ann Thorac Surg 22:278–283, 1976.

103. Leonardi HK, Shea JA, Crozier RE, Ellis FE Jr: Diffuse spasm of the esophagus. Clinical, manometric, and surgical considerations. J Thorac Cardiovasc Surg 74:736–743, 1977.

104. Orlando RC, Bozymski EM: Clinical and manometric effects of nitroglycerin in diffuse esophageal spasm. N Engl J Med 289:23–24, 1973.

105. Mellow MH: The effect of isosorbide and hydralazine on esophageal motility in symptomatic diffuse esophageal spasm. Gastroenterology 80:1229, 1981.

106. Henderson RD, Ho CS, Davidson JW: Primary disordered motor activity of the esophagus (diffuse spasm): diagnosis and treatment. Ann Thorac Surg 18:327–366, 1974.
107. Jekler J, Lhotka J: Modified Heller procedure to prevent postoperative reflux esophagitis in patients with achalasia. Am J Surg 113:251–254, 1967.
108. McCallum RW: Diffuse esophageal spasm and gastroesophageal reflux-induced esophageal dysfunction. In (ed): 2nd Internat Symposium on the Esophagus and Gastroesophageal Junction. Marion Laboratories, Ixtapa, Mexico, 1978.
109. Pope CE: Abnormalities of peristaltic amplitude and force—a clue to the etiology of chest pain. In Vantrappen G (ed): Proceedings of the Fifth International Symposium on Gastrointestinal Motility, Leuven. Typoff-Press, Herentals, 1976.
110. London RL, Ouyang A, Snape WJ Jr, et al.: Provocation of esophageal pain by ergonovine or edrophonium. Gastroenterology 81:10–14, 1981.
111. Herrington JP, Burns TW, Balart LA: Dysphagia in patients with prolonged peristaltic contractile duration—a clinical and manometric analysis. Gastroenterology 80:1173, 1981.
112. Orr WC, Robinson MG, Jaffe M: Hypertensive esophageal peristaltic contractions in the pathogenesis of chest pain. Gastroenterology 80:1244, 1981.

9 | Scleroderma and Associated Collagen Vascular Diseases

Ann Ouyang

INTRODUCTION

Progressive systemic sclerosis (PSS), or scleroderma, is a disorder of connective tissue that results in the excessive deposition of collagen in the skin, subcutaneous tissue, and other organs, particularly the gastrointestinal tract, lungs, heart, and kidney. The clinical spectrum is highly variable, ranging from widespread cutaneous and progressive visceral involvement to a more limited involvement manifested by the coexistence of calcinosis, Raynaud's phenomenon, sclerodactyly, telangiectasia, and, sometimes subclinically, esophageal involvement—the CREST syndrome.[1] The picture is confused further by the recognition that features of classical PSS can coexist with those of SLE and with polymyositis.[2,3] This mixed connective tissue disease is notable for the presence of high titers of a hemagglutinating antibody to an extractable nuclear antigen (ENA) that consists mainly of protein and ribonucleic acid. The syndrome appears to respond well to corticosteroid therapy and carries a favorable prognosis. This chapter will discuss the esophageal disease found in this spectrum of connective tissue disorders.

EPIDEMIOLOGY

Good epidemiologic studies of PSS and its variants are difficult to conduct because of the relative infrequency of the disease, its highly variable presentation, and the tendency for an overlap of features between PSS and other connective tissue disorders. Epidemiologic studies of PSS based on mortality analysis have reported an overall annual mortality of 2.1/million population with a female:male preponderance of 3:1.[4] A community-wide retrospective study in Tennessee reported a mean annual incidence of 2.7 new cases/million population over a 21-year period. The incidence rate was variable and increased to 4.5/million during the final 6 years of the survey, which may reflect a better recognition of the disease entity.[5] Again the F:M ratio was 3:1. A prospective study is being conducted by the American Rheumatism Association to develop clinical classification criteria for PSS. Its preliminary findings were reported in 1979.[6] There were more whites than blacks among patients with PSS, and the F:M ratio again approximated 3:1. The median age of onset of PSS is between 40 and 50 years, although this finding may reflect a delay in diagnosis, particularly in patients with the CREST syndrome.

ESOPHAGEAL AND GASTROINTESTINAL INVOLVEMENT

The extent of gastrointestinal involvement in PSS is variable. In a postmortem study histologic evidence of esophageal involvement was seen in 74% of cases, small-intestinal involvement in 46%, and large-intestinal involvement in 39%.[7] For comparison, the frequency of involvement of other organ systems is outlined in Table 9-1. The development of sensitive tests of physiologic function may reveal a higher percentage of patients with gastrointestinal involvement.

Table 9-1. Postmortem changes in 58 cases of scleroderma and 58 control cases without PSS[a]

Involved Organs	Percent of Pathologic Findings in PSS Cases against PSS-free Patients
Skin	98
Esophagus	74
Lungs	59
Kidneys	49
Small intestine	46
Pericardium	41
Muscles	41
Large intestine	39
Pleura	29
Myocardium	26

[a] Reproduced by permission from D'Angelo WA, Fries JF, Masi AT, Shulman LE: Pathologic observations in systemic sclerosis (scleroderma). A study of 58 autopsy cases and 58 matched controls. Am J Med 46:428, 1969.

Symptoms

Symptoms of esophageal involvement in PSS are less prevalent than the presence of esophageal dysfunction revealed by objective tests, such as manometry. Symptoms may be present in one-third to one-half of patients.[8-10] Complaints include pyrosis (heartburn) related to reflux esphagitis. If reflux is severe, the patient may notice regurgitation of food. Dysphagia may be present and can be seen in the presence of disordered esophageal peristalsis but more often results from a peptic esophageal stricture.[9] A stricture may develop in the absence of previous symptoms of pyrosis. Similar complaints are seen in patients with mixed-connective-tissue diseases.[11] Patients with polymyositis may have involvement of skeletal pharyngeal muscle, and this is manifested by difficulty in initiating swallows (pre-esophageal dysphagia).[9] This type of dysfunction is far less common than the esophageal smooth-muscle dysfunction in PSS.

Diagnostic Studies

Manometry. The characteristic manometric findings in scleroderma are two-fold: an incompetent lower esophageal sphincter (LES) and low-amplitude esophageal contractions in the smooth-muscle portion of the esophagus, which may initially be peristaltic and may in more advanced cases be aperistaltic (Fig. 9-1). The incompetent (LES) allows reflux of gastric acid from the stomach to the esophagus and the dysfunction of peristalsis of the lower smooth-muscle portion of the esophagus fails to clear the refluxed acid. The prolonged contact of acid with the esophageal mucosa results in severe esophagitis. Deterioration of esophageal function with time has been reported.[8] Aperistalsis affecting only the distal smooth-muscle portion of the esophagus appears fairly specific for PSS and is not seen in patients complaining only of Raynaud's phenomenon.[9] Dysfunction of the esophageal body may precede LES incompetence.[12]

The specificity of the esophageal motility disturbance for scleroderma has been debated in the past. Stevens et al.[13] described the incidence of distal esophageal aperistalsis in a variety of connective-tissue disorders and in a group of patients with idiopathic Raynaud's phenomenon. They concluded that whereas the esophageal dysfunction was found in 84% of patients with PSS, it was found in a variety of disorders and was related to the presence of Raynaud's phenomenon rather than to the cutaneous manifestation of PSS. The potential flaws in this study apply to all studies of patients with connective tissue diseases, namely in the criteria applied to categorize patients into disease entities. PSS may involve the viscera in the absence of skin lesions, and Raynaud's phenomenon may precede visceral involvement by years.[14] Others have indicated, by using different criteria, that esophageal aperistalsis is not associated with true idiopathic Raynaud's phenomenon.[15] With the recognition of the entity of mixed-connective-tissue disease it becomes apparent that reports of esophageal dysmotility in a variety of connective tissue diseases may have described patients with this overlap syndrome.[13,15-17] Conversely, however, patients with PSS or mixed connective-tissue disease who demonstrate esophageal dysmotility do suffer from Raynaud's phenomenon.[13,14]

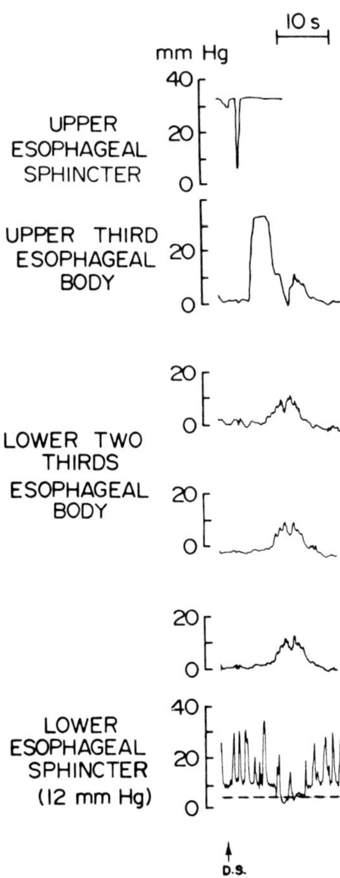

Fig. 9-1. Manometric tracing from a patient with scleroderma. Normal upper esophageal sphincter and normal amplitude of contraction of upper third of esophageal body. Loss of peristalsis with low-amplitude contraction of the lower two-thirds of the esophageal body and a hypotensive lower esophageal sphincter. (D.S. = dry swallow).

Polymyositis affects skeletal muscle, and dysfunction of pharyngeal contractions—of the cricopharynx and the skeletal-muscle portion of the esophagus—has been described, infrequently, in this disease entity.[9] The presence of dysfunction of the skeletal muscles of the pharynx and upper esophagus is associated with symptoms of pre-esophageal dysphagia.

Radiology. The routine chest x-ray may demonstrate air throughout the length of the esophagus in PSS. This finding tends to be seen late in the disease and may be related to easier visualization of air in the esophagus against a pulmonary fibrotic background. Air in the esophagus is not seen in other diseases that cause pulmonary fibrosis. Thus, in this setting it is fairly specific. An air esophagram itself can be seen in other conditions, including achalasia.[18-20]

Barium cineradiography studies demonstrate absence of peristalsis in the distal two-thirds of the esophagus and evidence of peptic esophagitis if there is an incompetent LES (Fig. 9-2). Double-contrast methods of studying the esophagus now allow detailed examination of the esophageal mucosa. The early radiographic signs of esophagitis include thickening of esophageal folds, limitation of distensibility, and irregularity of the esophageal margin. It is felt that good contrast studies of the

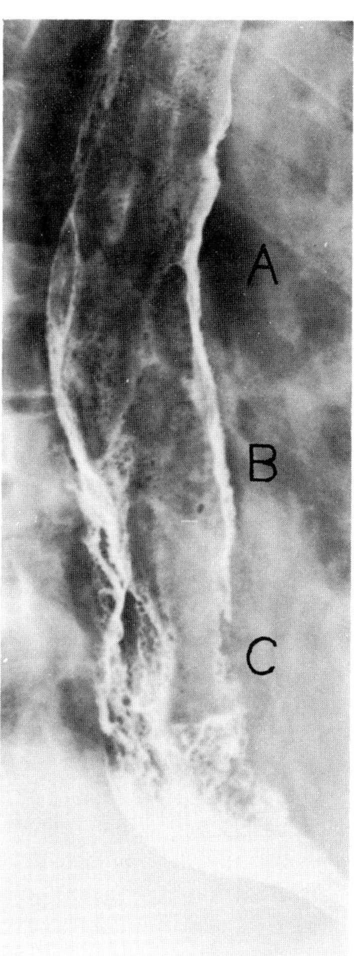

Fig. 9-2. Esophagram in patient with scleroderma. Dilated, atonic esophagus with fluoroscopic evidence of lack of primary peristalsis and free gastroesophageal reflux. The irregular appearance of the distal esophagus is due to moniliasis.

esophageal mucosa correlate with the stages of esophagitis as seen endoscopically.[21]

Early esophagitis, seen endoscopically as superficial erosions or ulcerations, is seen radiographically as streaks or dots of barium against the normally flat esophageal mucosal barium pattern. With chronic disease a finely nodular appearance may be seen. More advanced esophagitis may be seen endoscopically as deeper ulcers that can easily be demonstrated radiographically. The air-contrast method allows the ulcer to be identified even when it is not caught in profile. Single-contrast methods do not enable ulcers to be seen "en face." Peptic strictures may result, and moniliasis of the esophagus is not infrequent in patients with PSS. Dilation of the hypomotile esophagus can occur late in the disease.

As might be expected from manometric studies, evidence of skeletal muscle dysfunction may be seen on barium cineradiography in polymyositis.[22]

Esophageal Scintigraphy. Esophageal transit has been studied using a scintigraphic method to measure the clearance of a bolus of water labeled with ^{99m}Tc–

sulfur colloid.[23] In patients with scleroderma the quantity of labeled water cleared from the esophagus when the patient is supine is significantly reduced after either a single swallow or multiple swallows. During the day, transit may be normal, because patients maintain an upright posture. There is evidence that nocturnal gastroesophageal reflux, as documented by esophageal intraluminal pH recording, is a major factor in the development of esophagitis.[24] Thus the inability of patients with PSS to clear refluxed acid, which results from a combination of an incompetent LES and the distal esophageal motor abnormality, probably allows prolonged contact of acid with the esophageal mucosa at night.

Although esophageal scintigraphy is of great interest in measuring one of the major functions of the esophagus, it cannot distinguish between different causes of delayed esophageal transit such as achalasia and scleroderma.

Endoscopy.   Endoscopy is of value to evaluate mucosal disease in detail. It cannot diagnose scleroderma of the esophagus—a disease affecting the smooth muscle—but may be useful in evaluating the consequences of this motility abnormality. Esophagitis can be determined and strictures evaluated to determine whether they are benign or malignant. Barrett's columnar-lined esophagus can result from chronic peptic esophagitis and is thought to be a premalignant condition.[25-27]

Pathology and Pathophysiology

The pathophysiology of esophageal dysfunction in PSS is not well understood. The final pathologic changes are known because of autopsy studies. Direct physiologic studies of the esophageal smooth muscle in this disease are not available because of its inaccessibility and of the absence of any animal model. Most studies of collagen metabolism in patients with PSS have utilized skin biopsies.

At autopsy, the esophageal muscle demonstrates atrophy and/or fibrosis in 74% of cases, and 40% of the cases in one series showed mucosal disease with esophagitis and/or ulceration (Fig. 9-3).[7] The skeletal muscle of the esophagus is spared except in some advanced cases. Studies aimed at correlating physiologic dysfunction and pathologic changes suggest that the motility disturbances precede detectable histologic changes.[12]

Physiologic studies by Cohen et al. investigated the esophageal motility disturbances in patients with PSS.[14] Three groups of patients were described. One group had normal peristalsis and a mildly decreased LES pressure. These patients demonstrated a normal LES response to both methacholine and edrophonium, suggesting an intact muscle response to cholinergic agents and normal release of acetylcholine. There was a diminished response to the infusion of gastrin I (hexadecapeptide), suggesting latent cholinergic nerve dysfunction. The second group of patients had abnormal peristalsis. The LES in this group responded normally to methacholine but demonstrated a diminished response to edrophonium and to gastrin I. Thus nerve dysfunction was present although the muscle response was intact. This conclusion might explain the findings of Treacy et al. of physiologic dysfunction without evidence of smooth muscle atrophy.[12] Two patients were placed in a third group, in which there was a diminished LES response to all three agents, suggesting muscle failure. One of the patients was demonstrated to have marked smooth

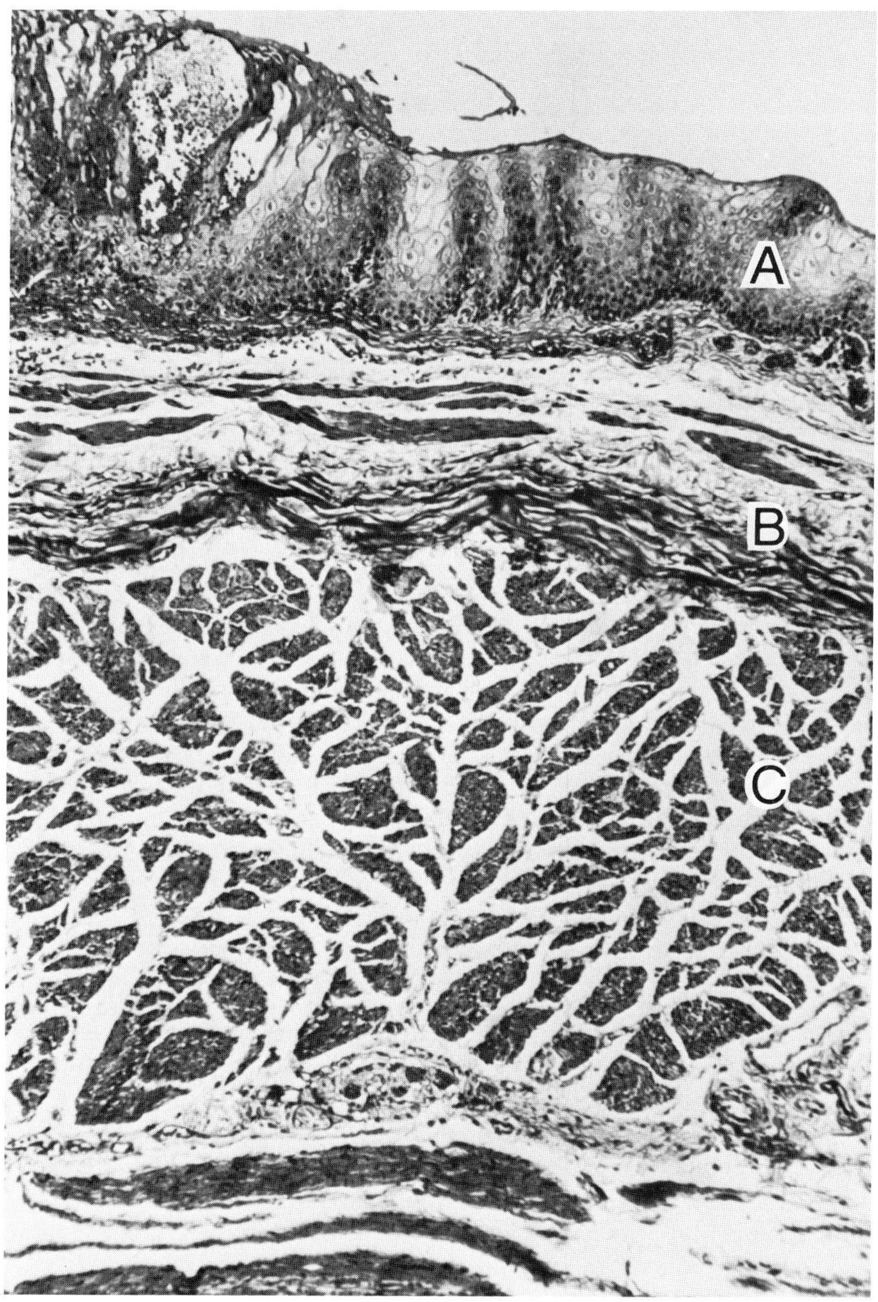

Fig. 9–3. Section of esophagus demonstrating scleroderma involvement. A. Mucosal changes of esophagitis with loss of squamous cell layer and elongation of rete pegs. B. Submucosa demonstrating fibrous tissue. C. Circular muscle layer demonstrating increased collagenous tissue. (Trichrome Stain. × 256).

muscle atrophy at subsequent autopsy. It appears from these data that neural dysfunction plays a role in early scleroderma. In the small intestine and colon a similar pathogenic mechanism appears to be involved in which initially a neural defect and later a failure of end-organ response to exogenous stimuli can be demonstrated.[28,29]

A neural dysfunction has also been postulated to explain the 80–90% prevalence of Raynaud's phenomenon in PSS.[30] Despite the relationship of esophageal motility disturbances and Raynaud's phenomenon in PSS, there is no correlation between the degree of motility abnormalities and the severity or duration of Raynaud's phenomenon.[31]

Since PSS is a systemic disease, one might expect a uniform pathologic process to affect all the involved organs. Most study, as mentioned above, has been directed at the skin changes because of their accessibility. Studies on the pathologic events underlying scleroderma have concentrated on three major areas, alteration in collagen metabolism, changes in the blood vessels, and abnormalities of the autoimmune regulatory process.

In the skin, fibrosis can be seen in the dermis and subcutaneous tissue in PSS. The dermal collagen stains normally with trichrome and van Gieson stains whereas that in the subcutaneous tissue is finer and stains lighter. Electron microscopy demonstrates large numbers of fine, immature collagen fibrils in the dermis, around the blood vessels, and in the fat trabeculae.[32] Evidence that these collagen fibrils are newly synthesized includes collagen solubility studies,[33] the electron microscopy findings of immaturity,[32] and the demonstration of increased collagen production by fibroblasts in scleroderma skin.[34] Degradation of collagen by collagenase may also be defective, as suggested by the demonstration of decreased collagenase activity in the skin of affected areas in patients with PSS. Interestingly, collagenase activity was normal when skin from unaffected areas was studied.[35] This defect in collagenase activity may therefore not be a unifying pathologic event in this systemic disease.

Vascular changes noted in PSS have been proposed as the primary lesion in this disorder. In the skin of patients with PSS, one finds a decrease in the number of capillaries of the papillary layer, but remaining capillaries appear normal. Crowding of the capillary lumen by endothelial cells has also been reported. Endothelial cell proliferation in the papillary and subpapillary plexus occurs, as demonstrated by in vitro ^{3}H-thymidine–uptake studies.[32] Thickening of arteriolar walls is frequent, resulting from an increase in endothelial cells, collagen, and mucopolysaccharides. Electron microscopy also reveals abnormalities in the blood vessels, namely reduplication of the basement lamina,[36] and abnormalities of the nucleus and mitochondria of capillary endothelial cells.[37] Thus structural vascular changes are present in addition to vasospastic changes thought to result in Raynaud's phenomenon.

In view of the overlapping of syndromes between scleroderma and systemic lupus erythematosis, an autoimmune disease, it has been thought that an autoimmune process might also underlie PSS. Immunologic studies have demonstrated the presence of a number of antibodies in patients with scleroderma, including rheumatoid factor, antinuclear antibodies (found in approximately half of the patients)[38] anti-N-DNA, cryofibrinogen, and anti-single-stranded RNA antibodies.[39] The antinuclear antibodies (ANA) may show homogeneous, speckled, or nucleolar patterns of fluorescence, alone or in combination. There is no correlation between the duration or severity of the disease and the titers of ANA or serum immunoglobulin. There is evidence of abnormalities in cell-mediated immune responses in PSS.[40] One study has demonstrated a decrease in a particular subset of T lymphocytes.[41]

One hypothesis that might tie all these abnormalities together would invoke an alteration of cellular and humoral immunity by an unknown factor; this alteration would result in vascular damage and subsequent fibrosis.[32] Whether such a sequence of events occurs in all organs affected in scleroderma and why neural dysfunction appears early in scleroderma that affects the esophagus remains unknown.

Complications of Esophageal Scleroderma

The complications of esophageal scleroderma are related to the presence of gastric acid reflux. Severe reflux may cause nocturnal aspiration with resultant nocturnal cough, pneumonitis, or lung abscess. This is rare. Prolonged esophagitis can result in hematemesis and stricture formation with or without mucosal changes to a Barrett's epithelium.

A benign peptic stricture is seen in approximately 11% of patients with idiopathic reflux but in 48% of patients with PSS.[42-44] Ahtaridis et al.[43] investigated patients with symptomatic reflux alone and those with peptic strictures. The LES pressure is lower in the group of patients with strictures. Of significance was the finding that 64% of patients with stricture had an esophageal motor abnormality whereas 32% of patients with reflux but no stricture demonstrated esophageal dysmotility. Thus a combination of acid reflux and poor esophageal clearance may increase the risk of developing a benign peptic stricture.

MANAGEMENT

Management of systemic sclerosis is aimed at preserving function, particularly of the hands and of vital organs such as the lungs and kidneys. Gastrointestinal involvement in scleroderma can include the entire intestinal tract. Discussion of affected areas distal to the esophagus is beyond the scope of this chapter, but such involvement can be crippling for the patient. Esophageal involvement per se does not need treatment except as needed to prevent complications or to treat the complications themselves.

As described above, the major motility disturbances of the esophagus in PSS are impaired or absent peristalsis of the distal two-thirds of the esophagus and a hypotensive LES. There is no medical or surgical treatment available to restore peristalsis. Initial treatment is therefore aimed at affecting the LES pressure and preventing the development of esophagitis. General therapeutic measures include avoidance of substances that decrease the LES pressure further, such as alcohol, chocolate and coffee;[45] avoidance of devices or maneuvers that increase the intra-abdominal pressure, such as tight belts and binders or lying supine immediately following large meals; and sleeping with the head of the bed elevated on blocks. Reduction of the acidity of gastric secretion will decrease the esophagitis incurred by reflux of gastric contents.

A double-blind randomized cross-over study[46] has demonstrated greater symptomatic relief of heartburn in patients with PSS, when they take cimetidine as compared with antacids. Patients were on each type of treatment for 8 weeks only, and antacids were permitted while patients were taking cimetidine. Significant improvement of esophagitis was also noted endoscopically. No improvement in strictures was found. Unfortunately, no gastric secretory studies were performed during either type of treatment. It is encouraging that short-term medical treatment with cimetidine and antacids can improve esophagitis when assessed objectively. Since the type of patient that appears to be at risk for developing strictures has been identified[43] and since strictures, once formed, do not appear to be amenable to medical therapy, it seems advisable that, once recognized, patients with PSS at risk for developing strictures should be treated long-term with vigorous medical therapy. Further studies are needed to determine the efficacy of long-term medical therapy initiated either early or late in the course of scleroderma involving the esophagus. In our experience, once strictures have developed, long-term relief may be obtained by bouginage followed by long-term cimetidine therapy.

Metoclopramide, a procaine amide derivative, has been reported to improve LES function in some patients with PSS.[47] It is a potentially useful drug in treating symptoms of reflux esophagitis. Patients may also have gastric involvement with scleroderma, and gastric atony and delayed gastric emptying may aggravate their symptoms of reflux. Metoclopramide may thus also be useful as a stimulant of gastric emptying.[48]

Esophageal moniliasis is seen in patients with PSS that involves the esophagus and is thought to be related to the altered esophageal motility that results in stasis of esophageal contents. Symptomatically patients may then complain of odynophagia, and mycostatin may be helpful.

The consequence of prolonged, severe reflux esophagitis is peptic stricture of the distal esophagus. Hiatal hernias are common in patients with scleroderma and may be related to shortening of the esophagus secondary to the fibrotic changes.

The usual indications for surgery in patients with sclerodermatous esophageal involvement are dysphagia related to peptic stricture and intractable esophagitis. The recommendations in the surgical literature are derived from data accumulated before the widespread use of H_2-receptor antagonists. A number of surgical procedures have been described; most are directed at preventing gastroesophageal reflux, and some are directed at the esophageal strictures. Bouginage of peptic strictures is usually successful initially. Surgery has been indicated in the past when bouginage becomes difficult. Most patients can be dilated intraoperatively, so that resection of the strictures is rarely needed.[49] Henderson and Pearson have recommended a combination of a modified Belsey fundoplication and a modified Collis gastroplasty after dilatation of the stricture. The addition of the Collis gastroplasty results in the fashioning of a gastric tube that enables less tension to be applied to the thoracic esophagus during the Belsey repair. Excellent results have been reported during a follow-up for an average of 13.5 months.[44] These authors have favored this surgical approach for benign peptic strictures from a variety of causes and report good 5-year results in this homogenous group of patients.[49] It is not clear, however, whether patients with scleroderma do as well in the long term. A major postoperative problem following a fundoplication in these patients is dysphagia because of the esophageal dysmotility even if the initial stricture is dilated. Care has to be taken to perform fundoplication over a dilator to allow an adequate orifice at the gastroesophageal junction.[50] Nonsurgical techniques using Grüntzig balloon catheters[51] are now available to dilate very narrow peptic strictures. With the availability of medical therapy in association with nonsurgical dilatation of strictures, further controlled studies are necessary to compare long-term efficacy of this combination therapy with that of surgical management. In any such study gastric secretory studies that objectively assess the efficacy of gastric acid suppression during medical therapy are important. The risk of postoperative dysphagia following fundoplication in patients with esophageal motor disorders is a rationale for performing manometry studies in any patient being considered for antireflux surgery. As has been emphasized earlier, the esophageal motility disturbances of scleroderma may precede obvious clinical involvement.

A number of therapeutic agents have been tried in patients who have evidence of rapidly progessive skin sclerosis and visceral involvement. There is evidence that the specific visceral organ involvement correlates with prognosis.[52] In one series, the 7-year cumulative survival was only 35%. However, 100% of patients with renal involvement and an elevated creatinine were dead within 10 months. Cardiac and pulmonary involvement were also correlated with a decreased survival. Gastrointestinal involvement apparently did not affect cures or survival data. Thus systemic treatment for esophageal scleroderma should not be considered unless there is evidence of severe skin or visceral involvement.

Systemic therapy is still under study in PSS. The rationale behind the treatments is based on the possible pathogenic mechanisms in scleroderma that were discussed above.

D-penicillamine has attracted much interest because of its chelating properties that may interfere with normal collagen maturation by preventing the formation of stable collagen crosslinks.[53] There is a resultant increase in soluble collagen in the skin that appears to correlate with clinical improvement in parameters of skin involvement.[54] Because of its method of action, D-penicillamine is ineffective on stable collagen and would be expected to be more efficacious in treating active disease. Complications related to this drug have been noted in 10–98% of cases,[55] the most frequently seen being allergic skin reactions. Other complications include nephropathy, which starts 6–12 months after the onset of treatment, thrombocytopenia, and the development of a lupus-like syndrome with the development of antibodies to double-stranded DNA. Penicillamine is initiated at low doses and slowly increased over several months to a dose of 1500 mg/day.[29] Careful evaluation of biochemical and hematologic parameters should enable early detection of complications and withdrawal of the drug. There are many reports of favorable improvement in skin involvement. There has been no good evidence that D-penicillamine will improve esophageal function in patients with PSS, but some authors have reported some improvement in symptoms.[56] In light of the good improvement obtainable with less toxic medical therapy, gastrointestinal symptoms alone are not an indication for the use of D-penicillamine.

Colchicine is known to stimulate the synthesis of collagenase and to disrupt microtubules that are necessary for the secretion of collagen. Its efficacy in treating PSS remains controversial. Corticosteroids and immunosuppressive agents have also been tried. There is no good evidence that these drugs affect the course of the disease.

SUMMARY

Gastrointestinal, and particularly esophageal, involvement is very common in PSS and is seen more frequently by objective testing of esophageal function than would be expected by symptoms. The current approach to managing esophageal symptoms is symptom-related. Symptoms of heartburn or evidence of esophagitis should be treated vigorously. The development of intractable esophagitis or peptic esophageal stricture has required surgical intervention in the past. Medical therapy can improve esophagitis, and this approach combined with nonsurgical dilatation of strictures remains to be compared in a controlled fashion with surgical management of patients who have complications of esophageal scleroderma.

REFERENCES

1. Rodnan GP, Medsger TA, Buckingham RB: Progressive systemic sclerosis—CREST syndrome: observations on natural history and late complications in 90 patients. Arthritis Rheum 18:423, 1975.
2. Sharp GC, Irven WA, Tan EM, et al.: Mixed connective tissue disease—an apparently distinct rheumatic disease syndrome associated with a specific antibody to an extractable nuclear antigen (ENA). Am J Med 52:148–159, 1972.
3. Sharp GC: Mixed connective tissue disease. Bull Rheum Dis 25:828–831, 1975.
4. Masi AT, D'Angelo WA: Epidemiology of fatal systemic sclerosis (diffuse scleroderma). Ann Intern Med 66:870–875, 1967.
5. Medsger TA, Masi AT: Epidemiology of systemic sclerosis (scleroderma). Ann Intern Med 74:714–721, 1971.
6. Masi AT, Medsger TA, Rodnan GP, et al.: Methods and preliminary results of the scleroderma criteria. Cooperative Study of the American Rheumatism Association. Clin Rheum Dis 5:27–48, 1979.
7. D'Angelo WA, Fries JF, Masi AT, Shulman LE: Pathologic observations in systemic sclerosis (scleroderma). A study of 58 autopsy cases and 58 matched controls. Am J Med 46:428–440, 1969.
8. Garrett JM, Winkelmann RK, Schlegel JF, Code CF: Esophageal deterioration in scleroderma. Mayo Clin Proc 46:92–96, 1971.
9. Turner R, Lipshutz W, Miller W, et al.: Esophageal dysfunction in collagen disease. Am J Med Sci 265:191–199, 1973.
10. Krejs GJ, Lobsiger RR, Bron BA, et al.: Esophageal function in progressive systemic sclerosis. Acta Hepatogastroenterol (Stuttg) 23:40–46, 1976.

11. Norman DA, Fleischmann RM: Gastrointestinal systemic sclerosis in serologic mixed connective tissue disease. Arthritis Rheum 21:811–819, 1978.

12. Treacy WL, Baggenstoss AH, Slocumb CH, Code CF: Scleroderma of the esophagus. A correlation of histologic and physiologic findings. Ann Intern Med 59:351–356, 1963.

13. Stevens MB, Hookman P, Siegel CI, et al.: Aperistalsis of the esophagus in patients with connective-tissue disorders and Raynaud's phenomenon. New Engl J Med 270:1218–1222, 1964.

14. Cohen S, Fisher R, Lipshutz W, et al.: The pathogenesis of esophageal dysfunction in scleroderma and Raynaud's disease. J Clin Invest 51:2663–2668, 1972.

15. Clark M, Fountain RB: Oesophageal motility in connective tissue disease. Br J Dermatol 79:449–452, 1967.

16. Dornhorst AC, Pierce JW, Whimster IW: Oesophageal lesion in scleroderma. Lancet 1:698, 1954.

17. Tatelman M, Keech MK: Esophageal motility in systemic lupus erythematosus, rheumatoid arthritis and scleroderma. Radiology 86:1041–1046, 1966.

18. Dinosis RE, Goodman D, Dreyfuss JR: The air esophagram: a sign of scleroderma involving the esophagus. Radiology 87:348–349, 1966.

19. Martinez LO: Air in the esophagus as a sign of scleroderma. J Can Assoc Radiologists. 25:235–237, 1974.

20. House AJS, Griffiths GJ: The significance of an air esophagram visualized on conventional chest radiographs. Clin Radiol 28:301–305, 1977.

21. Laufer I: Peptic esophagitis. In: Double Contrast Gastrointestinal Radiology. WB Saunders, Philadelphia, 1979, pp. 90–105.

22. Grünebaum M, Salinger H: Radiologic findings in polymyositis–dermatomyositis involving the pharynx and upper esophagus. Clin Radiol 22:97–100, 1971.

23. Tolin RD, Malmud LS, Reilley J, Fisher RS: Esophageal scintigraphy to quantitate esophageal transit (quantitation of esophageal transit). Gastroenterology 76:1402–1408, 1979.

24. Atkinson M, VanGelder A: Esophageal intraluminal pH recording in the assessment of gastroesophageal reflux and its consequences. Dig Dis 22:365–370, 1977.

25. Barrett NR: Chronic peptic ulcer of the esophagus and "esophagitis." Br J Surg 38:175–182, 1950.

26. Cho KJ, Hunter TB, Whitehouse WM: The columnar-lined lower esophagus and its association with adenocarcinoma of the esophagus. Radiology 115:563–568, 1975.

27. Naef AP, Savary M, Ozzello L: Columnar-lined lower esophagus: an acquired lesion with premalignant predisposition. J Thorac Cardiovasc Surg 70:826–835, 1975.

28. DiMarino AJ, Carlson G, Myers A, et al.: Duodenal myoelectric activity in scleroderma. New Engl J Med 289:1220–1223, 1979.

29. Cohen S, Laufer I, Snape WJ, et al.: The gastrointestinal manifestations of scleroderma: pathogenesis and management. Gastroenterology 79:155–166, 1980.

30. Winklemann RK: Classification and pathogenesis of scleroderma. Mayo Clin Proc 46:83–91, 1971.

31. Hurwitz AL, Duranceau A, Postlethwait RW: Esophageal dysfunction and Raynaud's phenomenon in patients with scleroderma. Dig Dis 21:601–606, 1976.

32. Fleischmajer R: The pathophysiology of scleroderma. Int J Dermatol 16:310–318, 1977.

33. Uitto J, Ohlenschaeger K, Lorenzen I: Solubility of skin collagen in normal subjects and in patients with generalized scleroderma. Clin Chim Acta 31:13–18, 1971.

34. LeRoy EC, McGuire M, Chen N: Increased collagen synthesis by scleroderma skin fibroblasts in vitro. J Clin Invest 56:880–889, 1974.

35. Brady AH: Collagenase in scleroderma. J Clin Invest 56:1175–1180, 1975.

36. Norton WL: Comparison of the microangiopathy of systemic lupus erythematosus, dermatomyositis, scleroderma, and diabetes mellitus. Lab Invest 22:301–308, 1970.
37. Fleischmajer R, Perlish JS, Shaw KV, Pirozzi DJ: Skin capillary changes in early systemic scleroderma. Arch Dermatol 112:1553–1557, 1976.
38. Rothfield NF, Rodnan GP: Serum antinuclear antibodies in progressive systemic sclerosis (scleroderma). Arthritis Rheum 11:607–617, 1968.
39. Alarcon-Segovia D, Fishbein E: Immunochemical characterization of the anti-RNA antibodies found in scleroderma and systemic lupus erythematosus. I. Differences in reactivity with Poly (U) and Poly (A) Poly (U). J Immunol 115:28–31, 1975.
40. Horwitz DA, Garrett MA: Lymphocyte reactivity to mitogens in systemic lupus erythematosis, rheumatoid arthritis and subjects with scleroderma. Clin Exp Immunol 27:92–99, 1977.
41. Inoshita T, Whiteside TL, Rodnan GP, Taylor FH: Abnormalities of T lymphocyte subsets in patients with progressive systemic sclerosis (PSS, scleroderma). J Lab Clin Med 97:264–277, 1981.
42. Palmer ED: Subacute erosive ("peptic") esophagitis: Clinical study of one hundred cases. Arch Intern Med 94:364–374, 1954.
43. Ahtaridis G, Snape WJ, Cohen S: Clinical and manometric findings in benign peptic strictures of the esophagus. Dig Dis Sci 24:858–861, 1979.
44. Henderson RD, Pearson FG: Surgical management of esophageal scleroderma. J Thorac Cardiovasc Surg 66:686–692, 1973.
45. Cohen, S: Pathogenesis of coffee-induced gastrointestinal symptoms. N Engl J Med 303:122–124, 1980.
46. Petrokubi RJ, Jeffries GH: Cimetidine versus antacid in scleroderma with reflux esophagitis. A randomized double-blind controlled study. Gastroenterology 77:691–695, 1979.
47. Ramirez-Mata M, Ibanez G, Alarcon-Segovia D: Stimulatory effect of metoclopramide on the esophagus and lower esophageal sphincter of patients with PSS. Arthritis Rheum 20:30–34, 1977.
48. Pinder RM, Brogden RN, Sawyer PR, et al.: Metoclopramide. A review of its pharmacological properties and clinical use. Drugs 12:81–131, 1976.
49. Pearson FG, Henderson RD: Long-term follow-up of peptic strictures managed by dilatation, modified Collis gastroplasty, and Belsey hiatus hernia repair. Surgery 80:396–404, 1976.
50. Henderson RD: Treatment of scleroderma. In: Motor Disorders of the Esophagus. Williams & Wilkins, Baltimore, 1976 pp. 177–182.
51. London RL, Trotman BW, DiMarino AJ, et al.: Dilatation of severe esophageal strictures by an inflatable balloon catheter. Gastroenterology 80:173–175, 1981.
52. Masi AT, Rodnan GP, Benedek TG, et al.: Survival with systemic sclerosis: a life-table analysis of clinical and demographic factors in 309 patients. Ann Intern Med 75:369–376, 1971.
53. Nimni ME, Bavetta LA: Collagen defect induced by penicillamine. Science 150:905–906, 1965.
54. Hansen M: Penicillamine research in rheumatoid disease. Symposium on Penicillamine Research in Rheumatoid Disease, Spåtind, Norway, March 7–10, 1976, p. 63.
55. Nassonova VA, Ivanova MM: Progressive systemic sclerosis: management; Part II: D-Penicillamine. Clin Rheum Dis 5:277–288, 1979.
56. Mellstedt H, Fagrell B, Bjökholm M: D-Penicillamine treatment in systemic sclerosis (scleroderma). Effect on nutritional capillary circulation. Scand J Rheumatol 6:92–96, 1977.

10 | Gastroesophageal Reflux Disease and Its Complications with a Critical Analysis of Treatment

Jose Behar

INTRODUCTION

Patients with symptomatic gastroesophageal reflux disease complain of heartburn and regurgitation. Heartburn, the most common symptom of this disease, is usually described as a substernal burning pain or discomfort characterized by motion from the subxyphoid area up towards the suprasternal notch. This pain may radiate up toward the neck and jaw, toward the back, and down into the epigastric area. Occasionally this burning pain may radiate into the arms and simulate the pain of cardiac origin.[1] Heartburn is frequently associated with the regurgitation of sour or bitter fluid. However, regurgitation of fluid or even of food may occur without the patient ever experiencing any burning pain. These symptoms are brought about by meals or postural changes although they can occur in the fasting stomach and without any obvious triggering causes. Severe substernal pain can be associated with water brash, that is, a sudden increase in watery salivary secretion. Most patients (84%) experience symptoms of reflux for more than 1 year before seeking medical attention.[2]

Progression of this disease can lead to intermittent dysphagia, which frequently occurs with the first swallow of every meal. This symptom is usually mild and nonprogressive with no associated weight loss. Often it is not caused by mechanical obstruction to the passage of food but is associated with a motility disturbance within the body of the esophagus, probably induced or aggravated by reflux of gastroduodenal contents.[3] Persistent and occasionally even progressive dysphagia for solids in patients with reflux esophagitis usually suggests the development of a stricture or even of carcinoma. Some patients may also complain of spontaneous chest pain experienced as a feeling of pressure or tightness or even colicky pain lasting for a few seconds to several hours. This pain is not readily relieved by ingestion of antacids. As with the intermittent dysphagia, chest pain is believed to be due to esophageal spasm.

Patients with severe reflux esophagitis can also develop anemia, which results from low-grade bleeding from erosions and ulcerations in the esophageal mucosa. Anemia is sometimes a presenting symptom. The incidence of this complication is approximately 5%.[4] However, major upper gastrointestinal bleeding that requires blood transfusion is uncommon. In these patients, major bleeding is usually preceded by ingestion of an exogenous caustic agent, by gastric intubation, or by retching and vomiting.

There is increasing evidence that aspiration of gastroduodenal contents into the respiratory tract or lung can occur in patients with reflux esophagitis. Some patients, particularly children, initially present with respiratory symptoms such as nocturnal coughing episodes, morning hoarseness, asthma-like syndromes, and occasionally recurrent pneumonitis. Although there is a strong suspicion that these respiratory complaints result from aspiration of gastroesophageal contents, objective demonstration of the actual aspiration has so far remained elusive. This relationship has been established by association and by increasing evidence that management of the underlying esophageal disorders brings these respiratory symptoms under control.[5-8] In addition, there is some indirect evidence that the upper respiratory tract may also be affected by gastroesophageal reflux, as shown by the presence of pharyngitis and posterior laryngitis in nonsmoking patients with reflux esophagitis.[9] Furthermore, a recent study has attempted to confirm aspiration of gastroduodenal contents in the respiratory tract. Lung scanning with the gamma camera following placement of radio-labeled technecium in the stomach was able to demonstrate the presence of this isotope in the lungs of patients with gastroesophageal reflux. Thus, use of the scanning technique may simplify the diagnosis of this complication and may help to elucidate its frequency and importance.[10]

PATHOGENESIS OF GASTROESOPHAGEAL REFLUX

Abnormal Anti-reflux Barrier

The high degree of association of a sliding hiatal hernia with reflux symptoms led to the view that the anatomic disruption of the gastroesophageal junction by the gastric herniation was the major pathogenetic mechanism in the production of gastroesophageal reflux. It was assumed that a sliding hiatal hernia interfered with or eliminated the action of mechanical factors that assisted the LES in controlling gastroesophageal reflux. It was suggested that the sliding hiatal hernia eliminated the acute esophageal angle of Hiss, avoided the compression of the distal esophagus by the diaphragmatic hiatus, and displaced the abdominal segment of the lower esophageal sphincter (LES) into the thoracic cavity with lower negative pressures.[11-14] The role of these mechanical factors, however, has not been verified by careful studies in dog models.[15,16] The creation of a hiatal hernia in dogs, for instance, does not result in esophagitis nor does it change resting LES pressures. Although there is an undeniably strong association between the presence of hiatal hernia and reflux esophagitis, it is not a simple one. Reflux symptoms tend to correlate better with the presence of an incompetent LES than with the presence or absence of a hiatal hernia.[17,18] Furthermore, this association does not necessarily imply a cause-to-effect relationship. The exact incidence of hiatal hernia in the general population is not known. There are difficulties in making the diagnosis with both radiologic and endoscopic techniques. Some studies suggest that up to 50% of subjects who undergo an upper gastrointestinal x-ray examination have a sliding hiatal hernia, and the incidence frequently depends on the radiologist's efforts to demonstrate this hernia.[19] Of interest is the observation that on the one hand patients with reflux esophagitis almost always have hiatal hernia, particularly when a stricture is present, and on the other hand, it is exceptional to find a patient with achalasia and hiatal hernia. These patients with severe reflux esophagitis tend to have a shortened esophagus as a result of chronic inflammation. Not only does the esophagus contract radially—forming a stricture—but longitudinally as well, thereby pulling the stomach up into the chest. Furthermore, because the association of achalasia, with its high LES pressures, and hiatal hernia is rare, it is possible to postulate that a sliding hiatal hernia would tend to occur in patients who have a weak LES.

It is now generally accepted that the major abnormality in patients with reflux esophagitis is a disorder of motor function of the smooth-muscle segment of the esophagus, especially an incompetence of the LES.[20-22] The causes of the LES incompetence are not known. Nevertheless, we can speculate that it may result from alterations of one or more mechanisms responsible for sphincter competence. We define LES competence as the ability of the LES to generate sufficient intraluminal pressures both under basal conditions and under a variety of physiologic conditions that prevent gastroesophageal reflux. The hypotheses that have been proposed to explain sphincter incompetence are based on still insufficient evidence obtained from experimental animal and human studies.

Sphincter tone or competence depends primarily on the strength of the circular muscle of the sphincter. The circular muscle layer of this region is considerably specialized. In vitro studies have shown that the circular muscle strips from this region develop greater active tension than adjacent strips of circular muscles in the esophagus or fundus and are not affected by complete denervation with tetrodotoxin.[23,24] These findings cannot be entirely explained by the greater muscle thickness of this region. In vivo animal studies show that the LES maintains a resting high-pressure zone that is either not affected at all (opossum) or is slightly reduced (cat) by complete denervation with neural poisons such as tetrodotoxin.[25,26] The myogenic mechanisms responsible for this state of closure at rest may be related to its lower membrane potential, which allows an influx of calcium in the LES muscle cells.[27] Furthermore, muscle cells from the LES but not from the body of the esophagus contain receptors for prostaglandins.[28] LES strips are also capable of converting arachidonic acid, a prostaglandin precursor, into contractile substances. This conversion can be prevented by agents that interfere with prostaglandin synthesis, for example, indomethacin, which causes a decrease in LES active muscle tension.[29] It is thus conceivable that endogenous prostaglandins may maintain a high resting tonic contraction of the circular muscle layer of the LES by acting locally at a specific receptor in the cell membrane that could facilitate the influx of calcium into these cells.

It has also been suggested that the innervation of the sphincter may participate in the genesis and/or regulation of this tone. This neural contribution, however, appears to vary considerably among species. In the opossum, the most important determinant of sphincter tone appears to be the circular muscle layer itself.[25] This also seems to be true for the cat sphincter although there is an important but small alpha-adrenergic contribution.[26] In dog and man, cholinergic mechanisms may be of importance, although their influence is not clear.[30-33]

The role of gastrointestinal neuropeptides in controlling LES competence is more controversial. Their potential role has been suggested by the following observations:[34] (1) the presence of receptors at the LES for certain neuropeptides that mediate either LES contraction or relaxation; (2) the presence of these neuropeptides at the autonomic nerve endings that innervate the esophagus as well as the LES; (3) the significant changes in basal LES pressures during the digestive process when these neuropeptides are released into circulation. However, the correlation between LES pressures and circulating levels of the few hormones studied is poor.[35] Nevertheless, it is conceivable that some neuropeptides may influence sphincter tone by acting at local levels either as neurotransmitters or as modulators of synaptic transmission. A great deal of additional work is needed to define whether or not there is a specific role for these hormones in the control of the LES tonic contraction. Marked elevation of the circulating levels of some of these hormones in physiologic and diseased states may cause changes in the strength of the LES circular muscle. An example of specific hormonal change causing LES incompetence and gastroesophageal reflux is observed during pregnancy.[36] Reflux symptoms are common in pregnancy and can be very severe. In the majority of these patients, these symptoms resolve after delivery. It has been suggested that the LES incompetence is induced by high circulating levels of progesterone and estrogens. These assumptions are supported by studies performed in young women taking oral contraceptives[37] and in experimental animals with pseudo-pregnancy induced by the administration of female hormones.[38]

Thus we can postulate that sphincter incompetence could result from abnormalities in the muscle, neural fibers, or gastrointestinal neuropeptides, alone or in combination. The LES circular muscle layer may be unable to maintain an adequate anti-reflux barrier if it is affected by (1) decreased tonic activity of excitatory nerves that in humans may very well be cholinergic or increased tonic influence of the noncholinergic, nonadrenergic inhibitory nerves, (2) atrophy of the circular muscle layer as found in advanced scleroderma, and (3) a functional disorder of the circular muscle layer of the LES, perhaps induced by circulating or local neuropeptides. These pathogenetic possibilities have some support from experimental or clinical observations. We have found two types of responses to bethanechol in patients with similar basal LES pressures. This drug is a cholinergic agonist that causes LES contraction by direct muscle action. In one subgroup of patients, LES pressures rose to normal levels in response to bethanechol. In the other subgroup, which consisted of patients who had severe esophagitis, frequently with evidence of stricture, the LES responded poorly, if at all, to bethanechol. This poor response may be due to an atrophy of the muscle layers or to an increased deposition of collagen fibers. This fibrosis may stiffen the esophageal wall, possibly interfering with the LES contraction.

Finally, we should also consider that in some patients the sphincter hypotension may be due to damage caused by gastroesophageal reflux on the sphincter itself.[39] This damage may be confined to the cholinergic innervation[40] or to the muscularis propria of the esophagus, including the LES circular muscle.[41] A vicious cycle may thus be established in some patients with idiopathic sphincter incompetence in whom gastroesophageal reflux could, in turn, cause further damage to the sphincter, leading to greater incompetence.

Although the hypothesis that sphincter incompetence is the major abnormality in patients with reflux esophagitis is an appealing and reasonably well-documented one, at least 25% of patients with reflux esophagitis have basal LES pressures that overlap with those of normal subjects.[4] There are a number of possible explanations for these unexpected findings. One is that basal LES pressures, as measured under laboratory conditions, may not always reflect the pressures that are present when gastroesophageal reflux occurs; these may be induced by a variety of factors such as dietary excesses, smoking, and alcohol, or by an abnormal LES adaptation in response to changes in intra-abdominal or intragastric pressures. Although the LES pressure changes after fatty meals,[42] smoking,[43] and alcohol ingestion[44] have been reasonably well documented, there is controversy concerning both the existence of the LES adaptive response and significance of the response in controlling gastro-esophageal reflux.[17,18,45] According to the initial observations, the LES responds with an excess of pressure to increases in intra-abdominal pressures, thus maintaining an adequate pressure barrier that impedes the development of reflux. Measurement of this adaptive LES response in man, however, has been clouded by technical difficulties, since it is difficult to maintain the pressure sensor in the same site within the LES before and during the performance of maneuvers. Initially, it was suggested that this response was the result of a neural reflex.[31,46,47] More careful human and animal studies, however, seem to suggest that this LES pressure change may result from mechanical compression by the diaphragm or by other anatomic structures.[49,50] Another explanation could be that resting LES pressures often vary substantially throughout the day, particularly during phase III of the interdigestive activity front.[51] In some patients, LES pressures may have been measured during the development of this front.

In an attempt to resolve these discrepancies, LES pressures and intraluminal esophageal pH were continuously monitored in normal subjects during sleep. Under these conditions, gastroesophageal reflux tends to occur during spontaneous and transient LES relaxations. These relaxations occur in subjects who have normal basal LES pressures. This transient LES relaxation accounted for 98% of the acid reflux episodes in these healthy subjects.[52] Transient LES relaxations occurred for approximately 5–30 sec, accompanied by gastroesophageal reflux approximately 60% of the time. Most reflux episodes, interestingly enough, were associated with an abrupt equilibration of intraesophageal and intragastric pressures, that is, the creation of a common cavity phenomenon. Most of this spontaneous LES relaxation occurs in the absence of a normal peristaltic sequence. Furthermore, some patients with reflux esophagitis who had normal resting LES pressures appeared to have reflux predominantly as the result of this mechanism of transient LES relaxation that seemed to operate in normal subjects.[53]

Abnormal Esophageal Clearance

The role of abnormal esophageal clearance in both the pathogenesis of gastroesophageal reflux and the determination of the severity of its consequences has now been fully recognized. The intraluminal acid clearance induced by repeated swallows is slower in the inflamed than in the normal esophagus.[54] The most obvious explanation for this delayed clearance is the presence of esophageal motor disorders with abnormal primary and spontaneous or secondary peristalsis. This assumption has been supported by the finding that patients with diffuse esophageal spasm and without esophagitis have an abnormal esophageal clearance of acid.[55] Patients with reflux esophagitis often exhibit mild to severe motor abnormalities of the body of the esophagus. Three abnormal motor patterns have been observed in our laboratory. First, the most frequently seen pattern is an increase in the number of nonperistaltic contractions. Second, in 15% of patients with reflux esophagitis the esophageal contractions are of extremely low amplitude or force (less than 30 mm Hg, compared with 50–150 mm Hg in normal subjects), a pattern indistinguishable from that observed in patients with scleroderma. These patients with reflux esophagitis, however, do not have any cutaneous, vascular, systemic, or serologic evidence of collagen disease. Some of these patients have been followed for up to 5 years without developing physical or laboratory findings suggestive of collagen disease. Most of these patients have a more severe course of esophagitis, similar to that observed in patients with fully developed scleroderma (Behar J: Unpublished Observations). Third, a few patients have a pattern of diffuse or localized esophageal spasm with high-amplitude, nonperistaltic contraction and frequent episodes of repetitive contractions. The correlation, however, between an abnormal esophageal motor pattern and delay in acid clearance is not always present. It is conceivable that the acid clearance tests are more sensitive than esophageal manometry in detecting motor abnormalities.

The pathogenesis of this abnormal esophageal clearance of acid and motor abnormality of the body of the esophagus remains unknown. It is possible that it is of the same nature as that of the LES, due to myogenic or neurogenic disorders. On the other hand, most patients with severe motor disorders of the body of the esophagus have severe esophagitis, and therefore it could be the result of damage to the esophageal muscles or neural plexus caused by the acid–pepsin complex or by bile salts. There are patients, however, who have a scleroderma-like pattern and yet whose esophagus is not markedly inflamed. These findings suggest that either mechanism could play a role in different patients; in some patients, the abnormal motor pattern could be part of the underlying motility disorder that results in esophagitis; in the others, it may be the result of the damage caused by gastroesophageal reflux.

Delayed Gastric Emptying

The finding that reflux symptoms and gastroesophageal reflux are more frequent in the postprandial state, particularly after large meals, suggests among other hypotheses, the possibility that the net gastric volume may contribute to the production of gastroesophageal reflux. It is thus natural to think that any delay in gastric emptying could worsen gastroesophageal reflux by inducing either more frequent episodes or episodes with larger volumes that might remain in contact with the esophageal mucosa for a longer duration. In most patients with reflux esophagitis, gastric emptying of liquids appears to be no different from that of normal subjects.[56,57] There is, however, some delay in emptying of solids in approximately 40% of the patients.[58] The significance of this finding is unclear. It is possible, however, that delayed emptying of solids could produce a longer stimulation of gastric acid secretion and result in larger liquid volume available for reflux.

It is thus possible to postulate that the disease entity known as reflux esophagitis is a heterogenous syndrome in which a variety of pathogenetic factors may cause various degrees of esophagitis. In addition, there may be several distinct subgroups of patients in whom some pathogenetic factors may be more important than others.

Consequences of Gastroesophageal Reflux

Repeated or prolonged episodes of reflux of gastroduodenal contents into the esophagus leads to the breakdown of the squamous mucosal barrier with increased desquamation of surface squamous cells. The damage of the squamous epithelium is related to the concentration and mutual potentiation of the causative agents such as hydrochloric acid, pepsin, and bile acids as well as to the duration of the gastroesophageal reflux episodes, that is, the time that the epithelium is bathed or exposed to these substances. The squamous epithelium appears to have a modest resistance to the damaging effect of the causative agents. This conclusion is based mainly on acute studies in animal models.[59] The squamous mucosal barrier is broken when the esophageal mucosa is exposed to moderate concentrations of hydrogen ion.[60] The acid effect is potentiated by pepsin[61] and/or bile acids.[62] At this concentration, hydrogen-ion back diffusion occurs across the cell membrane, which causes significant changes in the potential difference.[63,64] Frequently, however, patients with reflux esophagitis have gastric secretory rates with hydrogen-ion concentrations that are lower than those shown to damage the squamous epithelium in acute animal models.[65] It is believed that in these patients damage occurs because of either repeated episodes or prolonged reflux or perhaps because of the potentiation of the acid effect by pepsin and bile salts. The exact role of bile salts, however, has not been fully evaluated in clinical conditions. Once acid diffuses into the mucosa and submucosa, it sets off an inflammatory process in which prostaglandins may play a significant role. A recent study has revealed that indomethacin, an inhibitor of prostaglandin synthesis, ammeliorates the inflammatory response to radiation injury to the esophagus.[66]

The initial histologic lesion in the mucosa appears to be a dilatation of the mucosal capillaries and epithelial changes that consist of a thickening of the basal layer and an increase in the height of the submucosal projection or papilla.[67] This histologic appearance is the result of the relative changes in the dimensions of the basal layer and papilla with respect to the overall thickness of the mucosa. Increased length of the papilla has been interpreted as reflecting a greater desquamation of surface squamous cells, whereas the increase in the thickening of the basal layer is the result of a compensatory cell proliferation in an attempt to match the greater rates of cell loss. Increased cell proliferation in the basal layer has been demonstrated in patients with severe reflux esophagitis as compared with the normal squamous mucosa or with mucosa obtained from patients with treated reflux esophagitis.[68] Esophageal mucosal tissue samples obtained through suction biopsy were incubated with tritiated thymidine. The mucosa obtained from patients with severe reflux esophagitis takes up greater amounts of thymidine with a greater number of labeled cells in the basal layer compared with that from normal subjects and from patients with treated esophagitis.

Persistent or more severe reflux may cause progression of the mucosal injury with increased cellular desquamation that may not, under certain undetermined clinical situations, be matched by an increase in cellular proliferation, thus resulting in a mucosal erosion or even ulceration. The erosions are usually seen as linear or longitudinal mucosal abrasions covered by exudate and surrounded by a hyperemic halo.[4] Frequently, the adjacent mucosa appears to be grossly normal; however, reflux-like changes may be present. Complete breakdown of the squamous epithelium may allow the causative agents to penetrate into the submucosa or muscular layers, causing irritation of ganglion and/or muscle cells and leading to a variety of responses including the destruction of these cells. Severe esophagitis can cause spasm of the esophagus, which reverts after the esophagitis is treated. The ulcerations may also lead to one of two reactions that attempt to confine the inflammatory process: (1) an increase in the deposition of collagen fibers in the submucosa, muscularis propia, and periesophageal space, leading to fibrosis with subsequent narrowing of the esophageal lumen and stricture formation of variable lengths;[69] or (2) an epithelial response to heal the ulcerations. There are two types of epithelial responses depending on the presence or absence of gastroesophageal reflux.[70] If reflux is relatively controlled, the healing process is carried out by the adjacent squamous mucosa. However, if reflux persists unabated, the reparative process is performed by a mixed metaplastic epithelium in which gastric and intestinal glands restore the mucosal continuity. The epithelium generated by this process is called Barrett's mucosa because it includes a mixture of fundic, oxyntic, pyloric, and intestinal glands.[71,72] This metaplastic epithelium appears to be in dynamic equilibrium with the surrounding squamous epithelium. The Barrett's mucosa remains and may even extend further up in the esophagus as long as gastroesophageal reflux persists. Once gastroesophageal reflux is controlled by fundoplication, there is a gradual regression of the Barrett's mucosa.[73] Furthermore, there is increasing concern about this epithelium since it appears to be a premalignant lesion predisposing to a increased incidence of adenocarcinoma of the gastroesophageal junction.[74,75]

DIAGNOSIS

The diagnosis of reflux esophagitis depends on how we define this disease. In contrast to patients with episodic symptoms of reflux due to dietary excesses, patients with chronic gastroesophageal reflux have not only symptoms but also findings consistent with esophagitis and sphincter incompetence.[4] We have tests available that are designed to demonstrate the presence of both objective aspects of this disease.

Esophagitis can be demonstrated directly or indirectly by the acid infusion test, esophagoscopy, and esophageal biopsies. The acid infusion test elicits a substernal pain usually of a burning quality that resembles the patient's symptoms. The results are more specific for reflux esophagitis when the test is positive in the inital 15 min after the infusion of acid. It is useful in patients with atypical or vague chest discomforts.[76] Test results improve as the symptoms and esophageal lesions resolve. Therefore, the test should be performed before the treatment is started. Esophagoscopy detects unequivocal lesions of esophagitis such as erosions, linear ulcerations, punched out deep ulcers, stricture formation, and spontaneous friability with bleeding.[77] Erythema, however, is not specific since it cannot distinguish between active hyperemia and inflammation from passive hyperemia or congestion.[78] Esophagoscopy also is useful in assessing the severity of the esophagitis likely to develop complications. In approximately 40% of patients with chronic gastroesophageal reflux, esophagoscopy fails to reveal any gross lesions.[4] In these patients, suction biopsies with well-oriented histologic sections may reveal reflux changes in the mucosa. Since these abnormal histologic changes can be seen in some normal subjects in the most distal segment of the esophagus,[79] at least two biopsy specimens should be obtained 5 cm above the LES.[80] Neutrophils are seldom present in these biopsies (in 5%). Forceps biopsy instruments used through endoscopes can sample the mucosa under direct vision, and therefore they are indicated when carcinoma or Barrett's epithelia are suspected.

Sphincter incompetence can be assessed by esophageal manometry[81] or by demonstrating gastroesophageal reflux. Esophageal manometry can also provide information about the functional state of the esophagus, particularly the presence of nonperistaltic or low-force contractions. It can also determine the pressures of the upper esophageal sphincter. Symptoms of aspiration could be explained by a weak upper esophageal sphincter. Gastroesophageal reflux can be demonstrated by two different methods, the Tutle's test[4,82] and esophageal scintigraphy.[83] In the Tutle's Test, acid reflux is detected by a pH electrode in the esophagus placed

5 cm above the LES. Acid reflux can be demonstrated in the basal state or after the intragastric administration of 300 cc of 0.1N HCl. If reflux is observed in 90% of patients with chronic reflux symptoms.[4] A false-positive result occurs, however, in 10% of normal subjects. With esophageal scintigraphy reflux is demonstrated by measuring the radioactivity over the esophageal area with the gamma camera after the patient has ingested a bolus of water containing ^{99m}Tc-sulfur colloid. With this diagnostic technique, one can determine the presence of gastroesophageal reflux, irrespective of the pH, by a progressive increase in intra-abdominal pressures. The test has the additional advantage that it can estimate the esophageal transit time or clearance.[81] Although this latter method has obvious advantages, we consider that the Tutle's test is more sensitive since it can demonstrate free reflux or reflux in the basal state without any changes in intra-abdominal pressures.

The use of 12–24 hour pH electrode monitoring of the esophagus has also been proposed as a diagnostic test.[85] It is claimed that this test discriminates better between normal subjects and patients with reflux esophagitis by estimating the frequency and duration of gastroesophageal reflux. However, it is cumbersome, not cost effective, and difficult to perform in the majority of the hospitals. It is extremely useful, nevertheless, in studying the pathogenesis and treatment of this disease, particularly when used in combination with manometric techniques.

MANAGEMENT

The treatment of this disease entity attempts to achieve two major goals: to correct esophageal motor disorders and thereby improve the antireflux barrier and esophageal clearance, and to buffer or prevent the secretion of gastric acid and inactivate pepsin and, if possible, bile salts as well. In the process of achieving these objectives, we should consider the following: (1) patients should be properly selected and accurately diagnosed; (2) we are dealing with a chronic disease requiring some form of continuous therapy; (3) the esophagus is at higher risk when patients are asleep in the recumbent position because the gravity factor is absent, and the impaired esophageal acid clearance and unbuffered gastric contents result in prolonged acid reflux; (4) a severe inflammatory process might further damage the neuromuscular structures of the esophagus, worsen the sphincter incompetence, and perhaps impair the esophageal acid clearance; and (5) gross esophagitis can lead to complications that can be prevented and to a certain degree be reversed.

Medical Management

This therapeutic modality is an effective form of treatment in 80–90% of patients with reflux esophagitis. Intensive therapy is effective in relieving symptoms and presumably in increasing the rate of healing of the esophagitis lesion.

Measures that Prevent Gastroesophageal Reflux. Simple measures such as postural and dietary therapy can be extremely helpful. Elevation of the head of the bed 6–8 inches not only increases the gravity factor or pressure gradient between the stomach and the esophagus but also facilitates the clearance of the refluxed contents, thereby reducing the duration of gastroesophageal reflux.[86] Clinical observations have suggested that patients frequently complain of heartburn and regurgitation after large meals with a high fatty content and spices. In addition, some patients have specific food intolerances, and the ingestion of those food will cause symptoms of reflux. Presumably, the ingestion of small meals decreases the intragastric volume and might reduce the frequency and duration of episodes of gastroesophageal reflux. However, the correlation between the frequency and duration of reflux episodes and the size of the meal has not been investigated. Nevertheless, there is a significant symptomatic relief after patients follow these simple therapeutic suggestions. Additional dietary manipulations can also be helpful, since protein meals have been shown to increase LES pressures, whereas fatty meals, alcoholic beverages, and tobacco smoking—because of the nicotine content—reduce sphincter competence. Certain drugs can also be harmful, particularly anticholinergic drugs that not only reduce LES pressures but also slow gastric emptying.

Drug Therapy. If these simple maneuvers fail, drugs that improve LES competence and increase the magnitude or force of esophageal contractions—thereby facilitating esophageal clearance—can also be used. There are two drugs available that can accomplish both these objectives, bethanechol and metoclopramide. Bethanechol, a cholinergic drug, acts directly on the LES muscle. It is used in a dose of 25 mg ½ hour before each meal and at bedtime. In a double-blind cross-over study, bethanechol improved reflux symptoms and decreased the consumption of antacids when compared with placebo.[87] Its efficacy, however, is limited where it is needed the most, in patients with moderate-to-severe esophagitis. It is conceivable that the lack of dramatic therapeutic response in these patients may the result from duration of the pharmacologic action on the LES and esophagus. This has not been investigated carefully. Bethanechol also has some drawbacks, with a few patients complaining of abdominal cramps, constipation, or diarrhea. Furthermore, there may be some long-term effects since the drug stimulates gastric acid secretion in both normal subjects and patients with duodenal ulcer. It is not known, however, whether it increases gastric acid secretion in an average patient with reflux esophagitis.

Metoclopramide is an ideal drug on theoretical grounds. It reduces the duration of gastroesophageal reflux after a meal,[88] probably by improving the sphincter competence[89] and perhaps by increasing the esophageal acid clearance and gastric emptying.[90] It has also been suggested that metoclopramide causes pyloric contraction, thus preventing reflux from the duodenum.[91] The recommended doses of metoclopramide is 10 mg ½ hour before meals and at bedtime. In contrast to bethanechol, it neither causes abdominal cramps nor stimulates gastric acid secretion.[92] Although it has been used in Europe for a number of years, there is only one controlled clinical trial showing that this drug caused symptomatic relief and increased esophageal tolerance to acid when compared with placebo and moderate antacid ingestion.[93] Several controlled trials that have not yet been published have failed to find a significant difference between metoclopramide-treated and placebo groups and moderate ingestion of antacids. The drug's major disadvantage results from its effect on the central nervous system. Patients may complain of increased tiredness, anxiety, restlessness, and occasionally even agitation. Nevertheless, bethanechol or metoclopramide may find an important place in the therapy of this disease when used in combination with other forms of therapy.

Treatment of the Causative Agents.   The only dietary measure that may be important in controlling causative agents is the excessive ingestion of coffee. There is general agreement that coffee increases gastric acid secretion through caffeine and other factors not known at the present time.[94] Furthermore, our clinical experience indicates that patients with reflux esophagitis complain of heartburn after ingestion of coffee. The effect of coffee on the LES, however, is controversial.[94,95] One study indicated that coffee caused an increase in LES pressures; the other that it had no effect.

Until recently, the mainstay in the management of reflux esophagitis was antacid therapy. Antacids decrease the damaging effects of gastroesophageal reflux by at least three different mechanisms. First, they buffer the reflux contents present in the esophagus with immediate relief of the substernal burning pain. The buffering effect within the esophagus, however, is fairly brief because antacids are rapidly cleared by the esophagus. Second, they also buffer the intragastric contents, which prevents the recurrence of acid reflux and is probably the most important action as far as affecting the natural course of the disease. In the fasting state antacids are quickly emptied into the duodenum and their neutralizing effect does not last more than 1 hour. In contrast, in the postprandial state, the action of antacids may last for at least 2 hours.[96] Third, it has been suggested that antacids are able to increase LES pressures, improving sphincter competence.[97] This observation has not been confirmed by other workers. Although intensive antacid therapy can control symptoms of reflux over a short period of time, practical maintenance therapy with antacids—that is, 30 cc of an antacid 1 hour after each meal and at bedtime—is not sufficient to control the symptoms of reflux so as to maintain a normal quality of life in most (approximately 80%) patients.[98] They continue to have intermittent episodes of reflux that may be controlled again by intensive antacid therapy. We presume that the major limitation of maintenance antacid therapy occurs during the night when antacids are quickly emptied into the duodenum by the fasting stomach, with the gastric pH remaining acidic for the remainder of the night. The development of the H-2 receptor blockers has relegated the use of antacids either to treat patients with mild esophagitis or to supplement the effect of these newer drugs. Antacids can also be used when gastric acid secretion is extremely low or absent to treat bile-salt esophagitis.

In patients with moderate-to-severe esophagitis who continue to have symptoms of reflux despite adequate antacid therapy, H-2 receptor blockers such as cimetidine appears to be effective over at least an 8-week period. A controlled trial comparing cimetidine with placebo plus modest antacid therapy showed that 300 mg after each meal and at bedtime was more effective than placebo in relieving the frequency and severity of the heartburn, particularly at night, and in improving the tolerance of the esophagus to acid.[99] At the end of the treatment period, however, the endoscopic appearance of the esophagus did not improve. Furthermore, maintenance therapy that consisted of either 300 mg twice a day or 400 mg at bedtime failed to maintain the state of symptomatic remission in most patients.

Although these newer drugs appear to be promising, we need to determine whether or not they can change the natural history of the disease over a long period of time and if they can prevent the development of Barrett's mucosa, esophageal ulceration, or stricture. It is also important to know if improvement of esophagitis with these newer forms of therapy will improve the competence of the LES and acid clearance by the esophagus. Such studies would be extremely useful indeed.

Finally, both antacid therapy and, particularly, H-2 receptor blockers such as cimetidine may be useful in treating pulmonary aspiration induced by gastroesophageal reflux. Although cimetidine may not reduce the frequency and duration of reflux, it increases the pH of the refluxed content, thereby lessening the damaging effect on the respiratory tract. A recent study revealed that patients with nonallergic asthma treated with cimetidine around the clock have fewer respiratory symptoms than prior to therapy.[9] Further studies need to be performed to determine the effectiveness of this form of therapy on these pulmonary complications.

Nevertheless, despite these therapeutic developments, 10–20% of patients do not respond well to this therapeutic modality. There are four subgroups of patients with reflux esophagitis who appear to be particularly resistant to medical management: (1) patients with stricture; (2) patients who already have evidence of Barrett's epithelium or a punched out deep ulcer; (3) obese patients; and (4) elderly and debilitated patients. Patients who are acceptable surgical risks should therefore be referred for surgical management of this disease.

Surgical Treatment

It has been shown repeatedly that surgical management with an antireflux procedure is an effective form of treatment that prevents reflux, relieves symptoms, and promotes the healing of the esophagitis lesion.[100-102] It has also been shown that antireflux procedures improve patients with esophageal strictures[103] and induce the regression of the Barrett's mucosa.[73] Patients with esophageal strictures do not require any further esophageal dilatations after an antireflux procedure such as a posterior gastropexy of Hill.[103] In patients with well-established fibrotic strictures, however, there is an increased incidence of breakdown of these surgical procedures, with recurrence of the esophagitis and stricture. The effectiveness of these antireflux procedures depends a great deal on the experience of the surgeon and on the type of procedure performed. The general consensus is that the Nissen fundoplication[104] is probably the most effective antireflux procedure with the Hill posterior gastropexy and the Belsey Mark IV anterior fundoplication running a close second.[105,106]

It is also accepted that these surgical procedures not only repair the hiatal hernia but also create an antireflux barrier with a high-pressure zone.[107] This postoperative high-pressure zone corresponds to the previous or preoperative LES. However, this new high-pressure zone appears to be more asymetric with a sharp increase in pressures in a short segment within the LES. Nonetheless, it does not appear to be a passive structure, since this new high-pressure zone relaxes to its full extent during swallowing. In addition, the length–tension curves that are abnormal in the presurgery state become normal, indicating that the properties of the circular muscle layer of this zone have been affected by this surgical procedure.[108] Two hypotheses have been advanced to explain this phenomenon: (1) the surgical procedure shortens the circular muscle layer, thus increasing its length–tension characteristics by shifting the curve closer to the point of optimal tension development,[108] and (2) the fundal muscles re-enforce the LES since these muscles have physiologic and pharmacologic characteristics similar to that of the LES circular muscle layer.[109]

Nevertheless, the surgical management still needs considerable improvement. We need a better understanding of what is attained with the antireflux procedure in order to standardize it and perhaps improve it, creating a normal high-pressure zone without interfering with normal physiologic processes such as belching and vomiting. We also need to learn why these surgical procedures tend to break down within 6 years after operation.[110] Is this breakdown due to a progressive muscle disease that originally caused the LES incompetence, or is it due to the nature of the operation itself? There is some evidence that seems to indicate that the symptoms recur long before the repair breaks down, suggesting that they may be caused by progression of the LES incompetence.[111] If this were the case, perhaps, a second surgical procedure would be required. We must also learn to prevent the side effects that are most common with the most effective antireflux procedure, that is, the Nissen repair. Three types of complications have been observed: (1) the bloating syndrome with inability to belch and vomit; (2) dysphagia, which can be treated with a series of dilatations; and (3) a syndrome that is consistent with an incidental vagotomy, because gastric retention and diarrhea develop postoperatively. This syndrome can be persistent; however, in most cases, it is transient, lasting for 2–12 months.

REFERENCES

1. Bennett JR, Atkinson M: Oesophageal acid-perfusion in the diagnosis of precordial pain. Lancet 2:1150–1152, 1966.
2. Brunnen PL, Karmody AM, Needham CD: Severe peptic esophagitis. Gut 10:831–837, 1969.
3. Olsen AM, Schlegel JF: Motility disturbances caused by esophagitis. J Thorac Cardiovasc Surg 50:607–612, 1965.
4. Behar J, Biancani P, Sheahan DG: Evaluation of esophageal tests in the diagnosis of reflux esophagitis. Gastroenterology 71:9–15, 1976.
5. Euler AR, Byrne WJ, Ament ME et al.: Recurrent pulmonary disease in children: a complication of gastroesophageal reflux. Pediatrics 63:47–51, 1979.
6. Christie DL, O'Grady LR, Mack DV: Incompetent lower esophageal sphincter and gastroesophageal reflux in recurrent acute pulmonary disease of infancy and childhood, J Pediatr 93:23–27, 1978.
7. Kennedy JH: "Silent" gastroesophageal reflux: an important but little known cause of pulmonary complications. Dis Chest, 42:42–45, 1962.
8. Jolley SG, Herbst JJ, Johnson DG, et al.: Esophageal pH monitoring during sleep

identifies children with respiratory symptoms from gastroesophageal reflux. Gastroenterology 80:1501–1506, 1981.

9. Larrain A, Lira E, Otero M, Pope CE: Posterior laryngitis—A useful marker of esophageal reflux. Gastroenterology 80:1204 (abstr), 1981.

10. Chernow B, Johnson LF, Janowitz WR, Castell DO: Pulmonary aspirations as a consequence of gastroesophageal reflux: a diagnostic approach. Dig Dis Sci 24:839–844, 1979.

11. Dillard DH, Anderson HN: A new concept of the mechanism of sphincteric failure in sliding esophageal hiatus hernia. Surg Gynec Obstet 122:1030–1038, 1966.

12. Michelson E, Siegel CI: The role of the phrenico-esophageal ligament in the lower esophageal sphincter. Surg Gynec Obstet 119:1291–1294, 1964.

13. Bombeck CT, Dillard DH, Nyhus LM: Muscular anatomy of the gastroesophageal junction and role of phrenoesophageal ligament. Autopsy study of sphincter mechanism. Ann Surg 164:643–654, 1966.

14. Tocornal JA, Snow HD, Fonkalsrud EW: A mucosal flap valve mechanism to prevent gastroesophageal reflux and esophagitis. Surgery 64:519–523, 1968.

15. Sicular A, Cohen B, Zimmerman A, Kark AE: The significance of an intra-abdominal segment of canine esophagus as a component antireflux mechanism. Surgery, 61:784–790, 1967.

16. Lippa, FH, Thal AP: Experimental reflux esophagitis. Arch Surg 93:148–153, 1966.

17. Wankling WJ, Warrian WG, Lind JF: The gastroesophageal sphincter in hiatus hernia. Can J Surg, 8:61–67, 1965.

18. Cohen S, Harris LD: Does hiatus hernia affect competence of the gastroesophageal sphincter? N Engl J Med 284:1053–1056, 1971.

19. Wolf BS: Sliding hiatus hernia: The need for redefinition. Am J Roentgenol Radium Ther Nucl Med 117:231–247, 1973.

20. Pope CE II: A dynamic test of sphincter strength: its application to the lower esophageal sphincter. Gastroenterology 52:779–786, 1967.

21. Haddad JK: Relation of gastroesophageal reflux to yield sphincter pressures. Gastroenterology 58:175–184, 1970.

22. Winans CS, Harris LD: Quantitation of lower esophageal sphincter competence. Gastroenterology 52:773–778, 1967.

23. Christensen J, Conklin JL, Freeman B: Physiologic specialization at the esophagogastric junction in three species. Am J Physiol 225:1265–1270, 1973.

24. Biancani P, Zabinski MP, Kerstein MD, Behar J: Lower esophageal sphincter mechanics: anatomic and physiologic relationships of the esophago-gastric junction of cat. Gastroenterology 82:468–475, 1982.

25. Goyal RK, Rattan S: Genesis of basal sphincter pressure: effect of tetrodotoxin on lower esophageal sphincter pressure in opossum in vivo. Gastroenterology 71:62–67, 1976.

26. Behar J, Kerstein MD, Biancani P: Neural control of lower esophageal sphincter (LES) closure. Gastroenterology (submitted for publication).

27. Fox JE, Daniel EE: The role of calcium in the genesis of lower esophageal sphincter (LES) tone and contraction. Gastroenterology 74:1035 (abstr), 1978.

28. Daniel EE, Sarna S, Crankshaw J: Mechanisms of tetrodotoxin-insensitive relaxation of opossum lower esophageal sphincter. In Duthie HL (ed): Proceedings 6th International Symposium Gastrointestinal Motility, Edinburgh, 1977, MTP Press, Edinburgh, pp. 525–534.

29. Daniel EE, Crankshaw J, Sarna S: Myogenic control of esophageal motor function.

2nd International Symposium on Esophagus and Gastroesophageal Junction, Ixtapa, Mexico, 2:14–19, 1978.

30. Jacobowitz D, Nemir P Jr: The autonomic innervation of the esophagus of the dog. J Thorac Cardiovasc Surg 58:678–684, 1969.

31. Lind JF, Crispin JS, McIver DK: The effect of atropine on the gastroesophageal sphincter. Can J Physiol Pharmacol 46:233–238, 1968.

32. Behar J, Kastendieck J: Studies on sphincter competence. Gastroenterology 66:834 (abstr), 1974.

33. Dodds WJ, Dent J, Hogan WJ, Arndorfer RC: The effect of atropine on esophageal motor function in man. Gastroenterology 74:1028 (abstr), 1978.

34. Grossman MI: Chemical messengers: a view from the gut. Fed Proc 38:2341–2343, 1979.

35. Csendes A, Oster M, Brandsborg O, et al.: Gastroesophageal sphincter pressure and serum gastrin: reaction to food stimulation in normal subjects and in patients with gastric or duodenal ulcer. Scand J Gastroenterol 13:363–368, 1978.

36. Lind JF, Smith AM, Melver DK, et al.: Heartburn in pregnancy—a manometric study. Can Med Assoc J 98:571–574, 1968.

37. van Thiel DH, Gavaler JS, Stremple J: Lower esophageal sphincter pressure in women using sequential oral contraceptives. Gastroenterology 71:232–234, 1976.

38. Shulze K, Christensen J: Lower sphincter of the opossum esophagus in pseudo-pregnancy. Gastroenterology 73: 1082–1085, 1977.

39. Eastwood GL, Castell DO, Higgs RH: Experimental esophagitis in cats impairs lower esophageal sphincter pressure. Gastroenterology 69:146–153, 1975.

40. Higgs RH, Castell DO, Eastwood GL: Studies on the mechanism of esophagitis-induced lower esophageal sphincter hypotension in cats. Gastroenterology 71:51–57, 1976.

41. Biancani P, Dodds WJ, Storer E, et al.: Acute experimental esophagitis affects mechanical properties of the lower esophageal sphincter. Gastroenterology 76:1100 (abstr), 1979.

42. Nebel OT, Castell DO: Lower esophageal sphincter pressure changes after food ingestion. Gastroenterology 63:778–783, 1972.

43. Dennish GW, Castell DO: Inhibitory effect of smoking on the lower esophageal sphincter. N Engl J Med 284:1136–1137, 1971.

44. Hogan WJ, Viegas de Andrade SRT, Winship DH: Ethanol-induced acute esophageal motor dysfunction. J Appl Physiol, 32:755–760, 1972.

45. Lind JF, Warrian WG, Wankling WJ: Responses of the gastroesophageal junctional zone to increases in abdominal pressure. Can J Surg, 9:32–38, 1966.

46. Lind JF, Cotton DJ, Blachard R: Effect of thoracic displacement and vagotomy on the canine gastroesophageal junctional zone. Gastroenterology 56:1078–1085, 1969.

47. Crispin JS, McIver DK, Lind JF: Manometric study of the effect of vagotomy on the gastroesophageal sphincter. Can J Surg 10:299–303, 1967.

48. Kaye MD, Rein R, Johnson WP, Schowalter JP: Responses of the competent and incompetent lower oesophageal sphincter to pentagastrin and abdominal compression. Gut 17:933–939, 1976.

49. Csendes A, Oster M, Bradsborg O: The effect of vagotomy on human gastroesophageal sphincter pressure in the resting state and following increases in intra-abdominal pressure. Surgery 85:419–424, 1979.

50. Dodds WJ, Hogan WJ, Miller SJJ, et al.: Effects of increased intra-abdominal pressure on lower esophageal sphincter pressure. Am J Dig Dis, 20:298–308, 1975.

51. Diamant NE, Akin AN: Effect of gastric contractions on the lower esophageal sphincter. Gastroenterology 63:38–44, 1972.

52. Dent J, Dodds WJ, Friedman RH: Mechanism of gastroesophageal reflux in recumbent asymptomatic human subjects. J Clin Invest 65:256–267, 1980.
53. Dodds WJ, Hogan WJ, Helm JF, Dent J: Pathogenesis of reflux esophagitis. Gastroenterology (in Press).
54. Booth DJ, Kemmerer WT, Skinner DB: Acid clearing from distal esophagus. Arch Surg 96:731–734, 1968.
55. Stanciu C, Bennett JR: Oesophageal acid clearing: one factor in the production of reflux esophagitis. Gut 15:852–857, 1974.
56. Behar J, Ramsby G: Gastric emptying and antral motility in reflux esophagitis. Effect of oral metoclopramide. Gastroenterology 74:253–256, 1978.
57. Csendes A, Henriquez A: Gastric emptying in patients with reflux esophagitis or benign strictures of the esophagus secondary to reflux compared to controls. Scand J Gastroenterol 13:205–207, 1978.
58. McCallum RW, Berkowitz DM: The frequency of delayed gastric emptying in patients with gastroesophageal reflux (GER) and its response to metoclopramide (M) and bethanechol (B). Gastroenterology 74:1135 (abstr), 1978.
59. Kiriluk LB, Merendino KA: Comparative sensitivity of mucosa of various segments of alimentary tract in dog to acid-peptic action. Surgery 35:547–556, 1954.
60. Chung RSK, Johnson GM, DenBesten L: Effect of sodium taurocholate and ethanol on hydrogen ion absorption in rabbit esophagus. Am J Dig Dis 22:582–588, 1977.
61. Goldberg HI, Dodds WJ, Gee S: Role of acid and pepsin in acute experimental esophagitis. Gastroenterology 56:223–230, 1969.
62. Safaie-Shirazi S, DenBesten L, Zike WL: Effect of bile salts on the ionic permeability of the esophageal mucosa and their role in the production of esophagitis. Gastroenterology 68:728–733, 1975.
63. Orlando RC, Carney CN, Kinard HB, Powell DW: Structure-function alterations in the acid damage rabbit esophagus. Gastroenterology 76:1212 (abstr), 1979.
64. Kinard HB, Jones JD, Orlando RC, Powell DW: Esophageal potential difference (PD) measurements as an indicator of mucosal disease. Gastroenterology, 76:1169 (abstr), 1979.
65. Boesby S: Relationship between gastro-oesophageal acid reflux, basal gastroesophageal sphincter pressure, and gastric acid secretion. Scand J Gastroenterol 12:547–551, 1977.
66. Northway MG Libshitz HI, Osborne BM: Radiation esophagitis in the opossum: radioprotection with indomethacin. Gastroenterology 78:883–892, 1980.
67. Ismail-Beigi F, Horton PF, Pope CE II: Histological consequences of gastroesophageal reflux in man. Gastroenterology 58:163–174, 1970.
68. Livstone E, Sheahan DG, Behar J: Studies of esophageal epithelial proliferation in patients with reflux esophagitis. Gastroenterology 73:1315–1319, 1977.
69. Peters PM: The pathology of severe digestion esophagitis. Thorax 10:269–286, 1955.
70. Bremner CG, Lynch VP, Ellis FH: Barrett's esophagus: congenital or acquired? An experimental study of esophageal mucosal regeneration in the dog. Surgery 68:209–216, 1970.
71. Trier JS: Morphology of the epithelium of the distal esophagus in patients with mid-esophageal peptic strictures. Gastroenterology 58:444–461, 1970.
72. Paull A, Trier JS, Dalton MD, et al.: The histologic spectrum of Barrett's esophagus. N Engl J Med 295:476–480, 1976.
73. Brand DL, Ylvisaker JT, Gelfand M, Pope CE II: Regression of columnar esophageal (Barrett's) epithelium after anti-reflux surgery. N Engl J Med 302:844–848, 1980.
74. Haggitt RC, Tryzelaar J, Ellis FH, Colcher H: Adenocarcinoma complicating columnar epithelium-lined (Barrett's) esophagus. Am J Clin Pathol 70:1–5, 1978.

75. Berenson M, Riddell RH, Skinner DB, Freston, JW: Malignant transformation of esophageal columnar epithelium. Cancer 41:554–562, 1978.
76. Bernstein LM, Baker LA: A clinical test for esophagitis. Gastroenterology 34:760–781, 1958.
77. Kobayashi S, Kasugai T: Endoscopic and biopsy criteria for the diagnosis of esophagitis with a fiberoptic esophagoscope. Dig Dis 19:345–352, 1974.
78. Svoboda AC, Knauer CM, Gamble CN, et al.: Problems in the early diagnosis of peptic esophagitis. Gastrointest Endos 13:14–17, 1967.
79. Weinstein WM, Bogoch ER, Bowes KL: The normal human esophageal mucosa: a histological reappraisal. Gastroenterology 68:40–44, 1975.
80. Behar J, Sheahan DG: Histological abnormalities in reflux esophagitis. Arch Pathol 99:387–391, 1975.
81. Dodds WJ: Instrumentation and methodology for intraluminal esophageal manometry. Arch Intern Med 136:515–523, 1976.
82. Tuttle SG, Rugin F, Bettarello A: The physiology of heartburn. Ann Intern Med 55:292–300, 1961.
83. Fisher RS, Malmud LS, Roberts GS, Lobis IF: Gastroesophageal (GE) scintiscanning to detect and quantitate GE reflux. Gastroenterology 70:301–308, 1976.
84. Tolin RD, Malmud LS, Reilley J, Fisher RS: Esophageal scintigraphy to quantitate esophageal transit (quantitation of esophageal transit). Gastroenterology 76:1402–1408, 1979.
85. DeMeester TR, Johnson LF, Joseph GJ: Patterns of gastroesophageal reflux in health and disease. Ann Surg 184:459–470, 1976.
86. Babka JC, Hager GW, Castell DO: The effect of body position on lower esophageal sphincter pressure. Am J Dig Dis 18:441–442, 1973.
87. Farrell RL, Roling GT, Castell DO: Cholinergic therapy of chronic heartburn. A controlled trial. Ann Intern Med 80:573–576, 1974.
88. Behar J, Biancani P: Effect of oral metoclopramide on gastroesophageal reflux in the post-cibal state. Gastroenterology 70:331–335, 1976.
89. Cohen S, Morris DW, Schoen HJ: The effect of oral and intravenous metoclopramide on human lower esophageal sphincter pressure. Gastroenterology 70:477–480, 1976.
90. Connell AM, George JD: Effect of metoclopramide on gastric function in man. Gut 10:678–680, 1969.
91. Valenzuela JE, Defilippi C, Csendes A: Manometric studies on the human pyloric sphincter. Effect of cigarette smoking, metoclopramide, and atropine. Gastroenterology 70:481–483, 1976.
92. Meeroff JC: The effect of metoclopramide on human gastric emptying and secretion. Acta Gastroenterol Latinoam 6:55–58, 1974.
93. Winnan J, Avella J, Callachan C, McCallum RW: Double-blind trial of metoclopramide versus placebo-antacid in symptomatic gastroesophageal reflux. Gastroenterology 78:1292 (abstr), 1980.
94. Cohen S, Booth GH: Gastric acid secretion and lower esophageal sphincter pressure in response to coffee and caffeine. N Engl J Med 293:897–899, 1975.
95. Thomas FB, Steinbaugh JT, Fromkes JJ, et al.: Inhibitory effect of coffee on lower esophageal sphincter pressure. Gastroenterology 79:1262–1266, 1980.
96. Fordtran JS, Morawski SG, Richardson CT: In vivo and in vitro evaluation of liquid antacids. N Engl J Med 288:923–928, 1973.
97. Higgs RH, Smyth RD, Castell DO: Gastric alkalinization: effect on lower esophageal sphincter pressures and serum gastrin. N Engl J Med 291:486–490, 1974.
98. Behar J, Sheahan DG, Biancani P, et al.: Medical and surgical management of reflux

esophagitis: a 38-month report on a prospective clinical trial. N Engl J Med 293:263–268, 1975.

99. Behar J, Brand DL, Brown FC, et al.: Cimetidine in the treatment of symptomatic gastroesophageal reflux: a double-blind controlled trial. Gastroenterology 74:441–448, 1978.

100. Csendes A, Larrain A: Effect of posterior gastropexy on gastroesophageal sphincter pressures and symptomatic reflux in patients with hiatal hernia. Gastroenterology 63:19–24, 1972.

101. DiMarino AJ, Rosato E, Rosato F, Cohen S: Improvement in lower esophageal sphincter pressure following surgery for complicated gastroesophageal reflux. Ann Surg 181:239–242, 1975.

102. Bowes KL, Sarna SK: Effect of fundoplication on the lower esophageal sphincter. Can J Surg 18:328–333, 1975.

103. Larrain A, Csendes A, Pope CE II: Surgical correction of reflux: an effective therapy for esophageal strictures. Gastroenterology 69:578–583, 1975.

104. Bushkin FL, Neustein CL, Parker TH, Woodward ER: Nissen fundoplication for reflux peptic esophagitis. Ann Surg 185:672–677, 1977.

105. Skinner DB, Belsey RHR, Russell PS: Surgical management of esophageal reflux and hiatus hernia. J Thorac Cardiovasc Surg 53:33–54, 1967.

106. Hill LD: An effective operation for hiatal hernia. An eight year appraisal. Ann Surg 106:681–692, 1967.

107. Behar J, Biancani P, Spiro HM, Storer EH: Effect of anterior fundoplication on lower esophageal sphincter competence. Gastroenterology 67:209–215, 1974.

108. Biancani P, Zabinski M, Behar J: Pressure, tension, and force of closure of the lower esophageal sphincter and esophagus. J Clin Invest 58:476–483, 1975.

109. Siewert R, Jennewein HM, Waldeck F: Mechanism of action of fundoplication. In Daniel EE (ed): Proceedings 4th International Symposium Gastrointestinal Motility, Alberta, Canada, 1973, pp. 144–152.

110. Brand DL, Eastwood IR, Martin D, et al.: Esophageal symptoms, manometry and histology before and after antireflux surgery. A long-term follow-up study. Gastroenterology 76:1393–1401, 1979.

111. DeMeester, TR, Johnson LF, Kent AH: Evaluation of current operations for the prevention of gastroesophageal reflux. Ann Surg 180:511–525, 1974.

11 | Management of Esophageal Complications

Mark Mellow

INTRODUCTION

It is not without some trepidation that this gastroenterologist writes a chapter dealing with conditions that fall generally within the purview of our surgical colleagues. In many instances, opinions are given regarding procedures that have not been personally performed; I hope not to sound imperious in that regard. However, it would not appear to serve the readers' best interest merely to list, without comment, the myriad procedures that have been performed for the management of these entities. Therefore, I have attempted to include in each section an opinion on the course of action that I wish my surgical colleague would follow were we to be faced with the problem. Finally, I have attempted to mention those areas in which gaps in current knowledge of pathophysiology exist, in the hope that research will allow better treatment of these rather catastrophic conditions.

ESOPHAGEAL STRICTURES

Esophageal strictures are seen in association with, and as a consequence of, a variety of inflammatory processes, primary or secondary neoplasms, infections (e.g., candidiasis, tuberculosis, syphilis), as well as chemical or physical injury (e.g., lye ingestion, radiation). They most commonly occur as a result of primary esophageal carcinomas and reflux esophagitis. As with most mechanical lesions of the esophagus, dysphagia for solids is the primary symptom. The severity of dysphagia is dependent on the thoroughness of bolus mastication, the luminal diameter of the stricture, and whether or not an associated esophageal motility disorder is present.

Diagnosis

Although barium swallow demonstrates the stricture, its severity and character are best defined by esophagoscopy. It is often prudent to utilize a small-diameter pediatric-type endoscope in evaluating strictures. Examination of both the area of the stricture itself and the mucosa distal to it can be better accomplished with the narrow endoscope, allowing the diagnosis of carcinoma or columnar metaplasia (Barrett's epithelium) to be made. The need for obtaining multiple mucosal biopsies in order to make a satisfactory distinction between benign and malignant lesions cannot be overly stressed. Often dilation of the stricture must be performed before tissue distal to the stricture can be visualized and biopsies obtained for appropriate histologic examination.

Medical Management

Management of individual strictures should depend on several factors: the length of the stricture, the degree of luminal narrowing, and the associated pathology. The heterogenous nature of strictures must be borne in mind when comparing results of different approaches to stricture management. Regardless of etiology, initial management of strictures consists of attempting to widen the lumen by means of dilators (bougienage). This procedure may be performed using one of two basic types of dilators. Metal bougienage (Peustow type) is performed over a previously introduced wire. The wire should not be passed "blindly" but is best passed through the area of stricture under endoscopic visualization or, at least, with the aid of fluoroscopy. Metal bougienage is used for the initial management of strictures with marked luminal narrowing; strictures that compromise the lumen to a lesser degree can usually be managed by the passage of soft mercury-weighted bougies, which may have either a tapered (Maloney type) or blunt (Hurst type) distal end.

There is no standardized bougienage schedule. Flood recommends passing bougies of increasing diameters until slight bleeding or marked resistance is encountered and continuing treatment at weekly intervals until a size-40 French (12–13 mm) bougie is reached.[1] Gaskins suggests dilations in a graded fashion until the strictured area attains a diameter of at least 15 mm (size-45 French), with treatment sessions held daily or every other day and an advance of only two or three dilator sizes at each sitting.[2] Perforation, the infrequent but dreaded complication of bougienage, is probably best avoided by utilizing caution—not exerting undue force in bougie passage—regardless of treatment schedule. Although the procedure may be done conveniently on an outpatient basis, one must counsel the patient as to the signs of esophageal perforation (see section on perforation, below) and the need to report them promptly. The passage of bougies themselves cause irritation of the luminal surface, with resultant inflammation and edema that may lead to transient luminal narrowing. It is unknown if concurrent administration of anti-inflammatory agents would be beneficial. Once the stricture has been adequately widened, many authorities agree that prophylactic bougienage is unnecessary and that further treatment directed at the stricture itself need be done only if dysphagia recurs. The patient should be seen at regular intervals and questioned carefully with regard to recurrence of symptoms, with bougienage repeated at the earliest sign of return of dysphagia.

In general, if dilation of a benign stricture cannot be adequately performed and the patient's overall medical condition permits it, surgery should be performed. Stricture resection with re-anastomosis can be attempted in certain short severe strictures if adjacent esophageal tissue is suitable for anastomosis. If the stricture in question is a peptic stricture, an antireflux procedure must be performed concomitantly. Strictures that occur after radiation or chemical injury are often extensive and associated with considerable esophageal pathology. In these instances, colon interposition is generally the procedure of choice.[3]

In addition to bougienage, further management of malignant strictures is tempered by the general status of the patient and the extent of the carcinoma. Computed tomography, both thoracic and abdominal, has recently been shown to be extremely accurate in assessing spread of the tumor.[4] Unfortunately, in most patients, the tumor is considerably more widespread than clinical assessement indicated. Therefore, treatment is usually palliative. Although resection of distal esophageal carcinomas may be attempted in certain instances, radiation for midesophageal lesions is the generally accepted therapeutic regimen. The endoscopic placement of an esophageal prosthesis has been recommended for managing recalcitrant malignant strictures.[5] This technique is discussed in detail in the section on management of esophageal fistulae.

In gastroenterology, laser photocoagulation has been applied primarily to manage gastrointestinal bleeding. In seeking expanded application of the laser, some observers noted that whereas it has a coagulation effect at low densities (energy area), at higher energy densities it can vaporize tissue. At our institution, Fleischer has utilized this property of Nd:YAG lasers in treating obstructing esophageal carcinomas via a fiberoptic endoscope. Early results have been encouraging; luminal diameter has been increased significantly after a few esophagoscopic laser sessions, with no untoward complications, albeit in a small number of patients.

Management of Peptic Strictures

Although dilation combined with intensive antireflux therapy is said to yield good results in a majority of patients (60–85% in several series),[1,6] considerable question remains as to whether this approach should be universally applied to patients with peptic strictures. In this regard, it is worth noting that peptic strictures differ from other benign strictures in at least two respects. First, whereas the makeup of other benign strictures is almost exclusively fibrous tissue and, therefore, highly unlikely to revert to normal, there is evidence to suggest that a sizeable minority of peptic strictures consist primarily of inflamed and edematous tissue, and that if reflux can be properly controlled, the stricture may heal.[7] It is, therefore, not unreasonable to attempt a short course of dilations along with an intensive antireflux regimen in patients with peptic strictures. On the other hand, the insult responsible for the formation of nonpeptic strictures is past (corrosive, radiation injury), whereas in peptic strictures it is ongoing (gastroesophageal reflux). Therefore, one must not only be able to dilate the stricture but must prevent continued reflux.

Several observations made on patients with peptic strictures should severely temper one's optimism concerning long-term beneficial results of medical therapy. Most patients with peptic strictures have long histories of symptomatic reflux, have markedly hypotensive lower esophageal sphincter (LES) pressures, and often have an associated distal esophageal motor disorder, ranging from nonperistaltic repetitive contractions to contractions of markedly decreased amplitude.[8,9] Although I am unaware of any pharmacologic evaluation of LES responsivity in patients with peptic strictures, in general, magnitude of LES response to agonists correlates with resting LES pressure—i.e., those patients with the lowest resting LES pressures have the least response.[10] Therefore, not only does the markedly hypotensive LES favor reflux, but the chance of favorably altering the LES pressure pharmacologic is unlikely as well. In addition, the distal esophageal motor disorder impairs esophageal acid clearing. The morbidity of the numerous consequences of gastroesophageal reflux, namely heartburn, nocturnal aspiration, columnar meta-plasia with its malignant potential, and the discomfort of repeated bougienage should not be ignored either. Therefore, many clinicians (including this author) feel that, except in patients with mild strictures and readily manageable reflux or in patients whose general medical condition makes operation an unacceptable risk, a surgical approach to peptic strictures is preferable.

Surgical Therapy

Several antireflux procedures are now available. Although they vary in specific technique, the successful ones rely on two basic principles: strengthening the area of the gastroesophageal junction and increasing the length of the intra-abdominal "sphincter." Figures 11-1, 11-2, 11-3 briefly illustrate the techniques utilized in the Hill, Belsey, and Nissen-type repairs. Hill and Nissen antireflux procedures are done via an abdominal approach, the Belsey procedure via a thoracic approach. The reports of Skinner and Belsey, Hill, and Ellis et al. describe the procedures in considerable detail.[10-12]

Most surgeons advocate preoperative and intraoperative dilation of strictures, although in one series, a successful antireflux procedure alone resulted in healing a majority of the strictures.[7] Intraoperative stricture dilation carries a somewhat increased risk of perforation and of failure of early recognition, but, in experienced hands this risk is quite rare.

A gastroplasty (Collis procedure) is often added to the antireflux procedure.[13-15] In gastroplasty, a tube with the same luminal diameter as the normal esophagus is fashioned from the lesser-curvature side of the stomach, in continuity with the distal esophagus (Fig. 11-4). Although this does not increase the length of sphinc-

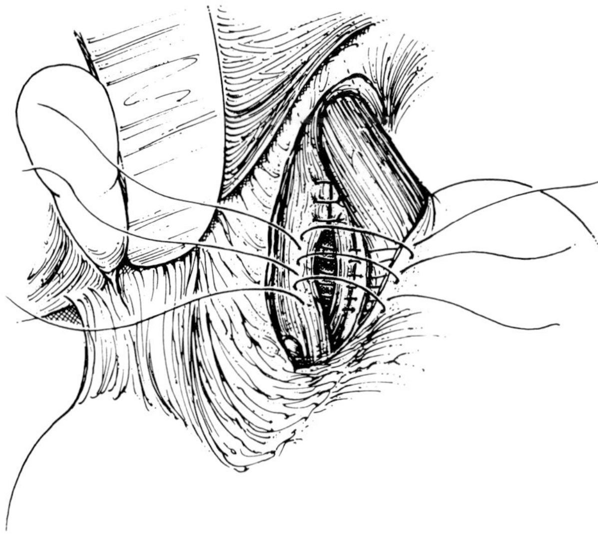

Fig. 11-1. Hill Procedure. Suturing of the lesser curvature of the stomach to the median arcuate ligament of the diaphragm and inclusion of anterior and posterior leaves of the lesser omentum, performed after closing of crura in region of esophageal hiatus. The gastric fundus is then sutured to the distal esophagus. Reprinted by permission from Bombeck CT, Nyhus LM: Esophageal hiatal hernia. In Nora PF (ed): Operative Surgery: Principles and Techniques, Lea & Febiger, Philadelphia, 1980, pp. 711–717.

teric zone exposed to intra-abdominal pressure (that could be accomplished by adequate fundoplication *above* the diaphragm),[16] the "esophageal" lengthening eliminates tension on both the repair and the intrathoracic esophagus in those patients with stricture and a somewhat shortened esophagus.

Recently, intraoperative LES pressure measurements have been reported.[17] Those employing the technique feel that it aids in establishing a proper high-pressure zone. Although this seems logical, the use of an undirectionally oriented catheter raises the question of sampling error due to pressure asymmetry, especially in a surgically constructed high-pressure zone. Even if a standard triple-lumen or multidirectional radially oriented catheter is used, it is not yet clear whether peak, mean, or lowest recorded LESP will best correlate with success of the antireflux procedure. In addition, the effects of various general anesthetic agents on LESP are not clearly defined; it is of interest that recorded intraoperative pressures are approximately twice that of early postoperative values.[17]

When we, as gastroenterologists, attempt to evaluate reports on the merits of the various antireflux procedures, we must bear in mind that these reports are of two general types. In one an expert surgeon performs the operations, which are all of the same type. The results obtained by that expert may not be applicable to surgeons in general. In the other, multiple surgeons (often relative surgical neophytes) perform a variety of antireflux procedures. In that experimental design, which operation is "best" may really mean which operation is easiest to perform.

It is important to evaluate patient selection criteria carefully. Studies should

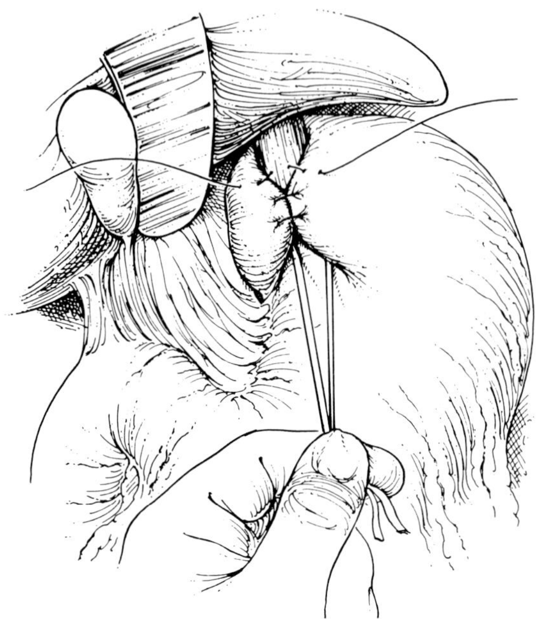

Fig. 11-2.   Nissen Procedure. Plication of fundus of the stomach around the distal esophagus. "Wrap around" is 360°. Reprinted by permission from Bombeck CT, Nyhus LM: Esophageal hiatal hernia. In Nora PF (ed): Operative Surgery: Principles and Techniques, Lea & Febiger, Philadelphia, 1980, pp. 711–717.

describe length and diameter of the stricture, whether or not an associated esophageal motility disorder is present, duration of preoperative symptomatology, and what medical therapy has been attempted. In addition, objective and subjective data pertaining to postoperative evaluation of the presence of reflux and its consequences should be presented, as well as problems arising from the surgical procedure itself. Current reports all indicate that antireflux operations of the Hill, Belsey, or Nissen type appear to be successful if performed properly.[12,13,17,18] However, there is, as yet, a paucity of data concerning long-term follow-up. The studies by Pearson and Henderson and by Brand and his group are most satisfactory in that regard.[18,19]

So: Hill vs Belsey vs Nissen? In general, patients undergoing Belsey repair have slightly longer hospital stays, somewhat fewer problems with diarrhea, and less impairment of the ability to belch or vomit.[15,16,17] Objectively, they have a somewhat greater chance of having post operative gastroesophageal reflux—at least as assessed by standard acid-reflux testing—somewhat lower mean resting LES pressure, and a shorter length of intra-abdominal sphincteric segment than do patients undergoing the Nissen repair.[12,15,17] Perhaps, in patients with severe distal esophageal motility disturbances (with or without associated progressive systemic sclerosis) the Belsey-type procedure is preferable. In the main, however, the choice of which antireflux procedure to perform may be less important than the choice of the surgeon to perform it.

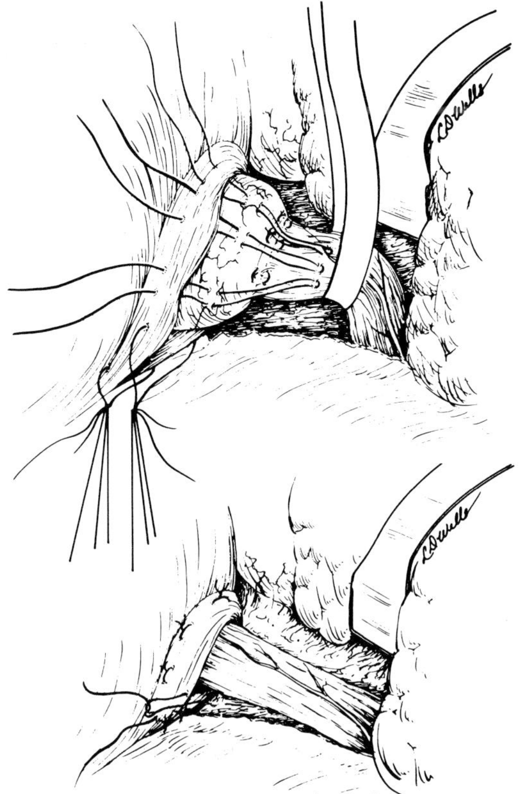

Fig. 11-3.   Belsey Procedure. Top. Suturing of the stomach to the anterolateral two-thirds of the esophagus. Sutures are placed first into the stomach wall several centimeters beyond the peritoneal reflection, then into the phrenoesophageal ligament and adjacent esophageal wall, and then carried back to the stomach wall. Bottom. The completed procedure. Reprinted by permission from Shields TW: The diaphragm. In Nora PF (ed): Operative Surgery: Principles and Techniques, Lea & Febiger, Philadelphia, 1980, pp. 271–279.

ESOPHAGEAL PERFORATIONS

Incidence and Etiology

Esophageal perforations are relatively uncommon, occurring at an incidence of 2–6 year in a large hospital population.[20-22] Table 11-1 lists the causes of esophageal perforations. Instrumentation, spontaneous perforation, and surgical injury make up the vast majority of cases. Since, in gastroenterological practice, instrumental and spontaneous perforations are seen most frequently, most of the ensuing discussion will be directed toward recognizing and treating these entities.

Instrumental perforations occur mainly after rigid endoscopy, at a rate of 0.25%–2%.[22,23] Endoscopy-related esophageal injury occurs at three sites: one in

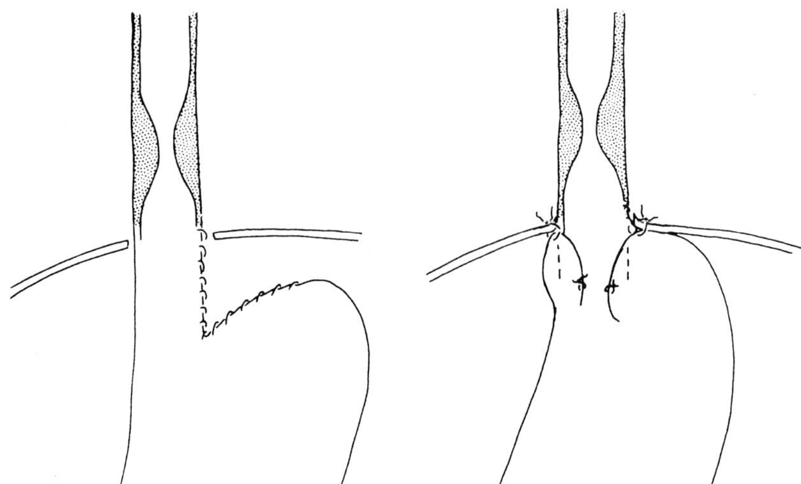

Fig. 11-4. Left. The gastric wall has been divided and the margins sutured separately. A gastric tube of esophageal diameter is created, in continuity with the distal esophagus. Right. A Belsey repair has been completed around the distal esophagus. From Pearson FG, Henderson RD: Experimental and clinical studies of gastroplasty in the management of acquired short esophagus. Surg Gynecol Obstet 136:737–744, 1973. Reprinted by permission from Surg Gynecol Obstet.

Table 11-1. Causes of esophageal perforations

Instrumental
    Bougienage
    Endoscopy
    Pneumatic dilation
    Blakemore tube

"Spontaneous"
    Postemesis
    Convulsions
    Straining-obstetrical
    Lifting

Postoperative
    Hiatal hernia repair
    Esophageal myotomy
    Esophageal reconstruction (including a colonic interposition)
    Local resection and anastomosis

Foreign bodies

Penetrating trauma

Nonpenetrating trauma

Corrosive injury

Esophageal ulcers

the cervical esophagus and two in the thoracic region. The most common site is the cervical esophagus, usually because of excessive extension of the neck—especially in an area of cervical osteophyte formation—and in patients with unsuspected pulsion diverticulae. The two major sites of thoracic esophageal perforation are at the point of esophageal narrowing at the aortic arch and in the distal esophagus, especially at a site of stricture or neoplasm. Perforations caused by fiberoptic endoscopies are extremely rare. Most commonly the gastroenterologist's instrumental perforation occurs as a result of dilation of a stricture or after pneumatic dilatation for achalasia.

Spontaneous (postemetic) perforations may occur in any patient who has experienced retching or vomiting and may, on occasion, occur without vomiting, usually as a result of straining or lifting heavy objects. Postemetic perforations are encountered most frequently in several clinical settings: after violent retching or vomiting during a bout of food poisoning or gastroenteritis, in hyperemesis gravidarum, in patients on chemotherapy, and in alcoholics. Although recognition is usually rather easy in the first three situations, it can be extremely difficult in the alcoholic. The site of postemetic perforation is almost always the left posterolateral wall just proximal to the gastroesophageal junction.[20]

DIAGNOSIS AND TREATMENT

Cervical Perforations

Perforations of the cervical esophagus occur most commonly after rigid endoscopy, although they are seen after ingestion of foreign bodies (e.g., animal bones) or after trauma. Major symptoms in a cervical esophageal perforation include pain in the neck and a "sticking" sensation in the throat. Fever, neck swelling, and crepitation may occur as well. The diagnosis is usually easily made, if one is alert to these symptoms, in a patient who has recently undergone endoscopy or endured trauma. However, the diagnosis may be quite subtle in bone ingestion, especially in the elderly (since dentures may inhibit tactile sensation) and in children. Plain films of the neck should be taken with the neck hyper-extended, since normally the clavicular shadow hides the esophageal inlet. Barium swallow with ingestion of small barium-soaked cotton balls may be necessary for detection of nonopaque foreign bodies.[20]

Perforations of the cervical esophagus generally involve only the adjacent retrovisceral space. Therefore, many surgeons believe that cessation of oral intake and prompt administration of antibiotics is sufficient.[21] The overall mortality from cervical perforations (0–15% in several series)[21,24] results from extension of inflammation and suppuration down the retroesophageal space into the mediastinum. Therefore, many authorities advocate that local drainage be instituted at the time the perforation is diagnosed even in the absence of evidence of caudad spread. Since this drainage procedure itself is relatively simple to perform and does not appear to add significantly to the morbidity or the length of the hospital stay,[24] this approach is not unreasonable.

Thoracic Perforations

The ease of diagnosis in a thoracic perforation depends upon extent of the perforation (i.e., whether or not it is confined to the mediastinum), the ability of the patient to verbalize his complaints, and, most importantly, a high index of suspicion on the part of the physician. Patients with esophageal perforations that are confined to the mediastinum may have chest pain as their only complaint. Postoperative patients may manifest perforation only by a low-grade fever, perhaps with a small pleural effusion. It is disconcerting, but not surprising, that a sizeable proportion of such patients are not diagnosed within 24 hours of the event, a fact that bears marked impact on subsequent morbidity and mortality. The overall mortality of thoracic esophageal perforations is 20–40% in most series, and the rate is markedly increased in patients in whom treatment is delayed more than 24 hours (13% vs 56% in the series by Sawyers et al.).[24] Patients suffering postemetic perforations have a higher mortality (approximately 35%) than those with postinstrumentation perforations (approximately 15%). This is thought to be related to delayed diagnosis of spontaneous perforations. Another contributing factor may be spillage of "unprepared" gastric contents, in contrast to the fasting gastric contents that enter the thoracic cavity after postinstrumental or postoperative perforations.

The typical patient with spontaneous perforation presents with an acute onset of severe chest and/or upper abdominal pain, often associated with dyspnea, which occurs after an episode of vomiting or retching. Physical examination reveals an acutely ill patient, hypotensive, with fever, subcutaneous emphysema, unilateral absence of breath sounds and/or evidence of pleural effusion. Although diagnosis in such a patient is not overly challenging, it is important to note that one-third of patients have clinically atypical presentations. The following hypothetical case report illustrates the difficulty in diagnosis.

Case Report

A 35-year-old male chronic alcohol ingestor is seen in the hospital emergency ward because of lower chest and epigastric pain. He states that he has been drinking heavily over the past 2 weeks and that on the morning of admission he had nausea and vomiting. Past history is positive for a previous admission for alcohol-associated pancreatitis and a questionable history of peptic ulcer disease. Physical examination reveals an acutely ill male complaining of pain. BP 110/70. Respirations 22. Chest examination reveals decreased breath sounds at the left base. He has epigastric tenderness and decreased bowel sounds. Chest x-ray reveals a left pleural effusion. Laboratory data: WBC 15,000, with a leftward shift, Hematocrit 48%. Serum amylase 200 units. The diagnosis of acute pancreatitis is made, and he is treated with intravenous fluids, nasogastric suction, and meperidine. Over the subsequent 24 hours, his condition worsens, with increasing pleural effusion, pain, and fever. The possibility of pancreatic abscess is considered. Blood cultures are obtained, and he is scheduled for abdominal sonography later that day. He develops venticular irritability and suffers a cardiorespiratory arrest. At autopsy the following is found: a perforation in the distal esophagus at the left postero-lateral wall just above the gastroesophageal junction; intense inflammation of the mediastinum and pleura, with involvement of the pericardial sac.

It is clear that this patient, while exhibiting typical features of acute alcoholic pancreatitis, in fact, suffered a postemetic esophageal perforation. Were there clinical clues to the presence of esophageal perforation? Perhaps more careful physical and x-ray examination would have revealed subcutaneous emphysema or a more subtle abnormality such as slight mediastinal widening (see below). Perhaps examination of the pleural fluid would have shown elevated amylase and an acidic pH (indicating acid contamination, via perforation). Since the procedures required to establish the diagnosis of esophageal perforation are without significant risk whereas the result of misdiagnosis is catastrophic, the clinical index of suspicion and willingness to act on that suspicion becomes paramount as a safeguard against misdiagnosis.

Careful examination of the chest radiograph is of extreme importance. Appleton has reported that 89% of 28 patients with esophageal perforation had a detectable abnormality on chest x-ray.[25] Table 11-2 lists the radiographic abnormalities noted.[25] Tears of the anterior and posterior wall generally are confined to the mediastinum. In lateral perforations the mediastinal pleura is breached, so that pleural spread occurs. In all thoracic perforations pleural fluid may occur secondary to mediastinal infection. Such fluid is sterile, without elevated amylase, and of neutral pH; these findings differentiate it from the composition of the fluid seen in direct pleural extension. A minority of esophageal perforations enter the abdomen, where they produce typical findings of an acute abdomen secondary to a perforated viscus. Again, preoperative diagnosis is of extreme importance, since the surgeon may be unable to repair the rupture through the original abdominal incision.

Esophageal studies with contrast material are necessary both to confirm the diagnosis and to establish other features relevant to surgical repair—e.g., the extent of the perforation, the extent of the associated abscess cavity, the associated primary esophageal pathology. Both water-soluble contrast materials and barium have their advocates. Those favoring barium consider that it is better tolerated in ill patients, gives better coating, and is less dangerous if aspirated.[25] James et al. have shown, in cats, that barium in the mediastinum is not particularly destructive, even in combination with bacteria.[26] He advocates the use of water-soluble contrast for the initial diagnostic exam but, if studies are negative, repeat evaluation with barium. All authorities agree that barium gives superior radiographic detail. Even with the use of barium, not all perforations are diagnosed radiographically. Reasons for missed perforations include closure of perforation, rapid passage of contrast through the esophagus, and improper patient positioning. Therefore, it is sometimes necessary to place the patient in prone, supine, and decubitus positions to demonstrate the leak. On occasion, diagnosis may need to be made by esophagoscopy.[27] I have stressed the difficulty of diagnosis, since the major factor relating to morbidity and mortality of thoracic esophageal perforations involves delay time between occurrence and recognition of the perforation.

Table 11-2. Plain radiographic features in 28 esophageal perforations

Site of Perforation	Number of Cases	Cervical Emphysema	Mediastinal Emphysema	Mediastinal Widening Without Emphysema	Pleural Effusion	Pneumothorax and/or Hydropneumothorax	Subdiaphragmatic gas
Cervical	7	6	1	—	—	1	—
Thoracic	18	5	7	1	2	8	—
Abdominal	3	—	—	—	—	—	2
Total	28	11	8	1	2	9	2

The type of treatment utilized in thoracic esophageal perforations (and its success) depends on several factors: time between perforation and recognition (since delay in diagnosis allows for development of suppurative mediastinitis and inflammatory involvement of esophageal tissue adjacent to the perforation site), size of the perforation, whether or not the perforation is confined to the mediastinum or has spread to the pleural space, the premorbid condition of the patient, and whether there is associated primary esophageal pathology.

It is difficult to evaluate the various published treatment protocols, since they are uncontrolled and retrospective, with each surgeon bringing a particular approach or skill to the problem that others, with less expertise, may find difficult to duplicate. The number of patients seen at any one institution is relatively small, and the differences between patients (e.g., site of perforation, recognition delay) make it difficult to attain a significant sample size for adequate randomization. However, several questions regarding pathophysiology and treatment would appear to be answerable on the basis of animal experimental models. These are as follows: What is the effect of individual components of extravasated material (gastric juice, bile, saliva)? Is there a time at which primary closure should not be attempted? Is there a role for nonsurgical treatment? What is the role of perioperative and postoperative total parenteral nutrition? Is there a role for corticosteroids vis-a-vis control of inflammatory mediastinitis and pleuritis? Is there a role for other potent nonsteroidal anti-inflammatory agents? How large an effect does operation time (which, in turn, will determine if major all-inclusive operations are done at time of initial thoracotomy) have on mortality? The answer to these and other questions are not simply of academic interest, since the overall mortality for thoracic esophageal perforation has not declined significantly in the last two decades.[28]

In general, instrumental perforations are associated with a somewhat more favorable outcome than are spontaneous perforations, and nonsurgical treatment (discontinuance of oral feedings, broad-spectrum antibiotics) has been advocated by some authors.[29-31] In Mengoli's series, only 1 in fifteen patients with instrumental thoracic perforation died after nonsurgical treatment.[29] Mean hospital stay was 18 days. Almost all perforations were diagnosed within 24 hours. Unfortunately, this is not a universal occurrence. Cameron et al. also treated selected patients with esophageal perforations nonsurgically.[30] Criteria for nonsurgical treatment were that disruption was contained in the mediastinum or between the mediastinum and visceral lung pleura, that there was drainage of the cavity back into the esophagus, and that symptoms and signs of clinical sepsis were minimal. A combination of gentamycin, clindamycin, and penicillin was used. Although results were encouraging, this group is not representative of those patients most likely to be seen by gastroenterologists. Five of the eight patients had a leak from an esophageal suture line secondary to surgery, a situation in which confinement of perforation is more likely to occur than with instrumental or postemetic perforations. These two studies demonstrate that some patients may recover from instrumental or postoperative thoracic esophageal perforations without being subjected to thoracotomy. However, many of the patients in whom iatrogenic perforation occurs in a gastroenterological practice need definitive surgery directed at their primary esophageal pathology (achalasia, recalcitrant peptic stricture). Therefore, nonsurgical treatment of perforations has not avoided operation; it has simply postponed it.

The majority of authors feel that, whatever the cause, surgical intervention is imperative in all cases of thoracic esophageal perforation. Even then, many differ as to what should be done in addition to primary closure if associated esophageal pathology exists. In addition, there is no consensus regarding the procedure of choice if primary closure cannot be performed at the time of initial operation. What follows is my conception of the surgical consensus regarding the course to follow for thoracic esophageal perforations.

With regard to instrumental perforations, the rare patient with early-diagnosed perforation, radiologically confined to the mediastinum and clinically benign, without associated esophageal pathology may be started on a nonsurgical regimen. Otherwise, patients with early-recognized instrumental perforations should undergo primary closure, with a definitive attack on the esophageal pathology performed at that time. Skinner recommends the latter approach. He advocates performing a myotomy, in a location away from the perforation, with an associated antireflux procedure in a case of perforation during pneumatic dilation for achalasia, and he advises carrying out primary repair in association with stricture resection or intraoperative dilation and antireflux procedure in the case of perforation during bougienage for stricture.[31]

With regard to instrumental perforations diagnosed late, if, at the time of operation, periesophageal inflammation and infection preclude primary closure, the most reasonable course of action would appear to be exclusion and diversion in continuity.[32] This procedure involves exclusion of the esophagus by ligating the cardia and diversion of oral secretions via a cervical esophagostomy, mediastinal and other appropriate drainage, and insertion of a gastrostomy tube for feeding. Such a procedure prevents gastroesophageal reflux, allows direct access to the mediastinum for drainage, and—in the event that healing of the esophageal wall inflammation occurs—permits subsequent use of the esophagus in definitive reconstructive procedures.

Although other authors might prefer resection of the intrathoracic esophagus with a cervical esophagostomy, that procedure involves considerable intraoperative time and eliminates the option of using the esophagus in future reconstructive surgery.

With regard to postemetic perforations, time is of the essence. Overall, mortality with postemetic perforations ranges from 25–50%. Early-recognized postemetic perforations require prompt operation with attempt at primary closure. Although the patient's premorbid cardiopulmonary and general status may play a role in decisions to operate, his current condition should not, insofar as his condition is a result of the perforation itself. In other words, a previously well but acutely ill patient is not too sick to undergo surgery. Patients with postemetic perforations recognized late should also be treated surgically. In such cases, although prognosis is grave, it appears that the best chance for survival involves a primary operative approach such as exclusion and diversion in continuity.

ESOPHAGEAL FISTULAE

Esophageal fistulae occur most commonly between the esophagus and the respiratory tract. The second most common location, between the esophagus and aorta, is, fortunately, relatively rare. Other fistulae (pericardium, stomach) occur with even less frequency.

Fistulae to the Respiratory Tract

Bronchoesophageal fistulae and tracheoesophageal fistulae in the adult are most commonly secondary to malignancies of the respiratory tract or the esophagus (see below). On occasion, they occur as a result of trauma or of inflammatory disease, most commonly chronic granulomatous inflammation such as tuberculosis, histoplasmosis, actinomycosis and syphilis.[33] The clinical presentation in benign inflammatory fistulae may be that of the classical paroxysmal coughing following ingestion of liquids, but, more often, symptoms are of a more indolent nature, including chronic cough, fever, and recurrent pulmonary infections, with or without associated dysphagia. Diagnosis is usually evident on performance of a barium esophagram. On occasion, bronchoscopy or esophagoscopy is required for fistula diagnosis. Once the fistula has been discovered, cultures and microscopic examination, including special staining for appropriate orgnisms, are necessary to establish the specific etiology.

Treatment of benign fistulae is generally considered to be surgical, with division of the fistula, closure of esophageal defects, excision of adjacent nodes and necrotic tissue, removal of irreversibly damaged lung tissue and placement of exogenous tissue (i.e., pleural or pericardial flap) between the esophagus and bronchus.[33] However, nonsurgical healing of a fistula has been reported in a patient with tuberculosis, with the use of antituberculosis therapy.[34]

Malignant Fistulae and Their Management

Malignant bronchoesophageal and tracheoesophageal fistulae generally occur during the course of clearly established malignancy. They are seen frequently, being noted in 5–10% of patients with esophageal carcinoma. Unlike benign fistulae, the diagnosis is usually ushered in by the acute onset of coughing that occurs after food ingestion. However, a chronic or subacute course may occur, as in benign fistulae, resulting in significant delay in diagnosis. Several therapeutic modalities have been employed in the management of malignant fistulae:[35]

Supportive Therapy without Surgical Intervention. This course is often considered in patients who appear to be suffering from marked inanition and far advanced disease. Although this may have some merit in patients with known advanced carcinomatosis, a clinical estimate of the extent of neoplastic involvement is unreliable and much of the "terminal" appearance of such patients is related to chronic, potentially reversible, suppuration. The use of thoracic and abdominal computed tomography is helpful in staging esophageal carcinoma.

Gastrostomy and Tracheostomy. Patients treated in this manner generally do very poorly, with mean time of survival less than a month, and are rarely able to leave the hospital.

Esophageal Diversion and Exclusion. This is a rather extensive procedure in a patient who is generally debiliated and malnourished. Wound healing is poor, and tissue breakdown and anastomatic leaks are common.

Colon Bypass with or without Esophageal Resection. This approach suffers from the disadvantages mentioned for other primary operations.

Permanent Endoesophageal Intubation. Such intubation can be accomplished from below, by introducing the tube through a gastrostomy under general anesthesia,[36] or from above. The concept of permanent tube placement is sound. Morbidity and mortality in esophageal carcinoma occur as a result of inanition and infection, which are caused by decreased oral intake and pulmonary aspiration (via either esophageal "overflow" or fistula formation). Tube placement prevents continuation of aspiration and allows ingestion of more nutrients through a better maintained lumen. Although the primary disadvantage of this procedure is irritation of already diseased tissue by the foreign body, with the potential for esophageal perforation, it is my opinion that the tradeoff is well worth it. Patients may live months to upwards of a year and are usually able to return home and to ingest relatively normal amounts of food. I can see no intrinsic advantages to pull-through intubation, however, and the exposure to general anesthesia and the morbidity accompanying a laparotomy are distinct disadvantages.

Placement of esophageal prostheses is discusses in detail by Peura et al.[37] For technical reasons, lesions must be at least 3 cm below the cricopharyngeus and 3–4 cm above the gastroesophageal junction. In brief, the narrowed fistulous area is first dilated progressively to accommodate a size-50-French dilator. The prosthesis is made of polyvinyl tubing, of a length exceeding tumor length by 6–7 cm to allow for a 2–3 cm flange above the tumor and to prevent tube occlusion by caudad tumor growth. A second polyvinyl tube is used to push the prosthesis through the tumor (Fig. 11-5 and 11-6). As stated previously, such a prosthesis usually permits the immediate ingestion of food, does away with the cough that accompanies oral intake, and promotes eventual healing of the pulmonary infection. Complications and failures relate to the presence of multiple fistulae that are located in a position where they are not occludable by prosthesis, formation of new fistulae through diseased tissue, erosion of the prosthesis through the esophageal wall into the mediastinum or aorta, tumor growth that results in occluding the prosthesis. In the series by Peura et al., mean survival after prosthesis insertion was 13 weeks. At least they were 13 weeks spent at home!

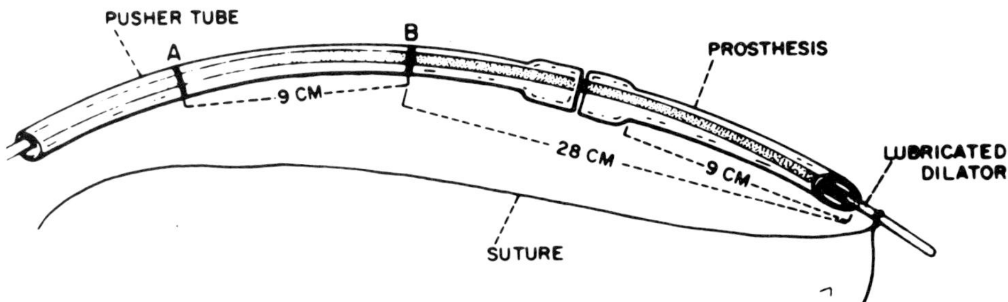

Fig. 11-5. The esophageal prosthesis assembly. The entire assembly is passed per os under fluoroscopic control to the orad tumor margin **(B)** and then through the tumor to the prosthesis flange **(A)**. Reprinted by permission from Peura DA, Heit HA, Johnson LF, Boyce HW: The esophageal prosthesis in cancer. Dig Dis Sci 23:796–800, 1978.

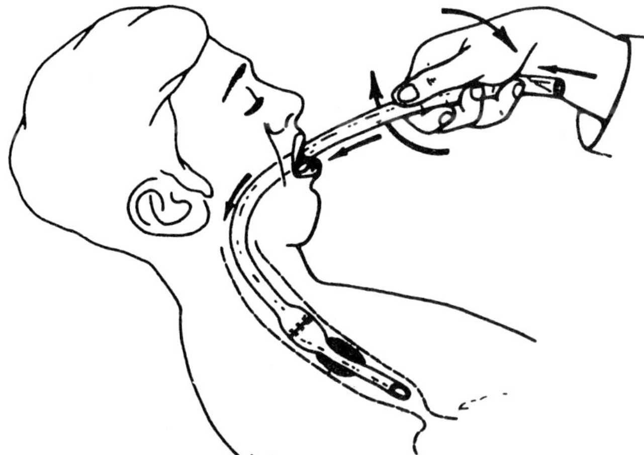

Fig. 11-6. The flange of the prosthesis is anchored above the tumor by gentle twisting pressure caudad on the pusher tube. The pusher tube is then removed. Reprinted by permission from Peura DA, Heit HA, Johnson LF, Boyce HW: The esophageal prosthesis in cancer. Dig Dis Sci 23:796–800, 1978.

Aortoesophageal Fistula

Aortoesophageal fistulae occur primarily as a result of foreign body ingestion, generally of sharp objects (e.g., animal bones), and are usually located at the area of the aortic arch.[38] They also occur secondary to esophageal carcinoma, penetrating injury, and aortic aneurysms, either as a primary outcome of the aneurysm or following its repair.[39,40] Fistulae that occur because of foreign body ingestion are initiated either by direct penetration or via pressure necrosis of the esophageal wall, with subsequent mediastinitis and localized aortitis resulting in the fistula formation. The latter sequence is probably more common, since the interval between foreign body ingestion and initial presentation is often delayed as much as 1–3 weeks. The patient is usually aware of having swallowed the object and of experiencing subsequent dysphagia. However, symptoms may be rather subtle, especially in the elderly. Usually the first sign of aortoesophageal fistula is the "signal" hemorrhage.[41] This is usually a minor bleeding episode. The time between this first bleeding episode and an eventual massive bleed is totally unpredictable. Since massive bleeding from aortoesophageal fistula almost always results in a fatal outcome, the most important aspect of management is early diagnosis of foreign body impaction. Since many such objects are not radiopaque, careful contrast studies need to be performed, in addition to plain roentgenographs of the chest. Swallowing of barium-soaked pieces of cotton may aid in localization. Once the foreign object is seen, initial management should consist of rapid endoscopy.[41] Even with successful removal of the object, a subsequent fistula may develop if delay time between ingestion and removal is sufficient to set off the process described above. Once "signal" hemorrhage has occurred, removal of the foreign body is hazardous; if the foreign body can be seen roentgenographically, direct surgical intervention without the potentially hazardous endoscopy may be warranted. If the patient presents with bleeding but no foreign body can be demonstrated, endoscopy is necessary for diagnosis. As with other aortoenteric fistulae, arteriography may be negative.

CHEMICAL INJURY

Chemical injury to the esophagus occurs most commonly in children, as a result of accidental ingestion of caustic substances, but may occur in adults as well, either accidentally or because of an attempted suicide. The extent of damage depends primarily on the chemical composition and the concentration of the ingested corrosive. Alkaline substances produce considerably more damage than do acids, since alkali result in liquefaction necrosis whereas acids cause coagulation necrosis, setting up a tissue barrier that prevents ongoing destruction.[42] It has been shown that, among alkali, pH is important in determining the extent of injury—the critical pH being $\geq$ 12.5.[43] This explains the prominence of lye on any list of corrosive agents that produce chemical damage, since all commercial lye products have a pH of 14.[43] The mucosal contact time may be incredibly brief; experimentally, a 10-sec contact with strong alkali may provoke a through-and-through lesion of the esophagus.

Diagnosis

Diagnosis of corrosive ingestion is usually obvious, but the question of whether or not esophageal injury has occurred requires direct mucosal visualization. Oropharyngeal damage does not necessarily imply esophageal damage and, more important, esophageal damage may (albeit rarely) occur without any visualized pathology in the oral cavity.[44] Many patients complain of dysphagia and chest pain, and drooling may be intense.

The acute and ultimate prognosis depend primarily upon the depth and extent of esophageal injury at the time of initial presentation. Therefore, in anyone suspected of corrosive ingestion, with or without visualized oral pathology, immediate endoscopy should be undertaken. A small-diameter pediatric-type endoscope should be used, as it may be less traumatic to the esophagus.

One may classify esophageal injury as follows: first degree, mucosal erythema and edema; second degree, erythema, blister formation, superficial ulceration, and fibrinous exudate; third degree, erythema, deep ulceration, and/or eschar formation. Using this classification, Webb[44] found that significant sequelae did not occur in eight patients with first degree burns but stricture formation occurred in some instances in patients with second degree burns. Risk of perforation is greatest in third degree burns. The endoscope should not be passed distal to a severe third degree burn because of risk of perforation, but passage may be attempted beyond less severely damaged mucosa.

Treatment

If esophagoscopy is normal, no treatment is indicated. Standard treatment of esophageal burns consists of the immediate parenteral administration of rather high-dose corticosteroids (usually 400–500 mg of hydrocortisone or its equivalent, daily in adults).[45-47] However, neither dosage nor length of treatment has been well established. Some authors gradually taper steroid dosages after the 1st week, discontinuing use at 3 weeks; others maintain steroids for months. The treatment schedule should probably be individualized vis-a-vis initial injury and response to therapy. However, since granulation-tissue formation and collagen deposition are not well advanced until at least 2 weeks after injury,[44] it would appear reasonable to maintain initial steroid dosage for at least that period of time.

It is customary to initiate steroid and broad-spectrum antibiotic treatment simultaneously.[44,47] Total parenteral nutrition should be initiated early in severe injury. The time for reinstituting oral feeding is also unclear. Marion et al.[48] and Guelrud and Arocha[49] have reported marked abnormalities in esophageal motor function in patients who suffered severe corrosive injury. In addition, LES pressure was significantly lower on initial testing than when patients were retested 1 month later. This combination would favor gastroesophageal reflux with poor esophageal clearing. Perhaps the prophylactic administration of H_2-receptor antagonists and/or antacids would prevent secondary acid-reflux-induced injury. With the availability of high-calorie liquid nutrients, it would appear prudent to avoid solids until clearcut evidence of healing exists. For this purpose, careful follow-up endoscopic examination, perhaps every 1 or 2 weeks, may be employed.

Unfortunately, there are relatively few experimental studies on which to base therapeutic decisions. The studies of Haller and Bachman,[50] in cats, and Rosenberg et al.,[51] in rabbits, both suggest that early administration of corticosteroids is helpful in preventing stricture formation. In the Haller–Bachman study, the concurrent administration of an antibiotic was not associated with mediastinal abscesses or fulminant pneumonias, as were seen in animals treated with steroids alone. To my knowledge, there have been no studies evaluating the effect of the new potent nonsteroidal anti-inflammatory agents in corrosive injury, but, in that regard, Northway and colleagues have reported that administration of indomethacin prevented radiation injury in the opossum esophagus.[52] The effect of antifibrinogenic agents, such as colchicine, on stricture formation in corrosive injury has not been evaluated. Studies examining new therapeutic approaches to caustic injury are sorely needed, since the rate of stricture occurrence in patients with significant esophagal injury at the time of initial clinical evaluation is still unacceptably high, in the order of 30–50% in patients with third degree burns. Even more important is education of parents with respect to the hazards of accidental corrosive ingestion in their children.

Complications of Corrosive Ingestion and Their Management

The most common complication of corrosive damage is stricture formation. Most authors agree that prophylactic bougienage is not helpful and may well be hazardous early in the course of esophageal injury. Strictures may occur in any part of the esophagus. They generally are noted a minimum of 3–4 weeks after ingestion. Eighty percent are recognized within 2 months, but some may not become evident until months or, rarely, years thereafter.[44] The passage of a weighted string at the time of diagnosis of severe mucosal injury has merit, since bougies may be passed over the string should a narrow tortuous stricture occur.[42]

Patients with severe damage must be observed carefully for signs of esophageal perforation. In fact, some physicians recommend emergency esophagogastrectomy in patients with third degree burns caused by lye ingestion.[53] If any question of perforation arises, radiocontrast examination of the esophagus is imperative. Tracheoesophageal fistulae may occur as well.

Once a stricture(s) has developed, management is dependent on its severity (see section on strictures). Often, especially in children with long, narrow strictures, colon interposition is necessary.[54] This may be accomplished with or without concurrent esophagectomy. The question of whether to leave the esophagus intact, with placement of a colon bypass (esophagectomy in patients with corrosive injury is often technically difficult, because of dense periesophageal scarring) or to remove the esophagus, with colon interposition—(because of the increased incidence of carcinoma in a previously corrosive-damaged esophagus) must be weighed in each individual case.

Evaluation of motor activity of the interposed colon has not been extensive, but Jones[55] noted progressive peristaltic contractions occurring every 4–6 min in several patients. Response to a water bolus was present in seven of nine patients, but with considerable delay. This study, and those by Sieber and Sieber[56] and by Rodgers et al.[57] indicate that the colon serves primarily as a passive conduit. Food with a thick consistency may remain in the interposed colon for over 30 min. Therefore, patients should be encouraged to drink considerable amounts of liquid with their meals and to avoid lying down soon after eating. For the most part, patients state that they are able to eat and swallow satisfactorily, and symptoms of reflux, though reported, are not common. Interestingly, Jones noted a colonic motor response in all nine patients within 1 min after the instillation of 0.1N hydrochloric acid. This response is postulated to aid colonic acid clearance and to prevent reflux-induced injury.

REFERENCES

1. Flood CA: Bougienage therapy for constrictive esophagitis. Gastrointest Endoscopy 25:130–132, 1979.
2. Gaskins RD: Peptic stricture. Gastroenterology 76:1021–1022, 1979.
3. Jones EL, Skinner DB, DeMeester TR, et al.: Response of the interposed human colonic segment to an acid challenge. Ann Surg 177:75–78, 1973.
4. Moss AA, Schnyder P, Theeni RF, Margulis AR: Esophageal carcinoma: pre-therapy staging by computed tomography. Gastroenterology 80:1235 (abstr), 1981.
5. Peura DA, Heit HA, Johnson LF, Boyce HW: Esophageal prosthesis in cancer. Dig Dis 23:796–800, 1978.

6. Lanza FL, Graham DY: Bougienage is effective therapy for most benign esophageal strictures. JAMA 240:844–847, 1978.
7. Lagradi A, Csendes A, Pope CE II: Surgical correction of reflux. An effective therapy for esophageal strictures. Gastroenterology 69:578–583, 1975.
8. Ahtardis G, Snape WJ, Cohen S: Clinical and manometric findings in benign peptic strictures of the esophagus. Dig Dis 24:858–861, 1979.
9. Henderson RD, Pearson FG: Preoperative assessment of esophageal pathology. J Thorac Cardiovasc Surg 72:512–517, 1976.
10. Skinner DB, Belsey RHR. Surgical management of esophageal reflux and hiatus hernia. J Thoracic Cardiovasc Surg 4:53–54, 1967.
11. Hill LD: An effective operation for hiatal hernia: an eight year appraisal. Ann Surg 166:681–692, 1967.
12. Ellis FH, Leonardi HK, Dabuzhsky L, Crozier RE: Surgery for short esophagus with stricture: an experimental and clinical manometric study. Ann Surg 188:341–350, 1978.
13. Pearson FG, Langer B, Henderson RD: Gastroplasty and Belsey hiatus hernia repair. An operation for the management of peptic stricture with acquired short esophagus. J Thoracic Cardiovasc Surg 61:50–63, 1971.
14. Pearson FG, Henderson RD: Experimental and clinical studies of gastroplasty in the management of acquired short esophagus. Surg Gynecol Obstet 136:737–744, 1973.
15. DeMeester TR, Wernly JA, Bryant GH, et al.: Clinical and in vitro analysis of determinants of gastroesophageal competence. Am J Surg 137:39–46, 1979.
16. Hill LD: Intraoperative measurement of lower esophageal sphincter pressure. J Thorac Cardiovasc Surg 75:378–382, 1978.
17. Pearson FG, Henderson RD: Long-term follow-up of peptic strictures managed by dilatation, modified gastroplasty and Belsey hiatus hernia repair. Surgery 80:396–404, 1976.
18. Brand DL, Eastwood IR, Martin D, et al.: Esophageal symptoms, manometry, and histology before and after anti-reflux surgery. Gastroenterology 76:1393–1400, 1979.
19. Fisher RS, Malmud LS, Lobis IF, Maier WP. Anti-reflux surgery for symptomatic gastroesophageal reflux. Mechanism of action. Dig Dis 23:152–160, 1978.
20. Loop FD, Groves LK. Esophageal perforations. Ann Thorac Surg 10:571–586, 1970.
21. Triggiani E, Belsey R: Oesophageal trauma: incidence, diagnosis and management. Thorax 32:241–249, 1977.
22. Sandrasagra FA, English TAH, Milstein BB: The management and prognosis of oesophageal perforation. Br J Surg 65:629–632, 1978.
23. Palmer ED, Wirts CW: Survey of gastroscopic and esophagoscopic accidents. JAMA 164:2012–2015, 1957.
24. Sawyers JL, Lance CE, Foster JH, Daniel RA: Esophageal perforation. An increasing challenge. Ann Thorac Surg 19:233–238, 1975.
25. Appleton DS, Sandrasagra FA, Fowler CDR: Perforated oesophagus: review of 28 consecutive cases. Clin Radiol 30:493–497, 1979.
26. Carter R, Hinshaw DB: Use of esophagoscope in the diagnosis of rupture of the esophagus. Surg Gynecol Obstet 2:1304–1306, 1965.
27. Mathewson C, Dozier WE, Hamill JP, Smith M: Clinical experiences with perforation of the esophagus. Am J Surg 104:257–266, 1962.
28. Mengoli LR, Klassen KP: Conservative management of esophageal perforation. Arch Surg 91:238–240, 1965.
29. Cameron JL, Kieffer RF, Hendrix TR, et al.: Selective nonoperative management of contained intrathoracic esophageal disruptions. Ann Thorac Surg 27:404–408, 1979.
30. Lyons WS, Seremetis MG, de Guzman VC, Peabody JW Jr: Ruptures and perforations

of the esophagus: the case for conservative supportive management. Ann Thorac Surg 25:346–350, 1978.

31. Skinner DB, Little AG, DeMeester TR: Management of esophageal perforation. Am J Surg 139:760–764, 1980.

32. Urschel HC, Razzuk MA, Wood RE, et al.: Improved management of esophageal perforation: exclusion and diversion in continuity. Ann Surg 179:587–591, 1974.

33. Spalding AR, Burney DP, Ritchie RE: Acquired benign bronchoesophageal fistulas in the adult. Ann Thorac Surg 28:378–383, 1978.

34. Wigley EM, Murray HW, Mann RB, et al.: Unusual manifestation of tuberculosis: TE fistula. Am J Med 60:310–314, 1976.

35. Lolley DM, Ray JF, Ransdell HT, et al.: Management of malignant esophagorespiratory fistula. Ann Thorac Surg 25:516–520, 1978.

36. Girardet R, Ransdell H, Wheat M: Palliative intubation in the management of esophageal carcinoma. Ann Thorac Surg 18:417–430, 1974.

37. Peura DA, Heit HA, Johnson LF, Boyce HW: Esophageal prosthesis in cancer. Dig Dis 23:796–800, 1978.

38. Nandi P, Ong GB: Foreign body in the esophagus. Review of 2394 cases. Br J Surg 65:5–9, 1978.

39. Sinar DR, DeMaria A, Kataria YP, Thomas FB: Aortic aneurysm eroding the esophagus. Dig Dis 22:252–254, 1977.

40. Smaha LA, Kilma T, Leatherman LL: Aortoesophageal fistula: late complication after repair of thoracic aortic aneurysm. JAMA 240:2077–2078, 1978.

41. Ctercteko G, Mok CK: Aorta-esophageal fistula induced by a foreign body: the first recorded survival. J Thorac Cardiovasc Surg 80:233–235, 1980.

43. Campbell GS, Burnett HF, Ransom JM, Williams GD: Treatment of corrosive burns of the esophagus. Arch Surg 112:495–500, 1977.

44. Vancura EM, Clinton JE, Ruiz E, Krenzelok EO: Toxicity of alkaline solutions. Ann Emerg Med 9:118–122, 1980.

45. Webb WR, Koutras P, Ecker RR, Sugg WL: An evaluation of steroids and antibiotics in caustic burns of the esophagus. Ann Thorac Surg 9:95–102, 1970.

46. Middelkamp JN, Cone AJ, Ogura JH, Higgins CR, Lowe GA: Endoscopic diagnosis and steroid and antibiotic therapy of acute lye burns of the esophagus. Laryngoscope 1354–1362, 1961.

47. Cardona JC, Daly JF: Current management of corrosive esophagitis. Ann Otol Rhinol Laryngol 80:521–527, 1971.

48. Haller JA, Andrews HG, White JJ, et al.: Pathophysiology and management of acute corrosive burns of the esophagus. J Pediatr Surg 6:578–584, 1971.

49. Marion L, Sanders B, Nayfield S, Zfass AM: Gastric and esophageal dysfunction after ingestion of acid. Gastroenterology 75:502–503, 1978.

50. Guelrud M, Arocha M: Motor function abnormalities in acute caustic esophagitis. J Clin Gastroenterol 2:247–250, 1978.

51. Haller JA, Bachman K: The comparative effect of current therapy on experimental caustic burns of the esophagus. Pediatrics 34:236–245, 1964.

52. Rosenberg N, Kunderman PHJ, Vroman L, Moolten SE: Prevention of experimental lye strictures of the esophagus by cortisone. Arch Surg 66:593–598, 1953.

53. Northway MG, Libshitz HI, Osborne BM, et al.: Radiation esophagitis in the opossum: radioprotection with indomethacin. Gastroenterology 78:883–893, 1980.

54. Ray JF, Myers WO, Lawton BR, et al.: The natural history of liquid lye ingestion. Arch Surg 109:436–439, 1974.

55. Schiller M, Frye TR, Boles ET: Evaluation of colonic replacement of the esophagus in children. J Pediatr Surg 6:753–760, 1971.
56. Jones ET, Skinner DB, DeMeester TR, et al.: Response of the interposed human colonic segment to an acid challenge. Ann Surg 177:75–78, 1973.
57. Sieber AM, Sieber WK: Colon transplants as esophageal replacement. Cineradiographic and manometric evaluation in children. Ann Surg 168:116–122, 1968.
58. Rodgers BM, Talbert JL, Felman AH: Functional and metabolic evaluation of colon replacement of the esophagus in children. J Pediatr Surg 13:35–39, 1978.

12 | Esophageal Cancer and the Premalignant Changes of Esophageal Diseases

John Jones Thompson

INTRODUCTION

In attempting to understand the clinical features of neoplastic esophageal lesions, a review of general principles that have emerged from research efforts in neoplasia is useful. The work of Clark et al.,[1-4] Farber and Cameron,[5] and Morson,[6] has suggested that the neoplastic process is a chronic one that develops slowly over many years. In well studied systems such as melanoma,[1-4] cervical carcinoma,[7] and adenomas of the colon,[6] neoplasia develops through a series of progressive stages that are well characterized morphologically but are still poorly defined at a basic molecular level. The term neoplastic system encompasses the concept that neoplasia develops sequentially through various "benign" stages, progressively acquiring biologic features that are associated with "malignancy." Four common features emerge from work done on melanoma, cervical carcinoma, and colonic adenomas:

1. Malignancies in experimental systems appear to develop sequentially from precursor lesions that are "biologically benign," not usually from de novo carcinoma.[1-7]

2. Only a small number of "benign" precursor lesions progress to "malignancy;" the remainder either remain stable or regress with time. At each stage in the neoplastic system these three options are available as potential pathways of differentiation.[1-7]

3. Local factors in the milieu surrounding neoplastic lesions ("cell contact," hormonal influences, growth factors), although poorly understood, appear to play a major role in growth regulation and differentiation of both benign and malignant lesions.[5,8,9]

4. At certain stages in neoplastic systems host immune function appears to be of major importance in growth regulation and differentiation.[1,10]

Current evidence suggests that all four of these features are characteristic of both squamous-cell carcinoma and Barrett's metaplasia with superimposed adenocarcinoma of the esophagus.

If neoplasia is viewed as a chronic process, then overt symptomatic cancer represents only the short, terminal, clinically visible phase. In most neoplastic systems, therapeutic attempts at cure are limited to this stage, usually because diagnosis depends on the occurrence of symptoms. The challenge for those interested in neoplasia is to define the developmental neoplastic systems for all cell types, devise sensitive epidemiologic and laboratory screening methods for diagnosing early lesions in asymptomatic people, and investigate the relevant growth regulatory factors operating that might permit simple therapeutic intervention.

NEOPLASTIC LESIONS OF THE ESOPHAGUS

Although there are numerous types of malignancy that are primary in the esophagus, precursor lesions have been investigated only for the two most common lesions: adenocarcinoma arising in Barrett's metaplasia and squamous carcinoma. Those interested in other lesions are referred to Enterline and Thompson.[11] The purpose of this chapter is to interrelate the "benign" and "malignant" lesions noted within the Barrett's metaplasia–adenocarcinoma sequence and the squamous-cell carcinoma sequence in the esophagus. Defining these neoplastic systems is a necessary first step in developing methods for early detection and eradication of asymptomatic disease.

BARRETT'S ESOPHAGUS AND ASSOCIATED NEOPLASIA

Definition

As stated by Barrett himself, columnar-lined esophagus "is a condition denied by some, misunderstood by others, and ignored by the majority."[12] As currently used, the term Barrett's esophagus refers to a *metaplastic* process in which a variable segment of the normal squamous epithelium above the physiologic sphincter is replaced with a complex mixture of columnar epithelium resembling that found in the small bowel, gastric body, and gastric cardia.[13,14] The process may be similar to the metaplastic "intestinalization" seen in early neoplasia of the gastric body.[15]

Etiology

A large amount of evidence suggests that Barrett's metaplasia is caused by reflux of acidic gastric juices[14-21] or bile-containing small bowel contents[22,23] into the distal esophagus. Such reflux presumably causes epithelial ulceration; subsequent regeneration of pluripotential basal cells under conditions in which trophic messages are mixed may cause the mosaic of various types of columnar epithelium that is seen.[13,14]

Experimental Model. Bremner, Lynch, and Ellis[16] have shown in dogs that ulceration, persistent reflux, and acidity of the gastric contents are all independent variables in the genesis of Barrett's metaplasia. Thus, in dogs that undergo only lower esophageal mucosal excision, reepithelialization almost always occurs toward normal squamous-cell differentiation; in dogs given mucosal excision, hiatal hernia, and histamine to stimulate gastric secretion, healing is almost always toward Barrett's metaplasia; and in animals given mucosal excision and hiatal hernia alone, healing is evenly split between normal squamous epithelium and Barrett's metaplasia. Hamilton and Yardley[22] and Meyer, Vollmar, and Bär[23] have observed Barrett's metaplasia in patients who have total gastrectomies but with reflux of small bowel contents. Thus reflux of acid gastric contents appear to be only one of several mechanisms for acquiring columnar metaplasia.

Clinical Data Supporting a Metaplastic Etiology. Studies in humans by Paull et al.[24] have shown that the metaplastic segment behaves manometrically as esophagus; the physiologic sphincter can be demonstrated distally; and the pressure in the segment is that expected in the lower esophagus. Peristaltic waves pass through the segment as they would in the lower esophagus.[25]

Anatomically, the segment in which Barrett's metaplasia is found can also be shown to be esophageal. Residual esophageal submucosal glands and squamous islands are frequently demonstrated within the metaplastic epithelium.[13,26] The underlying muscularis propria is continuous with the esophageal smooth muscle and is covered with adventitia rather than serosa.

Neoplastic Potential. Anatomic and clinical data strongly support the concept that Barrett's metaplasia is an acquired lesion with potential for neoplastic progression.[14,15,17-24] A correlation between columnar-lined esophagus and symptoms of reflux and hiatal hernia has been repeatedly shown. Transformation to Barrett's metaplasia and proximal progression of the process has been demonstrated in several series.[14,15,17] Although the figures vary,[14,15,17,27,28] somewhere between 2 and 11% of patients with reflux esophagitis are said to acquire Barrett's metaplasia, and between 0 and 8.5% are said to develop adenocarcinoma subsequently within the metaplastic segment. Numerous authors have observed this statistical relationship between adenocarcinomas of the esophagus and Barrett's metaplasia.[14,15,17,21,26,27,29-33] The study of Haggitt et al.[26] suggests that 86% of esophageal adenocarcinoma arises in a background of Barrett's metaplasia. Abnormal proliferative cell compartments have been documented by several authors,[32,33] and in addition the presence of dysplasia and carcinoma in situ (CIS) in association with Barrett's metaplasia[13,26,27,29] is well described.

In several studies,[13,31,34] a careful evaluation of carcinomas at the gastroesophageal junction has revealed that almost half contain minor foci of Barrett's metaplasia and CIS. This fact has suggested a common pathogenesis for adenocarcinomas of the lower esophagus and gastroesophageal junction to several authors.[13,31,34] Presumably in approximately half the cases, the invasive lesions overgrow the preexisting focus of Barrett's metaplasia that contains the precursor lesion. A similar mechanism of growth has been proposed for adenomas of the colon by Morson.[6]

Evidence in the literature is divided on the issue of reversion of Barrett's metaplasia to normal after various procedures, including fundoplication.[30,35,36] To date, no study has attempted to analyze the presence or absence of early neoplastic lesions versus the capacity to regress. Reversion to normal may in fact be a function of the degree of neoplastic progression present in an individual lesion. Further study of this question is needed.

Incidence and Epidemiology

Incidence figures for adenocarcinoma associated with Barrett's metaplasia vary considerably depending on the criteria used for acceptance of the diagnosis. Many authors exclude any case that involves the gastric cardia, ignoring other features such as the presence of early neoplastic lesions or of foci of columnar metaplasia in the adjacent esophagus.[31,37-39] If this definition is used, then adenocarcinoma in association with Barrett's metaplasia is relatively rare, varying from 2.4–4% of the total cases of carcinoma of the esophagus. Since the average incidence figures for carcinoma of the esophagus are only approximately 3/100,000 in the United States,[11] if restrictive criteria are used, incidence figures for adenocarcinoma arising in Barrett's metaplasia would be about 0.1/100,000. If all cases of adenocarcinoma of the lower esophagus and gastroesophageal junction are considered to be of common etiology, the incidence of adenocarcinoma arising in Barrett's metaplasia almost equals that of squamous carcinoma.[34,38]

As in squamous-cell carcinoma of the esophagus, a strong male predominance is noted in adenocarcinomas associated with Barrett's metaplasia, averaging approximately 3:1 in the literature.[14,15,19,28,34,38,39] It is of interest to note that carcinomas of the gastroesophageal junction show the same 3:1 ratio as esophageal carcinomas do.[13,34] Although incidence figures vary markedly, hiatal hernia and reflux esophagitis are strongly correlated with Barrett's metaplasia and carcinoma,[14,15,19,28,34,38,39] just as they are with carcinomas of the gastroesophageal junction.[13,34,40] Adenocarcinoma associated with Barrett's metaplasia is seen over a wide age range—varying over ages 23–86 years in the literature[13-15,19,26,28,31,34,38,39]—but most commonly occurs in the sixth and seventh decades. Although carcinomas associated with Barrett's epithelium may occur at any level in the esophagus, the vast majority are found in the lower esophagus and at the gastroesophageal junction.[13,21,31,34,38]

Microscopic Morphology

The types of columnar epithelium present in Barrett's metaplasia have caused considerable confusion in the literature, in part because of the use of biopsy studies which give only a limited sample for evaluation. Thus investigators have reported Barrett's metaplasia to be toward gastric fundic epithelium,[14,15,21,22,24,41,42] gastric cardiac or antral epithelium,[14,15,21,22,24] small intestinal epithelium,[14,43] and "specialized columnar epithelium."[21,24,44] The presence of paneth and neuroendocrine cells has also been reported.[43,45] In a careful study done by Ozello, Savary, and Roethlisberger,[14] and a study done on eight blocked, serially submitted esophagogastrectomy specimens by Thompson, Zinsser, and Enterline,[13] the examined epithelium was noted to be a "mosaic" of all the cell types reported. The histologic patterns observed are further complicated by the presence of varying degrees of mucosal

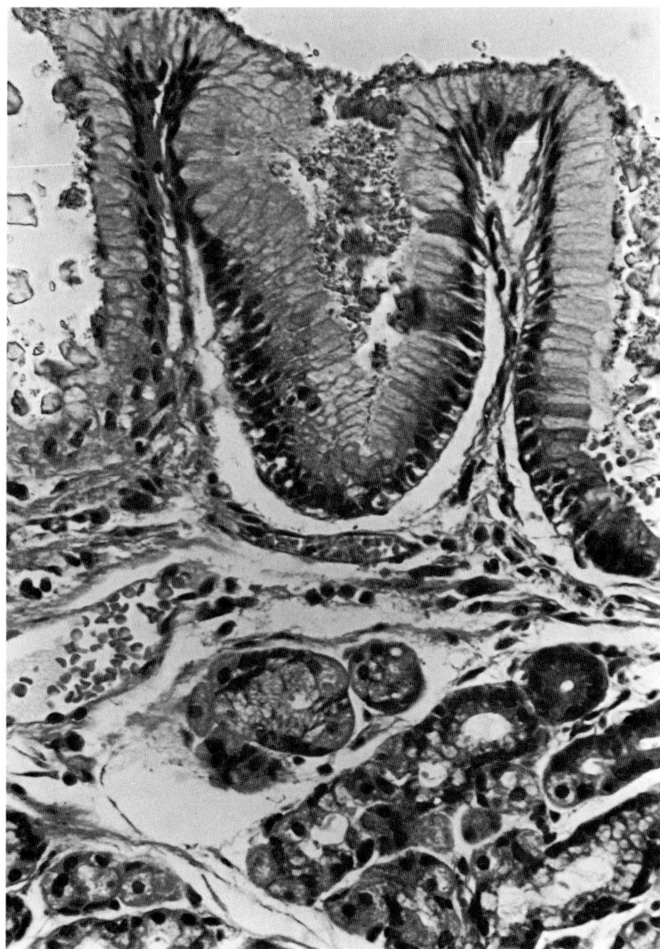

Fig. 12-1. Surface mucous and mucous neck cells: Note the surface mucous-type cells lining the uneven and slightly papillary surface. Gastric body glands, which contain both chief and parietal cells, lie beneath the surface (H and E × 297).

atrophy that is probably a consequence of continued esophageal reflux. The conflicting data in the literature on functional capacity and morphology of the columnar epithelium may in part result from the presence of atrophy. Barrett's metaplasia is perhaps best regarded as a complex and intimate mixture of epithelial cell types that are differentiating in a milieu in which there are diverse signals for pathways of differentiation.

Correlation of Microscopic and Macroscopic Features

In the study by Thompson, Zinsser, and Enterline,[13] eight esophagogastrectromy specimens of Barrett's metaplasia with associated neoplasia were available

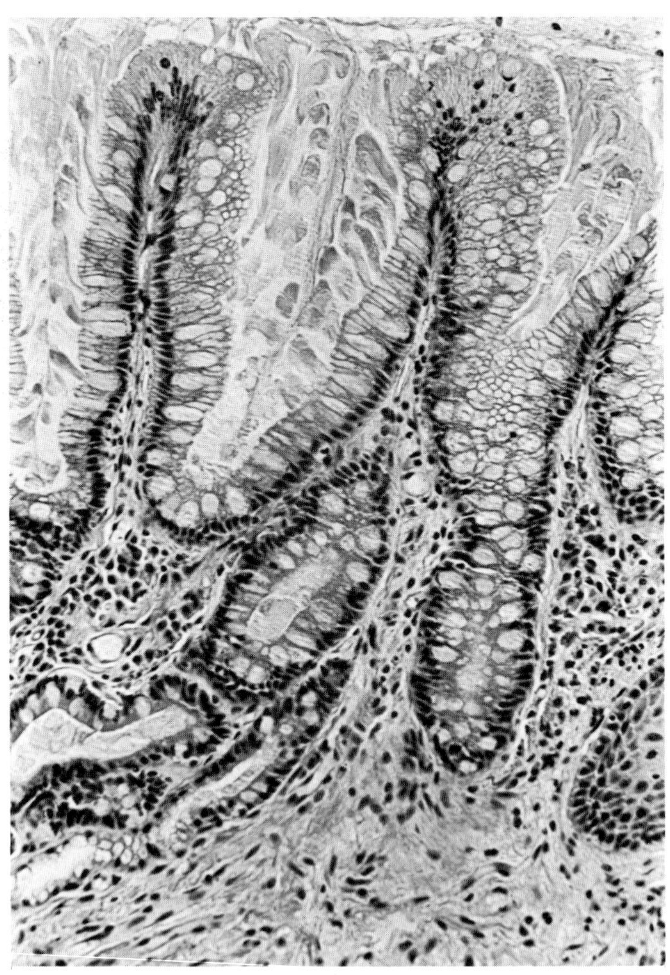

Fig. 12-2.   Intestinal goblet and absorptive cells. Both the villous surface and the underlying intestinal glands contain absorptive and goblet cells (H and E × 188).

for prospective evaluation. The mucosal surface was examined by dissecting-scope macroscopy with dye enhancement, by specimen radiography, and by gross inspection. Specimens were subsequently photographed, and a map was created of the observed epithelial patterns. The complete specimens were submitted for routine histologic evaluation and scanning electron microscopy. On the basis of the map, the histology, scanning-electron microscopy, dissecting-scope macroscopy, specimen radiography, and gross morphologic findings could be correlated with the specimen's level in the esophagus.

Specimens were evaluated histologically for cell and gland types, surface extensions (villi), and the degree and types of dysplasia. These parameters were all evaluated in relation to their distance from the esophagogastric junction. The cell types that were noted included gastric-type surface-mucous and mucous-neck cells (Fig. 12-1), intestinal-type goblet and absorptive cells (Fig. 12-2), chief and parietal cells (Fig. 12-3), and paneth (Fig. 12-4) and neuroendocrine cells (Fig. 12-5). Evaluation of the gland types revealed the presence of intestinal (Fig. 12-2), gastric body (Fig. 12-3), and gastric cardiac–antral glands (Fig. 12-6) and also that of residual esophageal submucosal glands (Fig. 12-7). The histologic and biochemical definition of these cells and glands are given by Ozello, Savary, and Roethlisberger.[14] The mucosal surface extensions noted above the level of gland orifices included a continuum from flat to a normal small-intestine villous pattern. This continuum was arbitrarily divided into five types: foveolar, ridged, rudimentary villar, villar, and villous (Fig. 12-8). These cell, gland, and villous types were found in almost every

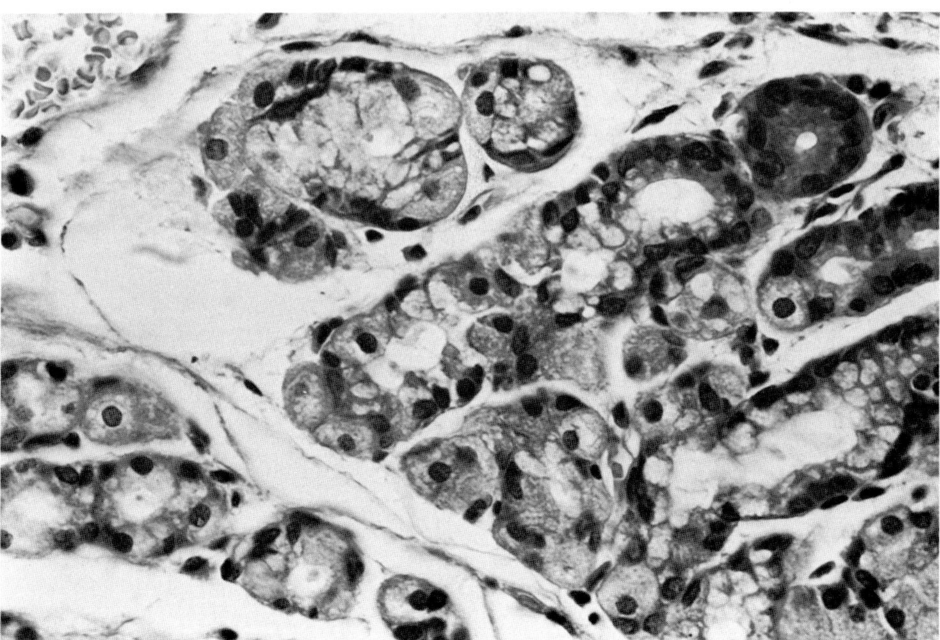

Fig. 12-3. Chief and parietal cells. Both chief and parietal cells can be seen in this gland (detail of Fig. 12-1, H and E ×463).

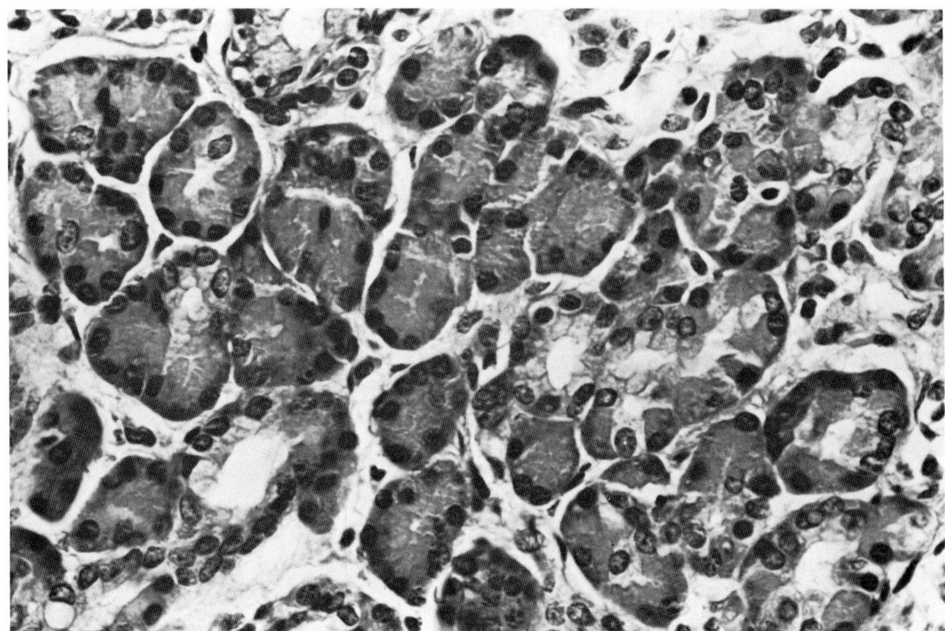

Fig. 12-4. Paneth Cells. The entire gland pictured is populated with Paneth cells that have a granular red cytoplasm on the *luminal* side of the nucleus (H and E × 463).

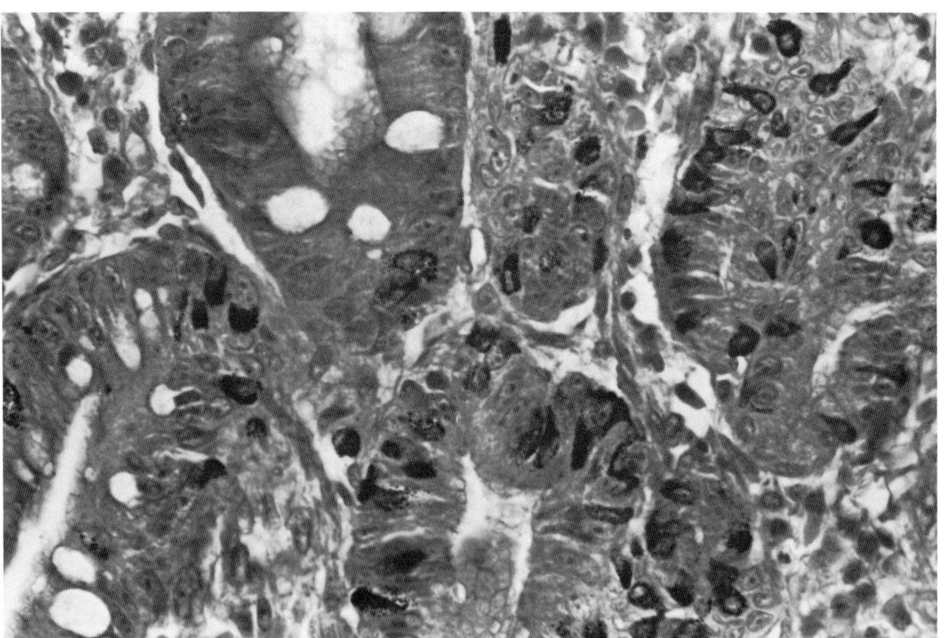

Fig. 12-5. Neuroendocrine cells. The dark granular areas in these glands are neuroendocrine cells (Grimelius technique × 463). Note that the granules tend to be found between the basement membrane and the nucleus, a feature that distinguishes them from Paneth cells on H and E staining.

conceivable mixture. However, the most commonly observed patterns included a villar or villous surface with goblet and absorptive cells and underlying intestinal glands (Fig. 12-2, 12-7), a ridged or rudimentary villar surface with surface mucous cells and intestinal or cardiac–antral glands (Fig. 12-6), and a flat-to-rudimentary villar surface with underlying gastric body glands (Fig. 12-1). In contrast to the findings of Paull et al.,[24] the mucosa did not appear to be oriented in progressive "zones." Although there was a tendency for gastric body glands to be located more distally, distribution of other cell, gland, and villous types was found to be a random mosaic. The differences noted in these studies are probably a result of the limited sampling inherent in biopsy studies.

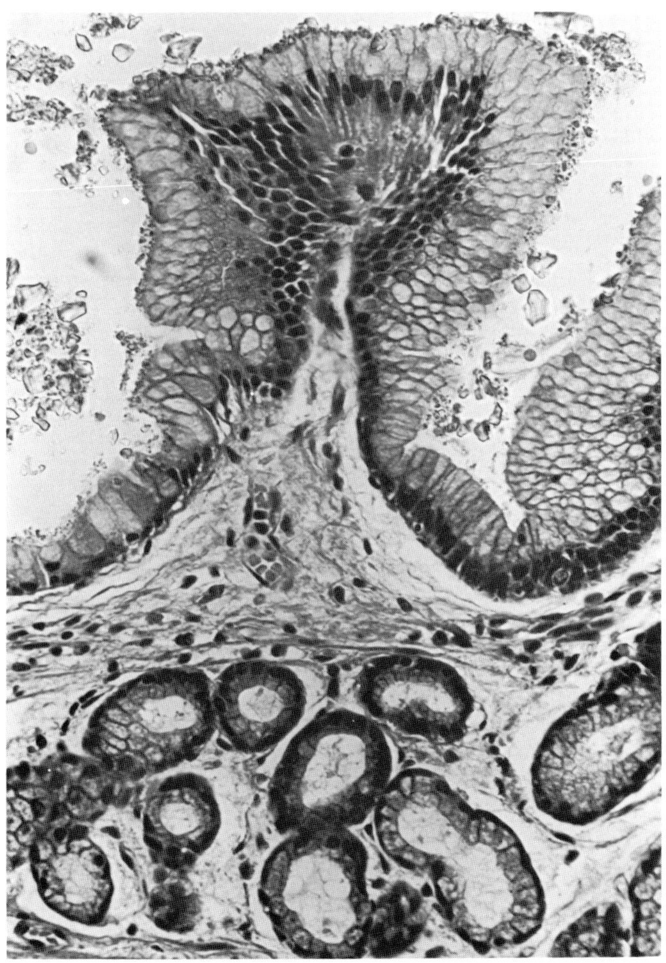

Fig. 12-6.   Cardiac antral glands. The epithelium has a villar surface covered with surface mucous and mucous neck cells. The underlying gland is of the cardiac–antral type (H and E × 297).

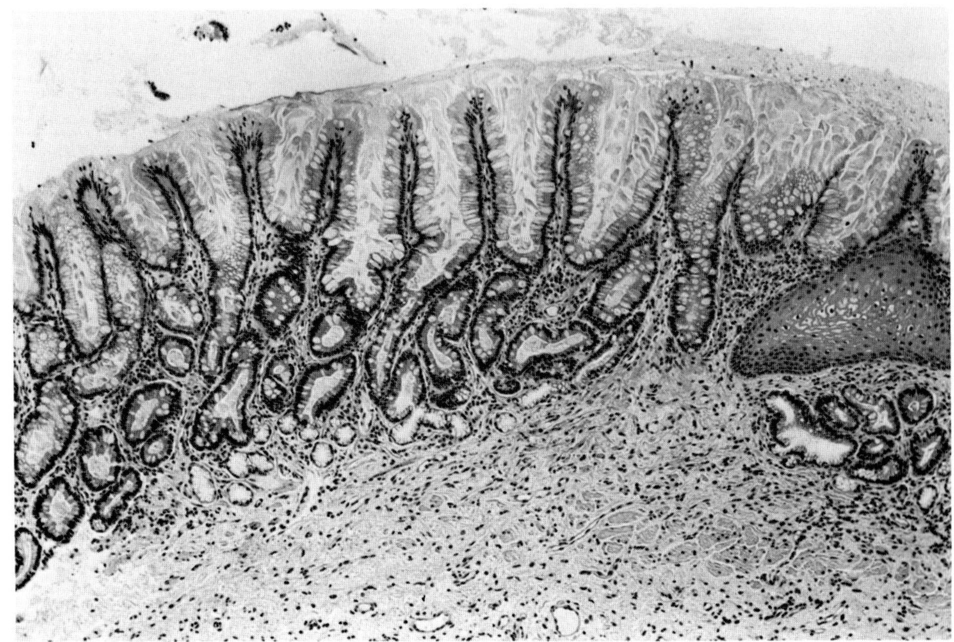

Fig. 12-7. Submucosal glands. Note the residual squamous island and underlying submucosal gland on the right, adjacent to epithelium that strongly resembles that of the small bowel (H and E × 72).

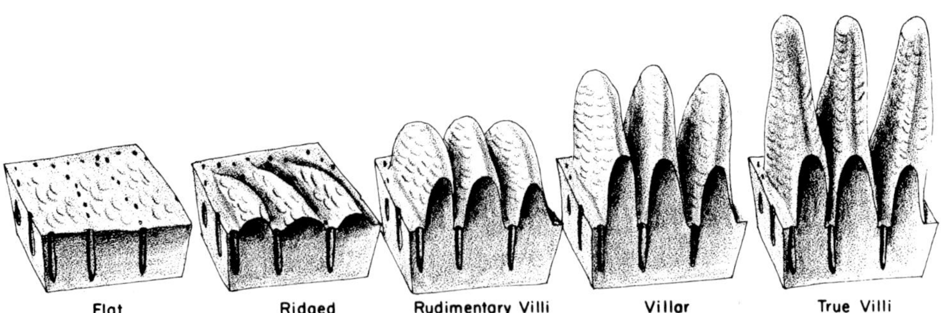

Fig. 12-8. The continuum of surface architecture seen in Barrett's metaplasia. The surface epithelium of Barrett's metaplasia may be flat, villous (as in the small bowel), or in any intermediate form. Intermediate forms appear to result both from differentiation toward flat types of mucosa and from atrophic changes secondary to continued reflux. When actually viewed (Figs. 12-11, 12-12), the surface is usually a complex mixture of architectural forms. (Drawing courtesy of Steven Giglotti)

Gross and Macroscopic Morphology. Barrett's metaplasia has a unique gross and macroscopic architecture which may become useful for developing radiologic and endoscopic diagnostic techniques. In the previously described study by Thompson et al.[13] these features were carefully correlated with microscopic assessment in order to evaluate their significance.

Gross examination of Barrett's metaplasia reveals several noteworthy features (Fig. 12-9):

1. The mucosa in areas of metaplasia is much deeper red in color than normal squamous epithelium.

2. The transition from columnar metaplasia to squamous epithelium is always sharp, and ulceration is frequently present at the junction.

3. The squamo-columnar junction usually does *not* show gross or microscopic evidence of fibrous stricture, suggesting that the "stricture" frequently seen radiologically is muscular in origin.

4. Focal ulcerations and residual squamous islands are frequent.

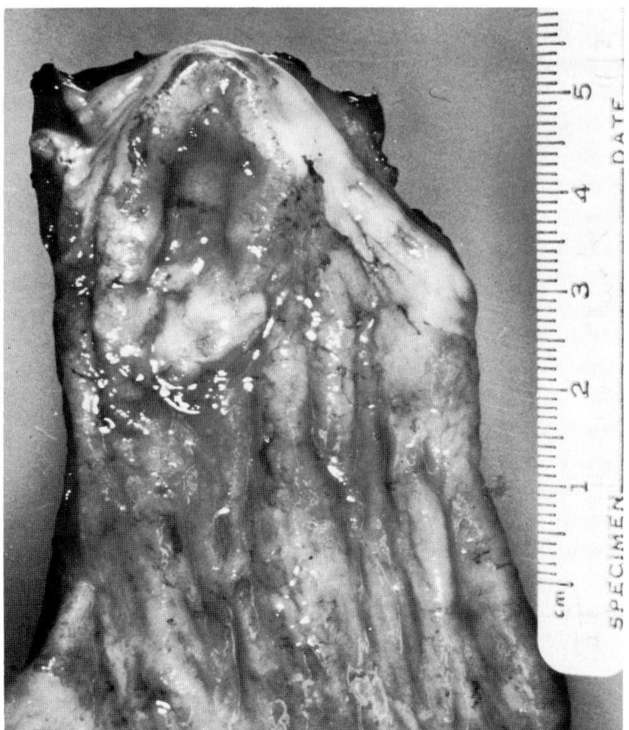

Fig. 12-9. Gross appearance. A large deeply invasive ulcerated carcinoma is in the upper left of the specimen. Across the top right, an irregular slanting patch of white represents residual squamous mucosa. The region beneath the tumor and squamous mucosa is darker and represents Barrett's metaplasia.

5.   Barrett's metaplasia occurs most frequently right at the anatomic junction of the esophagus and stomach and is often partly obscured by associated tumor; this suggests that Barrett's metaplasia or an allied process in the fundus is responsible for adenocarcinomas near the gastroesophageal junction.

Dissecting and Scanning-Electron Microscopy.   Use of the dissecting microscope with 1% tryphan-blue contrast enhancement and scanning-electron microscopy have demonstrated a surface pattern in Barrett's metaplasia that closely resembles the pattern described in nontropical sprue, in which varying degrees of mucosal atrophy obscure the villous pattern (Fig. 12-10–12-12).[13,46,47] The observed pattern is in sharp contrast to the normal featureless squamous mucosa (Fig. 12-10A) and to the extremely regular foveolar pattern with marginal grooves that is characteristic of normal fundic mucosa (Fig. 12-10B).[13,48] Within the region of Barrett's metaplasia, the surface is an intricate mosaic varying from a distorted flat, foveolar pattern to normal small-bowel villous architecture (Fig. 12-11, 12-12). The most common type of surface has a mixture of surface extensions from the mid-portion of the continuum shown in Fig. 12-8 (ridged, rudimentary villar, and villar).

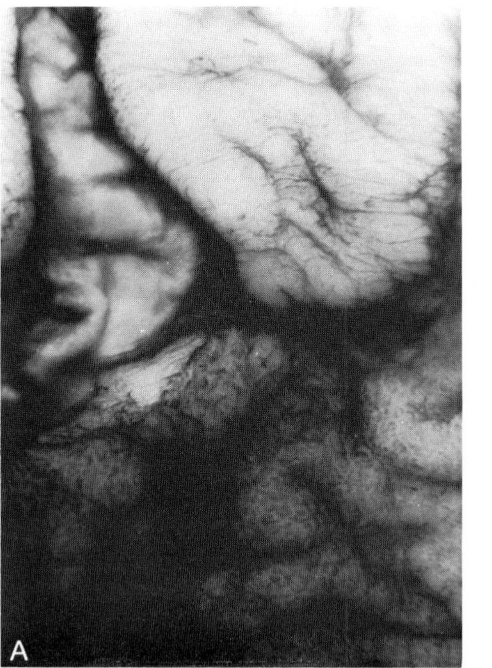
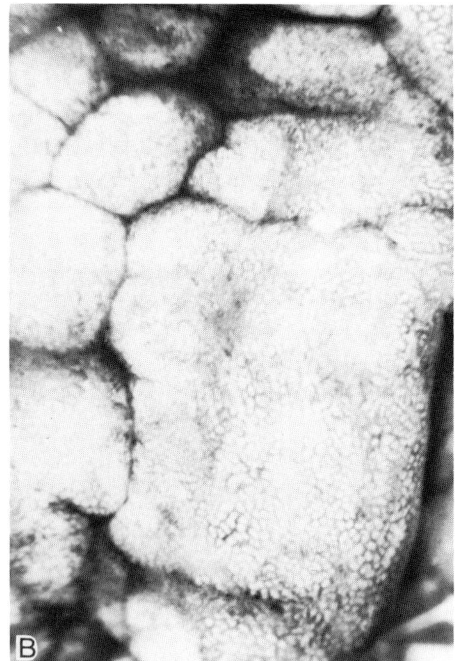

Fig. 12-10.   A. Normal squamous mucosa. An island of relatively featureless residual squamous mucosa is seen at the top right. At the bottom, ridges and foveoli of Barrett's metaplasia are present. Between the squamous island and Barrett's mucosa, a triangular-shaped area of ulceration (*top left*) can be seen (Tryphan Blue contrast × 5.2). B. Normal gastric mucosa. Normal gastric mucosa is divided into islands that are covered with numerous small pits or foveoli (Tryphan Blue contrast × 5.2).

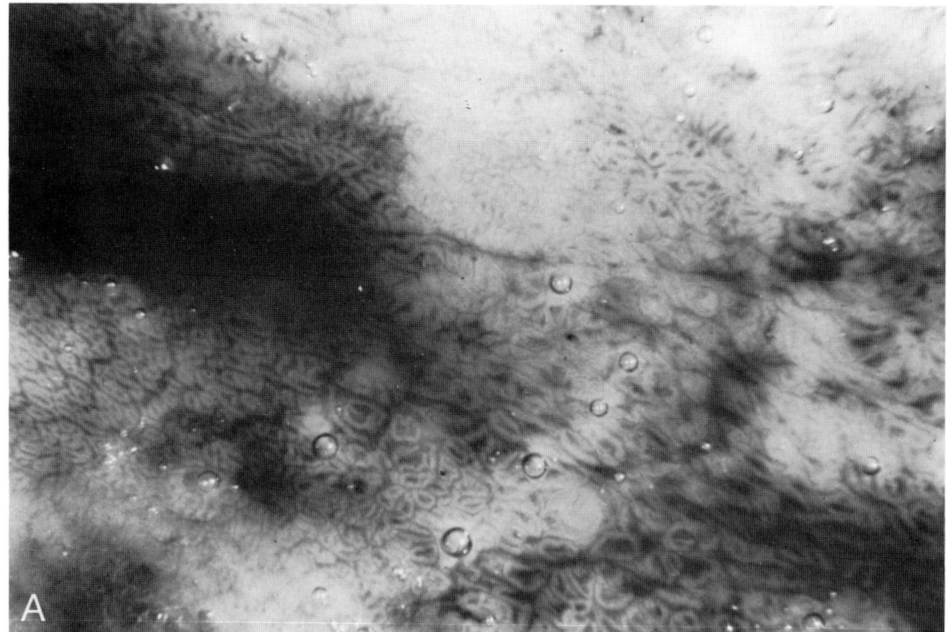

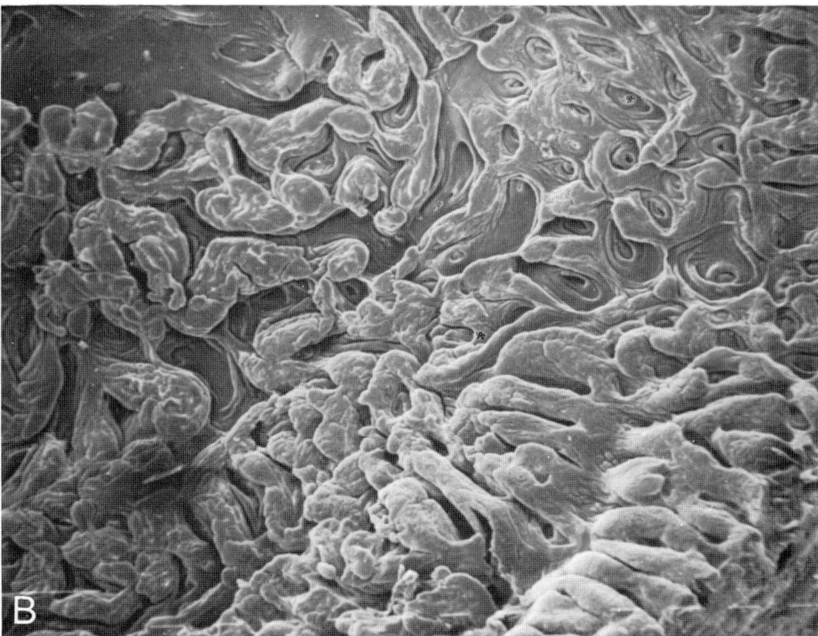

Fig. 12-11. Foveolar- to ridged mucosa. A. Dissecting-scope view of foveolar zone in Barrett's metaplasia. The pits vary markedly in size and contour. In addition, small ridges are just beginning to form in the center and bottom right (Tryphan Blue contrast × 22). B. Scanning-electron microscopy of foveolar- to rudimentary villar zone. In the upper right corner, numerous pits with surrounding concentric ridges can be seen. In the bottom right corner, ridges are prominent enough to obscure the pits. Toward the left side, surface extensions are becoming more prominent (rudimentary villi, SEM × 29).

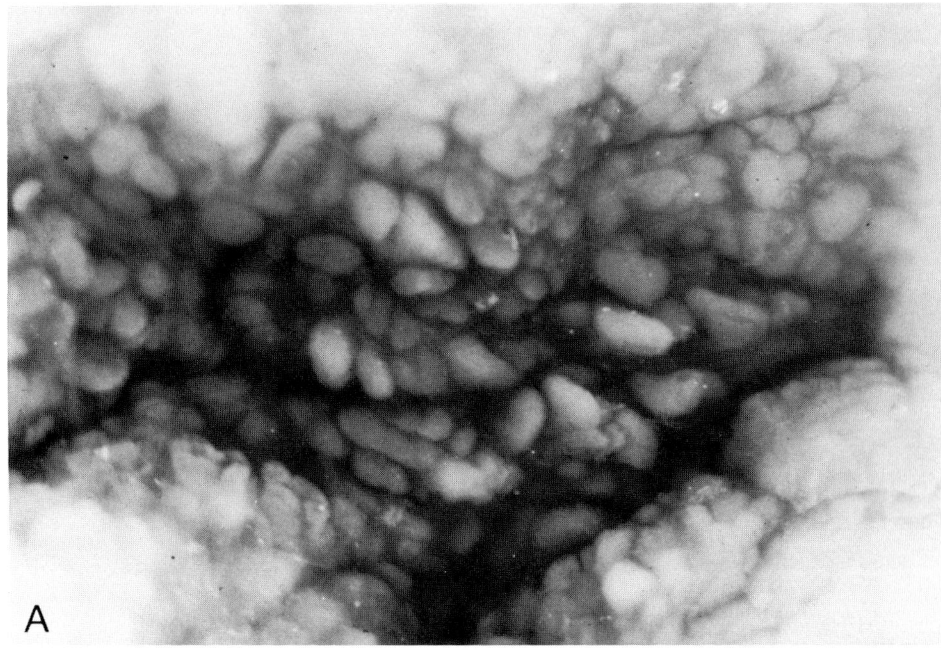

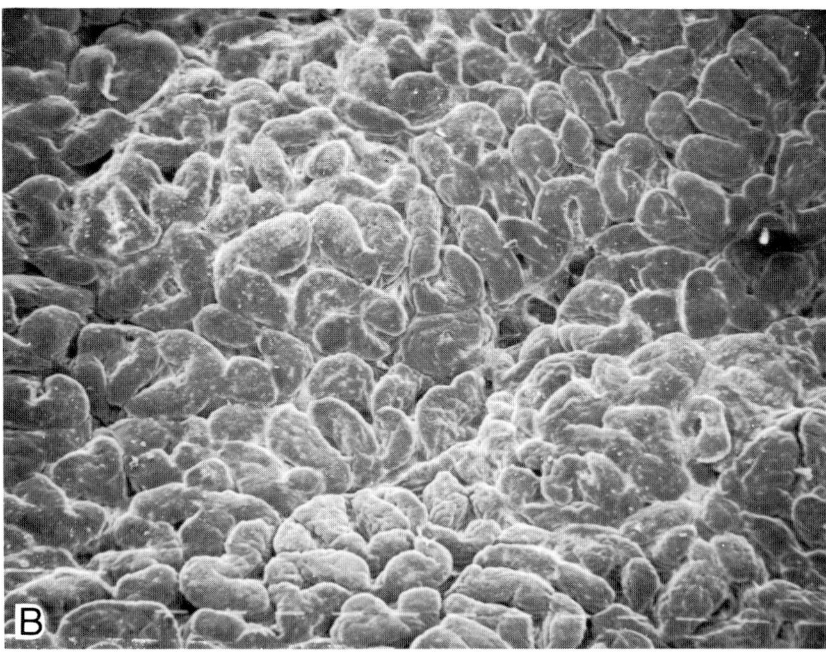

Fig. 12-12. Ridged- to villous mucosa. A. In the region seen here, prominent true villi and villar forms can be seen (Tryphan Blue contrast × 22). B. Scanning-electron microscopy of a variable area of Barrett's metaplasia shows an admixture of rudimentary villi, villar forms, and a few true villi (SEM × 29).

The observed macroscopic patterns accurately reflect the histology of the surface. Although regions that are defined macroscopically as villar and villous areas tend to show underlying intestinal glands under microscopic inspection, other gland types are occasionally seen. In a similar fashion, areas that appear flat or ridged when seen macroscopically usually but not invariably show underlying gastric fundic or cardiac–antral glands when viewed microscopically.

The surface in regions of dysplasia and carcinoma in situ tends to show an enlarged, irregular, and asymmetrically distorted villous pattern. Unfortunately, areas of marked acute inflammation may also show similar changes, making these findings nonspecific and not diagnostically useful. In regions with invasive carcinoma, surface ulceration is frequent. When seen in Barrett's metaplasia in conjunction with a mass, these features can be helpful in macroscopic diagnosis. Ulcers unassociated with a mass are more likely to be of the peptic type.[13]

Many of these features are below the resolution capability of currently used endoscopes. However, in the recent Japanese literature,[49,50] high-resolution instru-

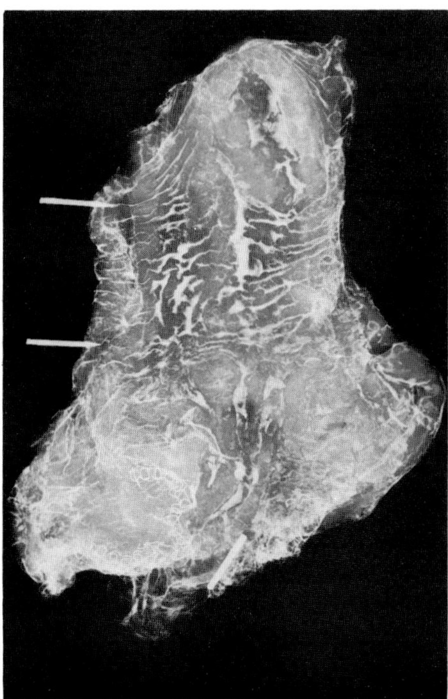
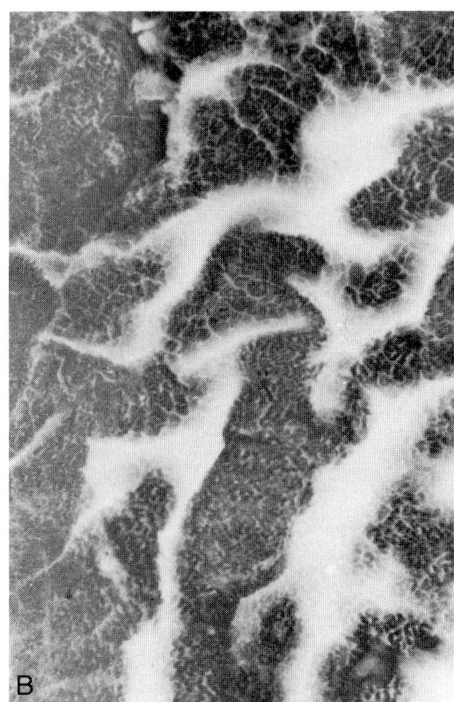

Fig. 12-13. Specimen radiography. A. The specimen seen in Fig. 12-9 was coated with high-density barium and radiographed. The tumor can be seen in the upper right corner of the photograph. Centrally, in the region between the two pins, the zone of Barrett's metaplasia shows a coarsely reticulated surface pattern. The lower pin is at the anatomic gastroesophageal junction. B. Two-fold magnification of specimen in A. Note the foveolar, ridged, and villar patterns that are just visible.

ments are described that can give excellent detail at up to 50 times magnification. When combined with dye-contrast enhancement,[20,49,50] the macroscopic features described should be diagnostically useful.

Specimen Radiography.   Specimen radiographs accurately image the macroscopic features of Barrett's metaplasia (Fig. 12-13A). When the radiographs are examined with a magnifying glass, the mosaic of surface extensions that were visualized macroscopically with the dissecting and scanning-electron microscopes can be fully appreciated (Fig. 12-13B). Unfortunately, the level of resolution possible with current double-contrast techniques does not permit most of these features

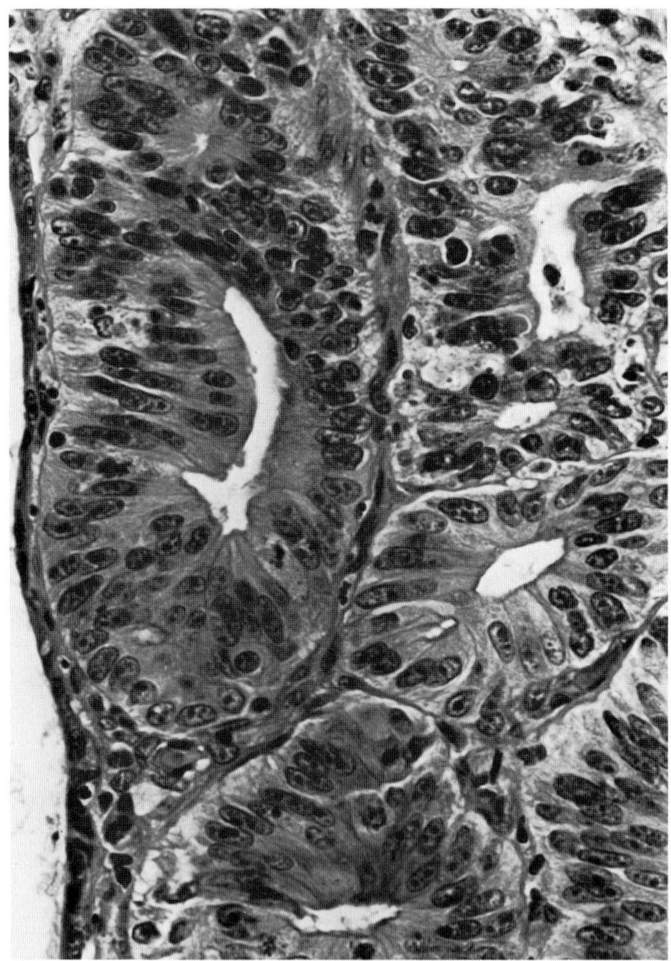

Fig. 12-14.   Severe dysplasia. Both the cytologic and the architectural features of these glands are markedly altered. The nuclei are large, variable in size and shape, and hyperchromatic. The glands are crowded and show loss of nuclear polarity toward the basement membrane (H and E × 470).

to be seen in vivo. In relatively atrophic and foveolar areas of Barrett's metaplasia, however, a reticulated pattern suggestive of "areae gastricae" can be seen (Fig. 12-13B).[13,51] In early cases of Barrett's metaplasia, before the typical high "stricture" is visible on x-ray, the presence of a reticulated pattern might be diagnostically useful. As double-contrast techniques improve, the other architectural features of Barrett's metaplasia that have been described may also become important.

Neoplastic Lesions.   If a careful search is made, multifocal areas of dysplasia and carcinoma in situ are common in the metaplastic Barrett's epithelium adjacent to adenocarcinomas of the esophagus (Figs. 12-14, 12-15).[13,26,27,29] The most commonly found dysplastic pattern consists of villi or glands lined by primitive, cytologi-

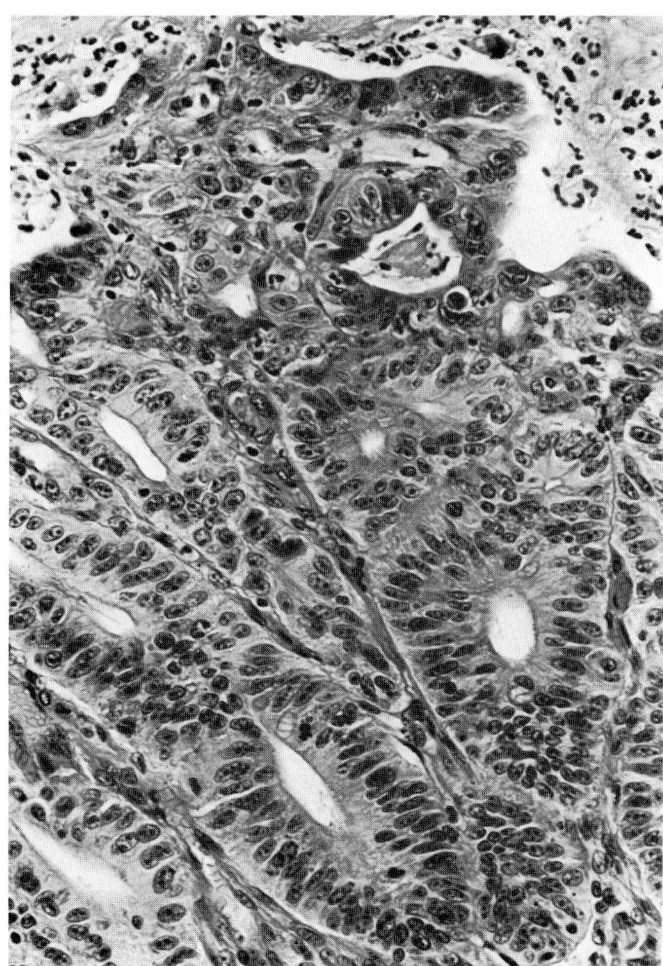

Fig. 12-15.   Carcinoma in situ (CIS). These glands show similar alterations to those seen in Fig. 12-14. In addition, areas of epithelial proliferation that are filling gland lumens and causing a "cribriform" pattern can be seen (H and E × 470).

cally atypical cells (Fig. 12-14). The degree of cellular and architectural atypia present can be used as in other tissue sites such as the colon to grade severity. An adenomatous type of dysplasia such as that found in colonic adenomas has also been reported in the literature (Fig. 12-16, A and B).[13,52]

As in other areas in which adenocarcinomas occur, differentiation may vary from good to moderate to poor. Subtypes of differentiation such as signet cell, mucinous, and papillary have been noted,[13,26,29,34] but these appear to have no significance in predicting survival.[28,34,37,38]

Biopsy and Cytologic Diagnosis

Based on the types of epithelium found in their study, Thompson, Zinsser, and Enterline[13] have suggested criteria for the biopsy diagnosis of Barrett's metaplasia. If inspection of an esophageal biopsy specimen reveals villiform surface architecture in conjunction with goblet and absorptive cells, the diagnosis of Barrett's metaplasia is warranted. The underlying glands are usually intestinal but may be cardiac–antral or gastric-body in type. If the surface is flat or shows some surface extension but is populated with surface mucous-type cells, then the biopsy is no longer diagnostic by itself. In this instance, correlation with the endoscopic site

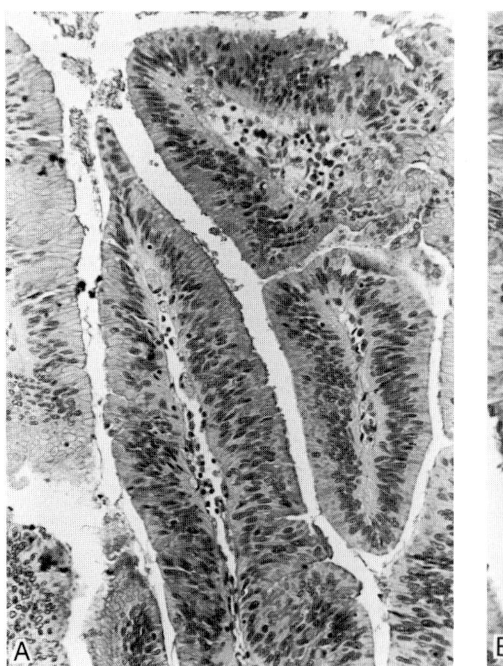
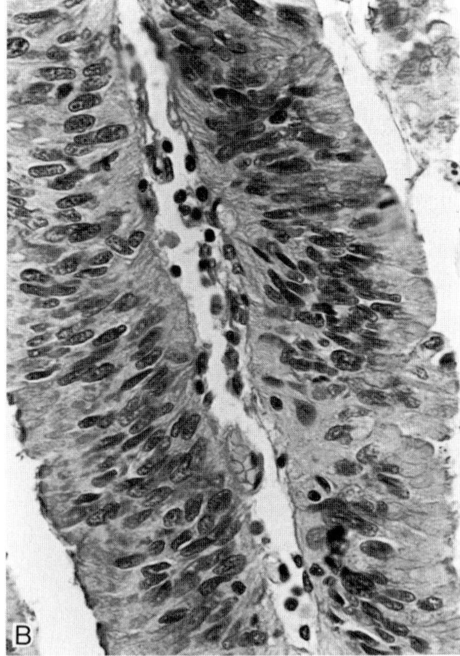

Fig. 12-16. Dysplasia in an adenoma. A. Note the villous structures that are lined by crowded cells with hyperchromatic, elongated cigar-shaped nuclei (H and E × 128). B. Note the hyperchromasia of nuclei and loss of nuclear orientation toward the basement membrane (detail of A, H and E × 320).

is necessary for diagnosis. Once again, the underlying glands may be intestinal, cardiac–antral, or gastric-body in type.

Although Barrett's metaplasia is not usually diagnosed cytologically, the presence of villiform tissue fragments with goblet cells should be diagnostic. Assessing the degree of dysplasia within a segment of Barrett's epithelium is likely to be inaccurate, since criteria for identifying dysplastic lesions within columnar epithelium at any site are unreliable.[53-55] The problem has not been adequately studied and deserves further attention.

Pattern of Spread and Survival with Associated Adenocarcinomas

Unfortunately, most adenocarcinomas of the esophagus and the gastroesophageal junction are deeply invasive at the time they are first discovered. In one series, only 44% of the diagnosed lesions were amenable to surgical resection.[34] Unlike the colon, the esophageal submucosa is rich in lymphatics, and early lymphatic spread is the rule.[11] Because of the intimate relationship of the esophagus to mediastinal structures, local spread may involve the tracheobronchial tree, lungs, aorta, or major vessels. The direction of lymphatic spread is a function of location within the esophagus. Thus tumors of the lower esophagus tend to drain toward the paraesophageal, celiac, and splenic groups, whereas tumors at a higher location usually drain to deep cervical, paraesophageal, posterior mediastinal, and tracheobronchial groups.[56,57] Metastatic disease most frequently involves the liver, but its occurrence in other organs such as lung and pleura, bone, pancreas, thyroid, adrenals, and skin has been reported.[34]

Overall survival in adenocarcinoma of the lower esophagus and gastroesophageal junction is dismal, varying from 0–7% at 5 years.[26,31,34,37-39] In most series, there was only one 5-year survivor. Thus, when an average value for all the series was calculated, only four 5-year survivors out of 152 patients could be found, a survival of 2.6%. It should be noted that survival figures for gastroesophageal adenocarcinomas do not differ from those found in lesions limited to the esophagus alone.

A variety of surgical, chemotheraputic, and radiologic therapies have been attempted.[26,31,34,37-39] As can be judged from the survival figures, none is particularly effective.

Summary and New Directions

Barrett's metaplasia appears to be a process that is caused by reflux of gastric or small-bowel contents into the esophagus. The metaplastic segment consists of a mosaic of columnar epithelial elements that have macroscopic and microscopic characteristics of both small bowel and stomach. Barrett's metaplasia is highly correlated with adenocarcinoma of the esophagus and appears to form the bridge between normal esophagus and fully developed invasive adenocarcinoma (neoplastic system). According to all but two reports in the literature, Barrett's metaplasia does not appear to regress either with or without therapy, but one might speculate that this is a function of the degree of neoplastic progression that has occurred. Currently, tumors that are diagnosed in association with Barrett's metaplasia are advanced lesions with almost no chance for cure.

Unlike many other tumor systems, the early neoplastic lesions (Barrett's metaplasia) of esophageal adenocarcinoma are symptomatic. Thus, many of the patients at risk for developing adenocarcinoma of the esophagus can be clinically identified by a long history of reflux esophagitis. The evolution of high-resolution macroscopic techniques for endoscopic and radiologic evaluation may allow the spectrum of Barrett's metaplasia and neoplasia to be defined more accurately. These new techniques may allow patients to be followed prospectively with the aim of primary prevention.

DYSPLASIA AND SQUAMOUS-CELL CARCINOMA OF THE ESOPHAGUS

Introduction

Until relatively recently, the neoplastic developmental sequence of squamous carcinoma of the esophagus was poorly defined. The detailed work of researchers in several provinces in Northwestern China,[58-63] combined with information gathered in other high-risk areas such as the littoral zone of the Caspian Sea in Russia and Northwestern Iran[64-66] and the Transkei region of Southern Africa[64,67,68] have generated a large body of relevant data. The pattern of disease progression that emerges from a synthesis of this data is remarkably similar to that seen in squamous-cell carcinoma of the cervix; a similarity that may suggest new directions for diagnosis and management. As with cervical carcinoma, the biologic potential of lesions comprising the developmental sequence of esophageal squamous-cell carcinoma form a continuous spectrum from "benign" to "malignant."

Incidence

Incidence figures for squamous carcinoma of the esophagus have a marked world-wide variation, a difference that has been useful in identifying epidemiologic variables of significance. In low-risk populations such as those in the United States (white), Canada,[11,64,69,70] Israel,[71] Nigeria,[64] and most of Europe (except for France),[64,72] the average incidence ranges from approximately 2–8/100,000. In these areas, peak incidence tends to occur in the seventh decade, and males are affected 1.5–3 times as frequently as females.[11,64] In regions of intermediate risk such as South Africa, Chile, Jamaica, Peurto Rico, Uruguay, Japan, India, parts of China, Russia, France, Switzerland, and the United States (blacks),[11,64-70,73] incidence figures vary from approximately 15–35/100,000. Once again, peak incidence tends to occur in the sixth to seventh decade and to be found with a male: female ratio that ranges from 1.5–15:1. In some areas of England, South Africa, Iran, Israel, and Scandanavia, the male:female ratio equals unity or is actually reversed.[11,64]

In three regions of the world, incidence for squamous carcinoma of the esophagus is remarkably high. In the provinces of Henan, Hebei, and Shanxi along the

Taihang Mountain range in Northern China, a survey of 62,000 people revealed a crude incidence of approximately 53/100,000.[58-61] In the counties of Yangcheng and Hebi within these provinces, crude rates are as high as 140/100,000.[60] If one considers the age range 60–69, the incidence is as high as 800/100,000. In this decade, squamous-cell carcinoma of the esophagus is the cause of death in 37–39% of the population.[60,61] As in other regions, a male:female ratio of 1.44:1 to 2.63:1 is noted.[60] In the counties of Hunyuan and Tatong, however, which are located in the same provinces in Northern China and are only several hundred miles from the high-incidence counties, rates are 1.43 and 2.80/100,000 respectively.[60] These geographic variations have suggested to numerous investigators that there are strong environmental influences on carcinogenesis.[58-63]

In the littoral zone surrounding the Caspian Sea in Iran and Russia, a second region of high incidence is found; crude incidence ranges as high as 110/100,000 in Russia and 195/100,000 in Iran.[64-66] As in China, peak incidence varies with age and in certain groups represents the major cause of death. Among males aged 35–64, the incidence in the Guriev district of Kazakhstan Province in Russia is as high as 547/100,000.[64] In most regions, the usual male predominance is noted. However, in one area of Northwestern Iran, the ratio is reversed.[66]

The third area of high incidence for squamous carcinoma of the esophagus is in the black population from Durban and the Transkei in South Africa.[64,67,68] Crude incidence values approximate 100/100,000 but reach as high as 357/100,000 in the age group 35–64.[64] Male:female ratios vary from 0.5:1 to 7.6:1 in South Africa, but in one region in central Africa 98% of the cases are in men.[11]

Factors Correlated with Occurrence

Analysis of the epidemiologic data on the occurrence of squamous carcinoma of the esophagus strongly suggests that environmental factors play a major role in carcinogenesis. Although no one factor or set of factors can explain the incidence figures presented, several types of influence appear to be important. These include dietary habits and deficiencies, smoking, alcohol consumption, genetic influences, conditions causing esophageal stasis, and possibly viral infection.

Dietary Considerations. In each of the high-incidence regions for squamous carcinoma of the esophagus, dietary patterns that appear to have etiologic significance have been identified. In China[59-61] the high content of trace elements and nitrosamines in food and drinking water and the consumption of moldy foods show a positive correlation with incidence. In the Caspian littoral zone and in South Africa, factors such as dietary habits and deficiencies and consumption of moldy foods also appear to be of importance.

A high concentration of nitrates, nitrites, secondary amines, and nitrosamines has been found in the drinking water and in foodstuffs from high-risk counties in Northern China. Investigations there suggest that nitrosamines can be formed in the stomach from nitrites and secondary amines. High concentrations of nitrosamines have been shown to produce esophageal carcinoma in Wistar rats.[60,61] Low concentrations of trace elements in the soil such as molybdenum, manganese, zinc, magnesium, silicon, nickel, bromium, iodine, chlorine, potassium, sodium, phosphate, and bicarbonate have also been shown to correlate positively with cancer incidence.[60] Molybdenum in particular has received attention because of its role as a cofactor for nitrate reductase, an important enzyme in the formation of nitrites, and thus ultimately nitrosamines. Other trace elements may also be shown to be cofactors that influence the concentration of carcinogens in foodstuffs, presumably by altering metabolism of plants grown on deficient soils. Dietary deficiencies in Vitamins A and C, riboflavin, protein, and overall caloric content also appear to be important variables.[60] Vitamin C has been shown to inhibit the formation of nitrosamines in the stomach, whereas deficiencies in Vitamin A, riboflavin, protein, and calories appear to raise the susceptibility of the esophageal mucosa to neoplastic transformation.[60] Contamination of pickled cabbage and other staple foods with geotrichum, candidum, and fusarium species has been shown to be significant.[59-61]

Similar dietary factors have been studied in the Caspian littoral zone.[66] Here too, deficiencies in Vitamins A and C, riboflavin, protein, and total caloric intake have been implicated. As in China, soils deficient in molybdenum and zinc have been suggested as important factors in generating foodstuffs that are high in nitrosamines and nitrites. Cereals and alcoholic beverages contaminated with fusarium species also may play a role.

In the black population in Durban and the Transkei, the use of extracts of the plant Solanum incanum to curdle milk has been shown to generate a high concentration of nitrosamines.[64] Although not as well studied as in China, soil deficiencies and contamination of food and drink with fusarium species also appears to be of significance.[64]

Alcohol and Tobacco. Although consumption of alcohol and tobacco does not appear to be an important variable in regions such as China and the Caspian littoral, in South Africa and in Western countries, their use appears to be of major significance.[11,58-64,66,69,70,72-76] Wynder and co-workers have shown in the United States and France that in people who drink heavily the risk of developing esophageal squamous carcinoma is increased approximately 12-fold.[69,75] Similar findings have been made by others in England,[74] France,[64,72] and South Africa.[64] Since alcohol by itself has not been shown to be a direct carcinogen, the mechanism of this interaction is not clear; suggestions include a solvent effect on coal tars derived from smoking and dietary deficiencies related to an alcoholic lifestyle.[11] In Seventh Day Adventists, a group known for abstinence from alcohol, risk of esophageal carcinoma has been shown to be lower.[11]

In the United States, smoking (including pipes and cigars) has been shown to increase the risk of developing esophageal carcinoma from two- to six-fold.[69,75] Similar findings have been made in Europe and South Africa.[64] In a carefully done autopsy study of 1,268 cases in the United States, Auerbach and associates showed a positive correlation between the various grades of esophageal dysplasia (including carcinoma in situ) and amount of smoking.[76]

In Iran and other regions, smoking opium and plant materials other than tobacco also has been implicated in the genesis of esophageal carcinoma.[64,66] Presumably carcinogens are released as a result of smoking a variety of substances.

Genetic Influences. A familial tendency to develop squamous carcinoma of the esophagus has been observed in seven families from Northern China and

1 from Northwestern Iran.[60,61,77] In both areas cases were noted at early ages (15 years of age in China) and in greater numbers than expected.

A familial association between esophageal squamous carcinoma, oral leukoplakia, and tylosis (hyperkeratosis of the interphalangeal epithelium) has also been noted.[78]

Esophageal Stasis. Conditions that lead to stasis in the esophagus or in some part of the esophagus are correlated with development of squamous carcinoma.[79,80] Joske and Benedict have estimated that the risk of carcinoma is increased 22 times for lye strictures, 9 times for esophageal webs, 7 times for achalasia, 6 times for peptic stenosis, and that it is also increased in various types of diverticula (Zenker's, pulsion, traction). Presumably these conditions all permit a more prolonged exposure of the esophageal mucosa to carcinogenic substances.

Other Associated Conditions. Risk factors for squamous carcinoma of the head and neck and for esophageal carcinoma appear to be similar.[73,81] Esophageal carcinomas are frequently (10%) associated with concurrent carcinomas of the pharynx, larynx, or oral cavity; in patients with esophageal carcinoma who develop second primary lesions, 60% will occur in the head and neck region.[81]

Plummer–Vinson syndrome appears to be associated with increased risk of developing squamous carcinoma, usually of the upper esophagus.[82,83] The dietary deficiencies of iron and other vitamins noted in this condition presumably lead to an increased susceptibility for neoplastic transformation.

Evidence for a Relationship between Dysplasia and Carcinoma

Although the occurrence of dysplastic lesions and carcinoma in situ (CIS) of the squamous mucosa of the esophagus has been reported numerous times in the American and European literature,[55,79,84-87] full characterization of the general incidence of dysplastic lesions, the significance of the histologic stage in the neoplastic sequence on survival, and progression within the sequence had not been adequately studied. Recent work in China,[58-63] and to a lesser extent in South Africa[67,68] and Iran[65] have clarified the squamous carcinoma developmental sequence, and have demonstrated its similarity to that found in the uterine cervix.

In two separate mass screenings done from 1961–1969 and 1971–1972, over 30,000 people were evaluated in three counties from the high-risk regions in Northern China.[58-63] In both studies, regions with a high incidence of carcinoma were noted to have a high incidence of dysplastic lesions. Furthermore, the average age of the patients with dysplastic lesions was noted to be approximately 7–8 years younger than the group with carcinoma, exactly what would be expected if dysplastic lesions are the precursors of carcinomas. All of the 67 early carcinomas noted in the screening had associated areas of CIS, dysplasia, and hyperplasia.

In a study done in Linxian County, 21,581 patients were studied over a 9-year period.[60,62] Results showed 12.7% had mild dysplasia, 11.2% had severe dysplasia, and 0.9% had CIS. These results are similar to those found in other neoplastic systems; relatively few carcinomas are found in relation to the number of dysplasias seen.

In a secondary study, 184 patients with mild and severe dysplasia were followed for an average of 4 years to determine the natural history of the process. Of the 79 patients with severe dysplasia, 26.6% proceeded to carcinoma in situ or invasive carcinoma, 32.9% varied from mild to severe dysplasia, and 40.5% either reverted to normal or to mild dysplasia. The subsequent incidence of carcinoma in the group with severe dysplasia was 140 times that noted in the normal population of the region. Of the 105 patients with mild dysplasia at the beginning, 15.2%progressed to severe dysplasia, 40% remained unchanged, and 44.8% reverted to normal. Thus it appears that at any stage of dysplasia, three options are possible: lesions can progress, remain stable, or revert to normal. Lesions toward

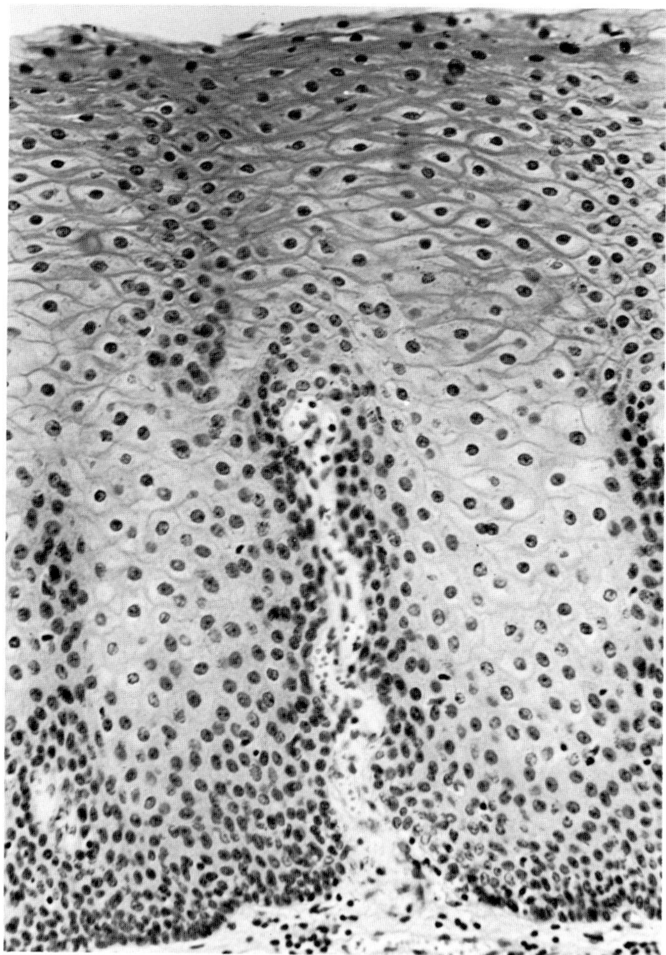

Fig. 12-17. Normal squamous mucosa. An orderly progression of cells from the basal proliferative zone to the glycogenated surface cells can be seen. The esophageal connective tissue papilla seen here centrally extends only slightly more than halfway to the surface (H and E × 188).

the severe end of the spectrum are more likely to progress than those at the mild end. As in other systems, progression appears to be a chronic process requiring many years for carcinoma to develop.

The results noted in Chinese studies have been partially confirmed in other areas of the world, although much less thoroughly studied. In South African Blacks, a similar distribution of dysplastic lesions and carcinoma in situ has been reported—dysplasia is much more common than more advanced lesions.[68] In Iran, a survey of 430 patients from a high-risk area revealed 80% with esophagitis, 16% with dysplasia, and 11% with CIS.[65] A similar distribution of dysplasia compared with CIS has been noted in two autopsy studies done in the United States.[76,86]

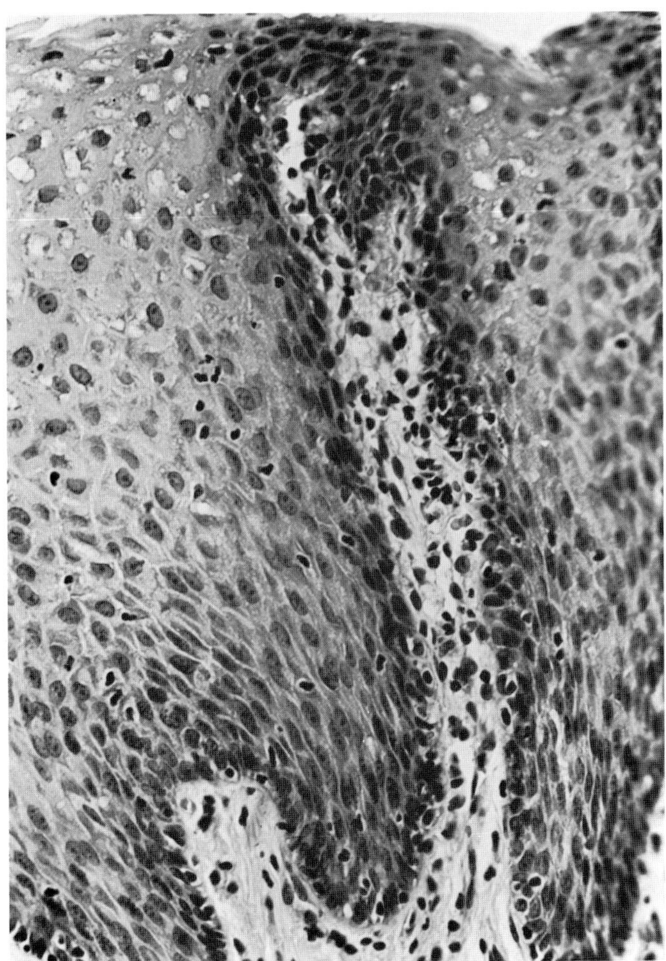

Fig. 12-18. Esophagitis. In contrast to the connective tissue papilla in Fig. 12-17, the one shown here extends almost to the surface. Fragments of polymorponuclear leukocytes can be seen within the epithelium. Also note that surface cells here do not become fully glycogenated, although maturation is orderly (H and E × 294).

Morphology of the Squamous Carcinoma Sequence

Microscopic Appearance.   In the Chinese experience, the first recognizable stage in the squamous carcinoma developmental sequence is the appearance of a few atypical cells (mild dysplasia) at the basal layer of hyperplastic or thinned esophageal mucosa.[61,63] These changes must be distinguished from those of esophagitis and regenerative atypia noted in areas of ulceration (Figs. 12–17 to 12–20). Cytologically, these cells are similar to those noted in mild dysplasia of the uterine cervix; they are polygonal in shape, have slight hyperchromatism, and demonstrate a slight increase in the nuclear-cytoplasmic (N:C) ratio.

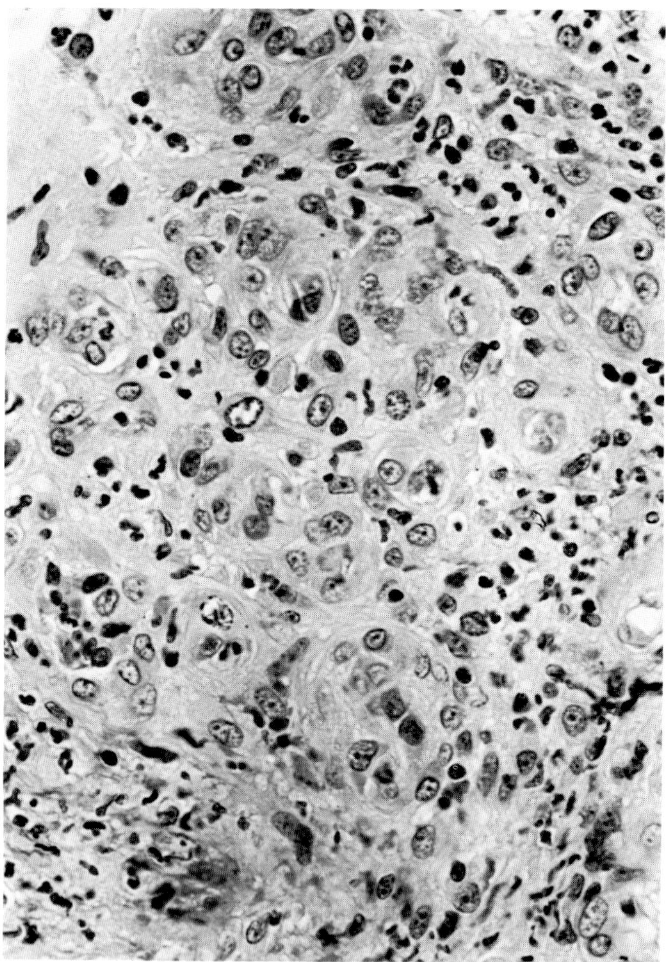

Fig. 12-19.   Atypia in an ulcer. Note the admixture of polymorphonuclear leukocytes and large somewhat atypical epithelial cells seen here. In contradistinction to dysplastic cells, the epithelial cells in this specimen show little variation in size, shape, or hyperchromaticity, even though a prominent chromatin pattern and nucleoli are visible (H and E × 470).

As the dysplasia progresses to moderate (Fig 12–21A), the proliferative zone with atpical cells becomes wider, encompassing from one-quarter to one-half of the mucosal width. The cells in this zone demonstrate mitotic activity throughout their expanded zone of proliferation. Although the surface layers of cells do mature, maturation is less complete and uniform than in normal mucosa. Cytologically, these cells no longer retain a polygonal shape, the nucleus is more hyperchromatic, and the N:C ratio is further increased.

In severe dysplasia (Fig. 12–21B), the expanded proliferative zone encompasses from one-half to three-quarters of the mucosa. Only a few layers of cells near the surface demonstrate a tendency to mature. Mitotic activity is seen at all levels except the most superficial. Cytologically, these cells are noted to have a very dense hyperchromatic nucleus, a relatively scant, frequently spindled cytoplasm, and a marked alteration in N:C ratio.

In CIS (Fig. 12–21C), the proliferative zone encompasses the entire mucosal thickness. Cells at the basal layer resemble those at the luminal surface, and mitotic activity can be seen in all layers. Cytologically, the cells show an extreme alteration of the N:C ratio, "salt-and-pepper" hyperchromatic nuclei, a scant rim of cytoplasm, and increased size. Microinvasive disease is frequently heralded by the appearance of prominent nucleoli in addition to the cytologic changes of CIS.

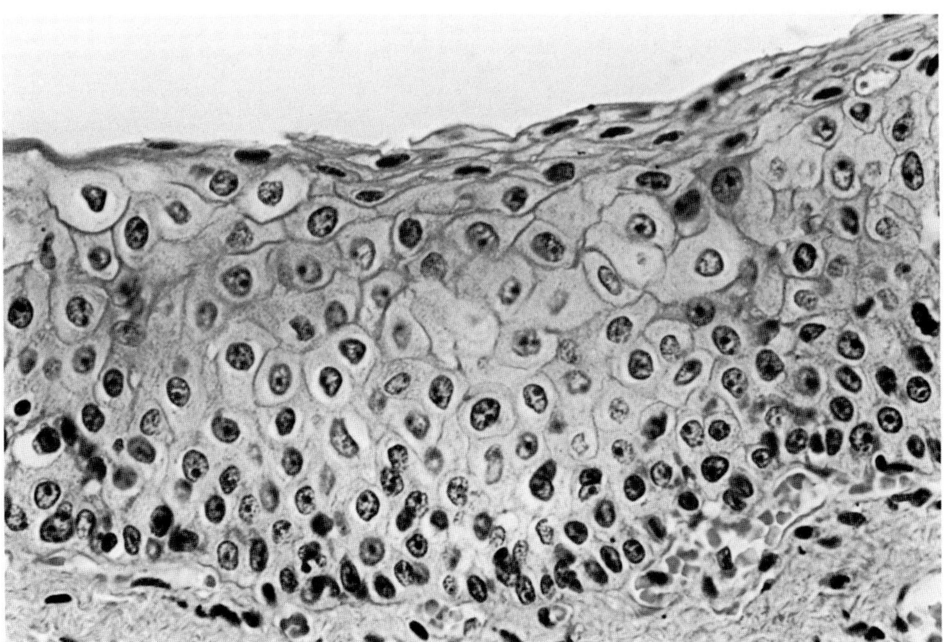

Fig. 12-20. Mild dysplasia. The basal cells seen in the bottom third of the epithelium are hyperchromatic, vary in size and shape, and demonstrate mitotic activity above the level of the basement membrane. Note also that maturation at the surface is somewhat decreased (H and E × 463).

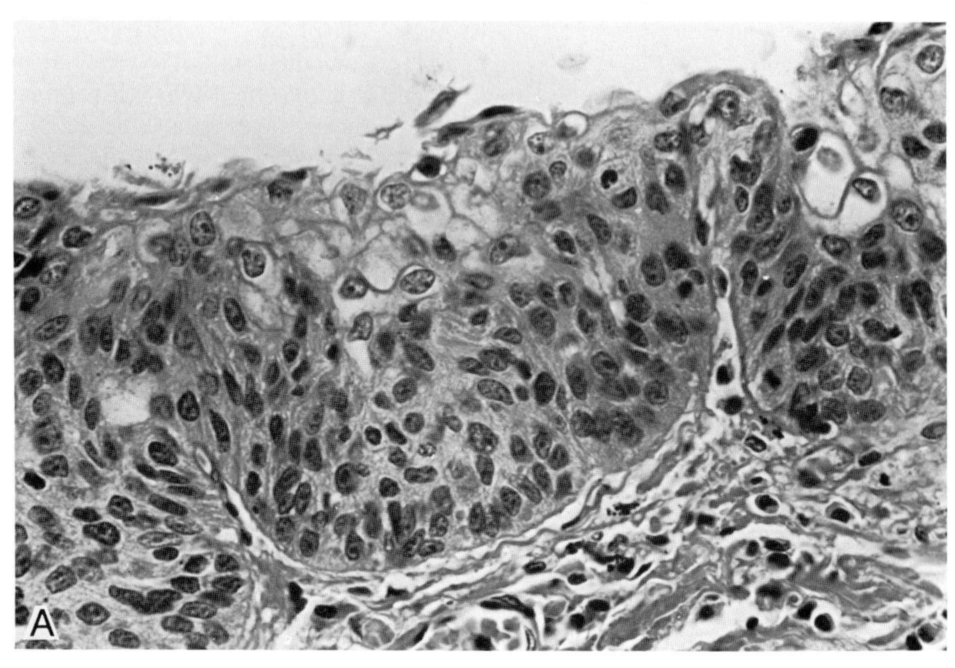

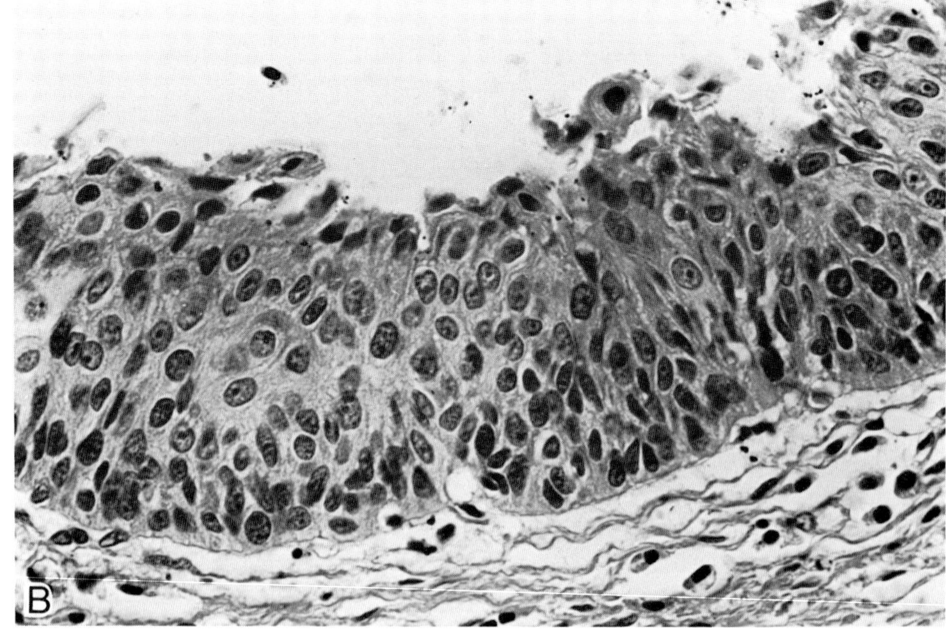

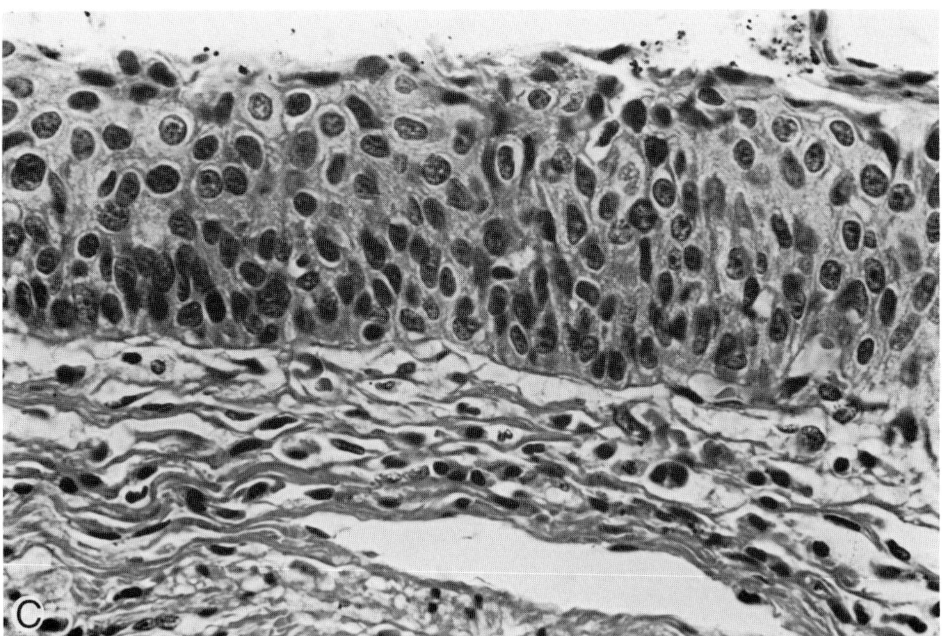

Fig. 12-21. Moderate (A) and severe (B) dysplasia, and carcinoma in situ (C). The cells visible in the bottom third of the epithelium in Fig. 12-20 can be seen to encompass progressively more and more of the total epithelial thickness (H and E × 463).

The definition of dysplasia and CIS based on the degree of expansion of the proliferative zone is similar to that used in the uterine cervix. The various grades of dysplasia and CIS tend to intergrade with one another and form a continuous spectrum of change. Although the grades of mild, moderate, and severe dysplasia, and CIS are arbitrary, they are easily recognized by pathologists because of their similarity to cervical dysplasias. Furthermore, the clinical studies done in China[58-63] have demonstrated the predictive value of such a classification.

If neoplastic progression is not halted, CIS tends to evolve into microinvasive and submucosal carcinoma.[61,63] Cells growing within the zone of CIS are usually clearly delimited from the underlying connective tissue by a basement membrane. In microinvasive carcinoma, single cells or groups of cells can be seen broaching the basement membrane but limited to the lamina propria. These cells have a tendency to keratinize and thus usually stand out from adjacent regions of CIS. The N:C ratio of these cells is much closer to normal—the nucleus fills much less of the total cell volume. In submucosal carcinoma, the same types of cells noted in microinvasive disease are seen in larger numbers, breaking through the muscularis mucosa and proliferating throughout the submucosal zone. Cytologically, these cells have ample amounts of spindled or angulated cytoplasm and dense nuclei with irregular areas of clearing (Fig. 12-22). As submucosal carcinoma

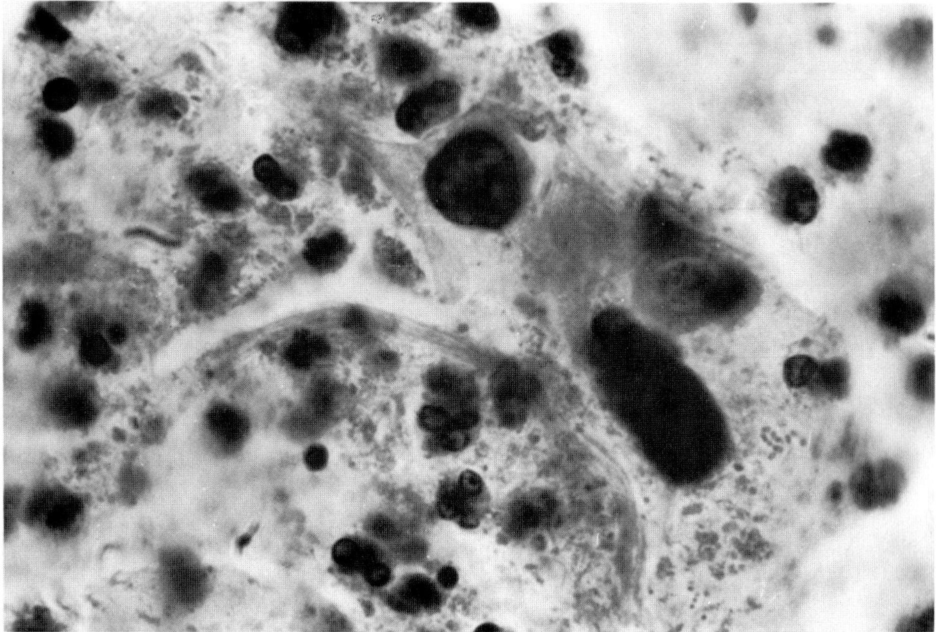

Fig. 12-22. Cytology of invasive squamous carcinoma. The nuclei seen with invasive squamous carcinomas are exceedingly dark and have irregular areas of chromatin clearing. The two large nuclei seen here in the center are from an invasive squamous carcinoma (Papanicolau stain × 1135).

progresses, it merges with the typical invasive carcinoma more frequently seen in Western countries.

Biopsy and Cytologic Diagnosis. The microscopic changes of early carcinoma are relatively easy to recognize in biopsy and cytology specimens. However, several problems present distinct difficulties. In the Chinese study describing pathologic changes in 100 cases of early carcinoma[63] all the cases of invasive disease were associated with varying degrees of dysplasia. Without a method to select the most fully developed area of disease for biopsy, underestimates of the degree of disease progression are likely to occur. In cytology preparations the wider sampling achieved may allow for a more accurate assessment of the degree of disease progression.[55,87] The tendency for esophageal carcinoma to reach submucosal lymphatic structures and cause stenosis early in the course of invasive disease also presents a problem. Lateral spread from a site of in-situ disease may be extensive. In cases where fibrosis near the site of origin prevents biopsy sampling in that area, superficial biopsies may miss the diagnosis, even though underlying lymphatics are involved (Fig. 12-23). Here again, cytologic wash techniques may provide a more accurate picture of disease progression, although the development of endoscopic techniques similar to those used in cervical colposcopy may allow biopsy sites to be chosen with a high degree of accuracy.

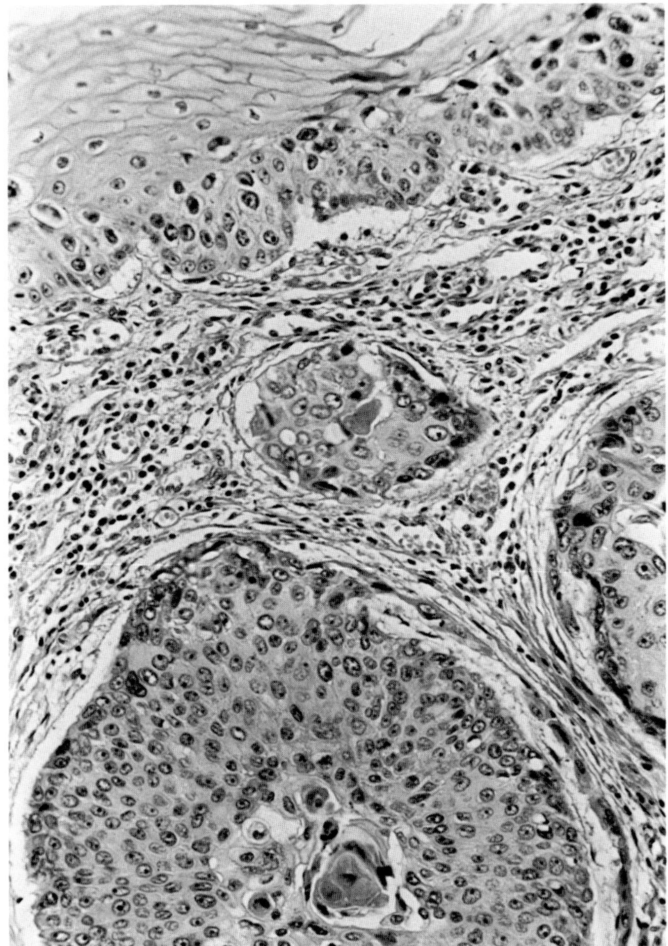

Fig. 12-23. Lymphatic spread. The surface epithelium is only slightly dysplastic in this case. In the underlying lymphatics, however, several large islands of invasive tumor can be seen. A superficial biopsy taken in a zone such as this would miss the diagnosis of invasive carcinoma (H and E × 188).

Gross Appearance. Fully developed invasive squamous carcinoma may take several gross forms of growth. Ming states that 60% are fungating (polypoid), 25% ulcerating, and 15% infiltrative (like a linitis plastica of the stomach).[56] These terms refer to the extremes that are useful for description; in reality, most cases present a mixture of growth forms (Fig. 12-24).

Early carcinoma has similar gross patterns of growth but has been studied only in China and Japan in sufficient numbers to allow accurate description.[63,88] In a study of 100 cases of early carcinoma (35 in situ, 41 microinvasive, and 24 submucosal), four patterns of growth were noted.[63] The first is the plaque type

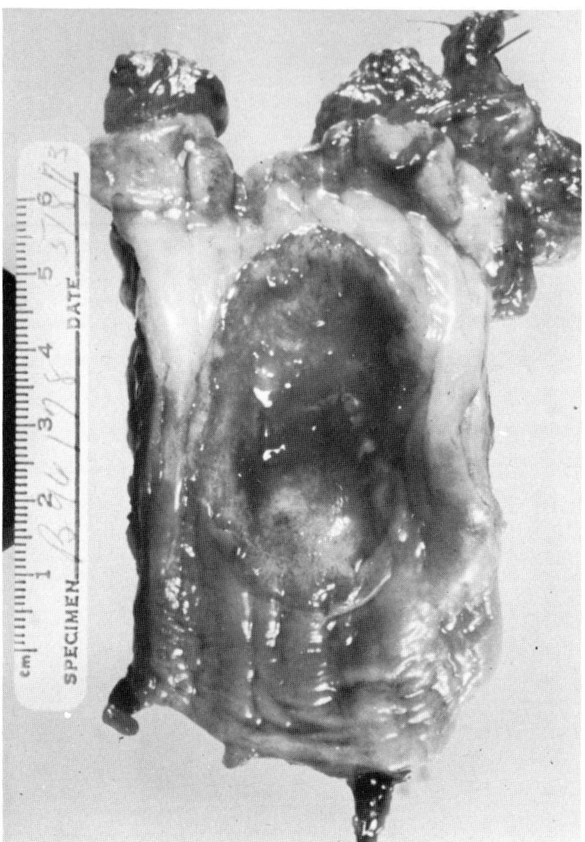

Fig. 12-24. Gross appearance. A typical ulcerating and infiltrating, well-advanced squamous carcinoma is seen. Diagnosis of tumors at this stage leaves little hope for cure.

(44 cases: 7 with CIS, 9 with microinvasion, and 28 with submucosal involvement). Here, the mucosal surface is slightly raised, coarsely granular, deeper in color, and lacks luster. Although both the longitudinal and transverse ridges that are normally seen tend to be obscured, no distinct mass is noted. The second form has been termed the erosive type (36 cases: 16 with CIS, 17 with microinvasion, and 3 with submucosal involvement). On examination, the mucosal surface is slightly depressed and is often partly eroded. The borders of these lesions tend to be serpiginous and sharply demarcated from neighboring mucosa by a distinctly darker color. Once again, the normal longitudinal and transverse esophageal ridges are interrupted, even though a distinct mass is not present. The third growth pattern is the papillary type (9 cases: 1 with CIS, and 8 with submucosal involvement). Here, the carcinoma presents as a small mushroom-like protrusion that may be partially eroded. The tumor is sharply separated from surrounding normal mucosa by a distinctly darker color. The last growth form is the occult type (11

cases, all CIS). In these lesions, the mucosa is neither raised or depressed but tends to be congested and darker in color. On routine gross examination, these lesions were almost unrecognizable.

In Western literature, symptoms of dysphagia and pain have been thought to occur only relatively late in the course of esophageal carcinoma.[11,56,71,89] In the Chinese series of 100 early cases, 96% were noted to have symptoms of dysphagia or chest pain. If verified in other series, the presence of symptoms may provide one means for screening patients at high risk for more extensive examination.

Macroscopic Appearance. The marked similarity between the pathology of squamous carcinoma of the cervix and that of the esophagus has suggested that the macroscopic approaches that have been so helpful in managing cervical disease might be adapted to use in esophageal endoscopy.[79,90-92] Endoscopes are now available that have similar resolution and magnification to colposcopes.[49,50] One article even reports that the vascular changes noted with early squamous carcinoma of the cervix are also present in the esophagus.[92] The use of diagnostic criteria based on vascular pattern, intercapillary distance, surface pattern, color, degree of opacity, and clarity of demarcation is accurate approximately 96% of the time in colposcopy.[93-95.] These criteria should be just as useful in endoscopy when performed with the Schiller test and appropriate filters.

Spread and Complications

The proximity of the esophagus to mediastinal structures makes local spread the most significant single factor in determining prognosis.[56] In addition, the rich submucosal lymphatic network of the esophagus makes early nodal dissemination common.[56] In one series of operable cases (roughly 40% of total cases), 38% had extra-esophageal spread, and 41% had positive nodes.[56] Common complications include fistulas to the aorta and lungs and metastasis to the liver, lungs, adrenals, and kidneys. Lymphatic spread is dependent on the site of the tumor within the esophagus. Lesions located within the lower esophagus tend to involve nodes in the paraesophageal, celiac, and splenic groups; those in the midesophagus the para-esophageal, posterior mediastinal, and tracheobronchial nodes; and those in the cervical region the deep cervical, paraesophageal, and posterior mediastinal nodes.[11,56]

In Western series, prognosis appear to be most closely related to size of the tumor and extent of spread; the degree of differentiation of the tumor appears to have little significance.[11] Nonetheless, if one considers all patients with the disease, *overall* 5-year survival only varies from 5.8–12%.[11] Most series exclude large numbers of patients. Thus, a comparison of surgery, radiation, chemotherapy, or a combination of these modalities is difficult.[11]

In the Chinese series of 100 early carcinomas limited to CIS, microinvasion, or submucosal disease, all but one patient were cured by surgery.[63] The early stage of disease in these cases made surgery relatively simple, and mortality from this cause represented the only death. Thus it appears that early diagnosis can have a marked impact on the current prognosis of esophageal carcinoma.

CONCLUSIONS

A review of the literature suggests that patients at risk for developing squamous carcinoma of the esophagus can be defined by a combination of history and symptoms. The presence of dysphagia, chest pain, or esophageal stasis, and risk factors such as age, locale, smoking, drinking, and dietary habits are important. Recently, the neoplastic developmental sequence for esophageal squamous carcinoma has been well described. Furthermore, macroscopic techniques that were originally designed for the prospective management of those at risk for cervical carcinoma appear to be applicable to esophageal disease and should also allow accurate directed biopsies to be performed. Since early carcinoma of the esophagus appears to be a curable disease, the ability to diagnose patients in an early neoplastic phase of their disease may allow for a marked change in the current grim prognosis.

REFERENCES

1. Clark WH Jr, Folberg R, Ainsworth AM: Tumor progression in primary human cutaneous malignant melanomas. In Clark WH Jr, Goldman LI, Mastrangelo MJ (eds): Human Malignant Melanoma, Grune & Stratton, New York, 1979.
2. Clark WH Jr., Mastrangelo MJ, Ainsworth AM: Current concepts of the biology of human cutaneous malignant melanoma. Adv Cancer Res 24:267–338, 1977.
3. Clark WH Jr., Ainsworth AM, Bernadino EA: The developmental biology of primary human malignant melanomas. Semin Oncol 2:83–103, 1975.
4. Elder DE, Bondi EE, Greene MH, Clark WH Jr.: The relationship of nevi and melanoma: the dysplastic nevus syndrome. In Ackerman AB (ed): Pathology of Malignant Melanoma, Masson, New York, 1981, pp. 185–216.
5. Farber E, Cameron R: The sequential analysis of cancer development. Adv Cancer Res 31:125–226, 1980.
6. Morson BC: The Pathogenesis of Colorectal Cancer. WB Saunders, Philadelphia, 1978.
7. Richart RM: Natural history of cervical intraepithelial neoplasia. Clin Obstet Gynecol 10:748–784, 1968.
8. Illmensee K: Reversion of malignancy and normalized differentiation of teratocarcinoma cells in chimeric mice. Basic Life Sci 12:3–25, 1978.
9. Illmensee K, Stevens LC: Teratomas and chimeras. Sci Am 240:120–132, 1979.
10. Winchester RJ, Kunkle HG: The human Ia system. Adv Immunol 28:221–292, 1979.
11. Enterline HT, Thompson JJ: Surgical pathology of the esophagus. In Silverberg SG (ed): Principles and Practice of Surgical Pathology, John Wiley & Sons, New York, 1982 (in Press).
12. Barrett NR: The lower esophagus lined by columnar epithelium. Surgery 41:881–894, 1957.
13. Thompson JJ, Zinsser K, Enterline HT: Barrett's metaplasia and adenocarcinoma of the lower esophagus and gastroesophageal junction. (submitted for publication).
14. Ozello L, Savary M, Roethlisberger B: Columnar mucosa of the distal esophagus in patients with gastroesophageal reflux. Pathol Annu 12:11–86, 1977.
15. Borrie J, Goldwater L: Columnar cell-lined esophagus: assessment of etiology and treatment. J Thorac Cardiovasc Surg 71:825–834, 1976.
16. Bremner CG, Lynch VP, Ellis FH Jr.: Barrett's esophagus: congenital or acquired?

An experimental study of esophageal mucosal regeneration in the dog. Surgery 68:209–216, 1970.

17. Naef AP, Ozello L: Columnar-lined lower esophagus: an acquired lesion with malignant predisposition. J Thorac Cardiovasc Surg 70:826–835, 1975.

18. Robbins AH, Hermos JA, Schimmel EM, et al.: The columnar-lined esophagus—analysis of 26 cases. Radiology 123:1–7, 1977.

19. Burgess JN, Payne WS, Andersen HA, et al.: Barrett esophagus: the columnar-epithelial-lined lower esophagus. Mayo Clin Proc 46:728–733, 1971.

20. Burbige EJ, Radigan JJ: Characteristics of the columnar-lined (Barrett's) esophagus. Gastrointest Endosc 25:133–136, 1979.

21. Messian RA, Hermos JA, Robbins AH, et al.: Barrett's esophagus: clinical review of 26 cases. Am J Gastroenterol 69:458–466, 1978.

22. Hamilton SR, Yardley JH: Regeneration of cardiac type mucosa and acquisition of Barrett mucosa after esophagogastrectomy. Gastroenterology 72:669–675, 1977.

23. Meyer W, Vollmar F, Bär W: Barrett-esophagus following total gastrectomy. Endoscopy 2:121–126, 1979.

24. Paull A, Trier JS, Dalton MD, et al.: The histologic spectrum of Barrett's esophagus. New Engl J Med 295:476–480, 1976.

25. Johnston JH Jr.: Gastric lined esophagus associated with rings and stenoses. Ann Surg 173:641–648, 1971.

26. Haggitt RC, Tryzelaar J, Ellis FH, Colcher H: Adenocarcinoma complicating columnar epithelium-lined (Barrett's) esophagus. Am J Clin Pathol 70:1–5, 1978.

27. Belladonna JA, Hajdu SI, Bains MS, and Winawer SJ: Adenocarcinoma in situ of Barrett's esophagus diagnosed by endoscopic cytology. New Engl J Med 291:895, 1974.

28. Poleynard GD, Marty AT, Birnbaum WB, et al.: Adenocarcinoma in the columnar-lined (Barrett) esophagus. Arch Surg 112:997–1000, 1977.

29. Berenson MM, Riddell RH, Skinner DB, Freston JW: Malignant transformation of esophageal columnar epithelium. Cancer 41:554–561, 1978.

30. Radigan LR, Glover JL, Shipley FE, Shoemaker RE: Barrett esophagus. Arch Surg 112:486–491, 1977.

31. Hawe A, Payne WS, Weiland LH, Fontana RS: Adenocarcinoma in the columnar epithelial lined lower (Barrett) esophagus. Thorax 28: 511–514, 1973.

32. Herbst JJ, Berenson MM, McCloskey DW, Wiser WC: Cell proliferation in esophageal columnar epithelium (Barrett's esophagus). Gastroenterology 75:683–687, 1978.

33. Pellish LJ, Hermos JA, Eastwood GL: Cell proliferation in three types of Barrett's epithelium. Gut 21:26–31, 1980.

34. Webb JN, Busuttil A: Adenocarcinoma of the oesophagus and of the oesophagogastric junction. Br J Surg 65:475–479, 1978.

35. Brand DL, Ylvisaker JT, Gelfand M, Pope CE: Regression of columnar esophageal (Barrett's) epithelium after anti-reflux surgery. New Engl J Med 302:844–848, 1980.

36. Mangla JC: Barrett's epithelium: regression or no regression. New Engl J Med 303:529, 1980.

37. Turnbull ADM, Goodner JT: Primary adenocarcinoma of the esophagus. Cancer 22:915–918, 1968.

38. Bosch A, Frias Z, Caldwell WL: Adenocarcinoma of the esophagus. Cancer 43:1557–1561, 1979.

39. Lortat-Jacob JL, Maillard JN, Richard CA, et al.: Primary esophageal adenocarcinoma: report of 16 cases. Surgery 64:535–543, 1968.

40. Adler RH, Rodriguez J: The association of hiatus hernia and gastroesophageal malignancy. J Thorac Surg 37:553–569, 1959.

41. Dalton MD, McGuigan JE, Camp RC, and Goyal RK: Gastrin content of columnar mucosa lining the lower (Barrett's) esophagus. Dig Dis 22:970–972, 1977.
42. Mangla JC, Schenk EA, Desbaillets L, et al.: Pepsin secretion, pepsinogen, and gastrin in "Barrett's esophagus." Gastroenterology 70:669–676, 1976.
43. Schreiber DS, Apstein M, and Hermos JA: Paneth cells in Barrett's esophagus. Gastroenterology 74:1302–1304, 1978.
44. Berenson MM, Herbst JJ, Freston JW: Enzyme and ultrastructural characteristics of esophageal columnar epithelium. Dig Dis 19:895–907, 1974.
45. Dayal Y, Wolfe HJ: Gastrin-producing cells in ectopic gastric mucosa of developmental and metaplastic origins. Gastroenterology 75:655–660, 1978.
46. Whitehead R: Mucosal Biopsy of the Gastrointestinal Tract, 2nd Ed, WB Saunders, Philadelphia, 1979.
47. Mangla JC, Lee CS: Scanning electron microscopy of Barrett's esophageal mucosa. Gastrointest Endosc 25:92–94, 1979.
48. Fallah E, Schuman BM, Watson JHL, Goodwin J: Scanning electron microscopy of gastrointestinal biopsies. Gastrointest Endosc 22:137–144, 1976.
49. Okazaki Y, Sakaki N, Takemoto T: Magnifying endoscopic observation and pathophysiology of the gastric mucosa. Jap J Stom Intest 13:605–614, 1978.
50. Hiratsuka H, Gocho K, Tanaka M, et al.: Examination of the magnified mucosal surface and pathophysiological changes of the human small intestine. Jap J Stom Intest 13:615–624, 1978.
51. Laufer I: Double Contrast Gastrointestinal Radiology with Endoscopic Correlation. WB Saunders, Philadelphia, 1979.
52. McDonald GB, Brand DL, Thorning DR: Multiple adenomatous neoplasms arising in columnar-lined (Barrett's) esophagus. Gastroenterology 72:1317–1321, 1977.
53. Prolla JC: Histopathology and cytology in detection. JAMA 226:1554–1556, 1973.
54. Prolla JC, Reilly RW, Kirsner JB, Cockerham L: Direct-vision endoscopic cytology and biopsy in the diagnosis of esophageal and gastric tumors: current experience. Acta Cytol 21:399–402, 1977.
55. Schickendantz GA, Sabagh RA, Ramos Mejia MM, Terzano G: Cytologic-histopathologic correlation in esophageal cancer. Acta Cytol 11:64–67, 1967.
56. Ming SC: Tumors of the esophagus and stomach. Armed Forces Institute of Pathology, Fascicle 7, Washington D.C., 1973.
57. Morson BC, Dawson IMP: Gastrointestinal Pathology, 2nd Ed, Blackwell Scient Pub, Oxford, 1979.
58. Li FP, Shiang EL: Screening for oesophageal cancer in 62,000 Chinese. Lancet 2:804, 1979.
59. Miller RW: Cancer epidemics in the People's Republic of China. J Natl Cancer Inst 60:1195–1203, 1978.
60. Yang CS: Research on esophageal cancer in China: a review. Cancer Res 40:2633–2644, 1980.
61. The Coordinating Group for Research on Etiology of Esophageal Cancer in North China: The epidemiology and etiology of esophageal cancer in North China. Chin Med J 1:167–183, 1975.
62. The Coordinating Groups for the Research of Esophageal Carcinoma, Honan Province and Chinese Academy of Medical Sciences: Studies on relationship between epithelial dysplasia and carcinoma of the esophagus. Chin Med J 1:110–116, 1975.
63. Tumor Prevention, Treatment and Research Group, Chengchow, Honan; Esophageal Cancer Research Group, Chinese Academy of Medical Sciences, Peking; and Linhsien

County People's Hospital, Honan: Pathology of early esophageal squamous cell carcinoma. Chin Med J 3:180–192, 1977.

64. Warwick GP, Harrington JS: Some aspects of the epidemiology and etiology of esophageal cancer with particular emphasis on the Transkei, South Africa. Adv Cancer Res 17:81–229, 1973.

65. Crespi M, Grassi A, Amiri G, et al.: Oesophageal lesions in northern Iran: a premalignant condition. Lancet 2:217–220, 1979.

66. Mahboubi E: The epidemiology of oral cavity, pharyngeal and esophageal cancer outside of North America and Western Europe. Cancer 40:1879–1886, 1977.

67. Wolpowitz A, Van Heerden J, Punt AM, et al.: Carcinoma of the esophagus. South Afr Med J 56:1043–1044, 1979.

68. Dreyer L: The incidence of dysplasia and associated epithelial lesions in the oesophageal mucosa of South African Blacks. South Afr Med J 58:406–408, 1980.

69. Wynder EL, Mabuchi K: Etiological and environmental factors. JAMA 226:1546–1548, 1973.

70. Fagelman KM, Jager R, Polk HC: Esophageal carcinoma: trends in incidence, treatment methods and prognosis. J Ky Med Assoc 77:637–642, 1979.

71. Shani M, Modan B: Esophageal cancer in Israel: selected clinical and epidemiological aspects. Dig Dis 20:951–954, 1975.

72. Faivre J, Milan C, Martin F, et al.: Cancer of the esophagus: an incidence study in Cote d'Or (Burgundy). Oncology 38:1–3, 1981.

73. Norton GA, Postlethwait RW, Thompson WM: Esophageal carcinoma: a survey of populations at risk. South Med J 73:25–27, 1980.

74. Chilvers C, Fraser P, Beral V: Alcohol and oesophageal cancer: an assessment of the evidence from routinely collected data. J Epidemiol Community Health 33:127–133, 1979.

75. Wynder EL, Bross IJ: A study of etiological factors in cancer of the esophagus. Cancer 14:389–413, 1961.

76. Auerbach O, Stout AP, Hammond EC, Garfinkle L: Histologic changes in esophagus in relation to smoking habits. Arch Environ Health 11:4–15, 1965.

77. Pour P, Ghadirian P: Familial cancer of the esophagus in Iran. Cancer 33:1649–1652, 1974.

78. Tyldesley WR: Oral leukoplakia associated with tylosis and esophageal carcinoma. J Oral Pathol 3:62–70, 1974.

79. Mandard AM, Tourneux J, Gignoux M, et al.: In situ carcinoma of the esophagus: macroscopic study with particular reference to the Lugol test. Endoscopy 12:51–57, 1980.

80. Joske RA, Benedict EB: The role of benign esophageal obstruction in the development of carcinoma of the esophagus. Gastroenterology 36:749–755, 1959.

81. Goldstein HM, Zermosa J: Association of squamous cell carcinoma of the head and neck with cancer of the esophagus. Am J Roentgen 131:791–794, 1978.

82. Wynder EL, Hultberg S, Jacobsson F, Bross IJ: Environmental factors in cancer of the upper alimentary tract. Cancer 10:470–487, 1957.

83. Shamma'a MH, and Benedict EB: Esophageal webs: A report of 58 cases and an attempt at classification. N Engl J Med 259:378–384, 1978.

84. Khan MY, Maltzman B, Jonnard R: Carcinoma of esophagus. NY State J Med 11:575–579, 1980.

85. O'Gara RW, Horn RC: Intramucosal carcinoma of the esophagus. Arch Pathol 60:95–98, 1955.

86. Postlethwait RW, Musser AW: Changes in the esophagus in 1,000 autopsy specimens. J Thorac Cardiovasc Surg 68:953–956, 1974.
87. Bishop D, Lushpihan A: The cytology of carcinoma in situ and early invasive carcinoma of the esophagus. Acta Cytol 21:298–300, 1977.
88. Seifert E, Borst HH, Ostertag H: Carcinoma-in-situ of the esophagus (early esophageal carcinoma). Endoscopy 5:147–153, 1973.
89. Ellis FH, Lane FWJ, Boyce HW Jr.: Cancer of the esophagus. Hosp Pract 80: 63–67, 1976.
90. Toriie S, Kohli Y, Akasaka Y, Kawai K: New trial for endoscopical observation of esophagus by dye scattering method. Endoscopy 7:75–79, 1975.
91. Miller G, Maurer W, Savary M, et al.: A case of oesophageal cancer limited to the mucosa and submucosa. Endoscopy 3:175–178, 1979.
92. Geboes K, Desmet V, Vantrappen G, Mebis J: Vascular changes in the esophageal mucosa. Gastrointest Endosc 26:29–32, 1980.
93. Kolstad P, Stafl A: Atlas of Colposcopy, 2nd Ed, University Park Press, Baltimore, 1977.
94. Cartier R: Practical Colposcopy. Karger, Basel, 1977.
95. Stafl A, Mattingly RF: Colposcopic diagnosis of cervical neoplasia. Obstet Gynecol 41:168–176, 1973.

13 | Infections of the Esophagus

Harvey M. Friedman
Stephen J. Gluckman

Many different viruses, bacteria, fungae, and mycobacteria can on occasion cause infection of the esophagus. However, for most agents infection of the esophagus is rare, and when it occurs, the esophagus is one of many organs involved in a generalized illness. Two organisms, Candida and herpes simplex virus, however, can produce infection limited to the esophagus and, in fact, are the commonest causes of esophageal infection. The resulting types of esophagitis will be discussed in detail in this chapter.

HERPES SIMPLEX VIRUS ESOPHAGITIS

In 1943 Pearce and Dagradi described four cases of esophageal ulcerations in which intranuclear inclusion bodies were detected at the ulcer margins.[1] The disease was ascribed to a virus infection of unknown type. Nine years later, Fingerland et al. noted five similar cases and isolated herpes simplex from the ulcers by animal inoculation.[2] Since then a number of investigators have examined esophageal tissue at autopsy and noted ulcerations caused by herpes simplex virus (HSV).[3-6] In these autopsy studies almost all cases went unrecognized during life; however, that HSV esophagitis can cause illness is apparent from the growing number of reports in recent years describing the clinical features of the infection.[7-13]

The available information is rather limited in defining the incidence of HSV esophagitis. The most complete studies are from autopsy series. These are retropective analyses and must be considered approximations, in part because only grossly involved areas of esophagus were sampled for histologic studies and also because herpes simplex virus cannot be distinguished from varicella zoster virus by histologic means. Berg studied 455 cancer patients at autopsy and detected herpes virus in 11 of 121 (9%) noncancerous esophageal ulcerations.[3] Nash and Ross reviewed 55 cases of esophageal ulcerations detected at autopsy over a 3-year period at a general hospital. In 14 cases (25%) the ulcers were caused by HSV, in 21 (38%) by Candida, and in 3 (5%) by mixed infection with herpes and Candida. No specific diagnosis was made in the remaining cases.[5] Buss and Scharyj analyzed 3,911 consecutive autopsies and found evidence of herpes virus esophagitis in 50 patients (1.3%).[6] The esophagus was the most commonly involved organ in those patients with visceral herpes simplex infection. From these reports, the incidence of herpetic esophagitis ranges from 0.3–0.6% among all autopsies. When esophageal ulcerations are detected at autopsy, 9–30% are caused by HSV.

Although bacteria and yeast commonly colonize the gastrointestinal tract, HSV is not part of the normal flora. Factors that appear to predispose to herpes infection of the esophagus include esophageal trauma by nasogastric intubation, malignancy—especially lymphomas and leukemias—chemotherapy, radiation therapy to the mediastinum, corticosteroid administration, and immunodeficiency states.[6-14]

Two mechanisms have been proposed for the development of esophageal infection. In some patients infection probably occurs by contiguous spread of virus from the oropharynx to the esophagus.[14] It is of interest, however, that most patients with herpetic esophagitis do not have active infection in the oropharynx, so this route of infection is probably rare. A second mechanism involves reactivation of HSV from latently infected sensory ganglion cells. This is the presumed mechanism for virus reactivation at other sites such as oral and genital mucosa.[15,16] HSV has been detected in a latent form in the jugular portion of the vagus ganglion.[17] Reactivation of virus from this site would permit virus to spread axonally to the esophagus, the end organ innervated by the ganglion.

The earliest lesion to develop is a vesicle. As is typical in locations that lack a keratin "roof," the vesicle rapidly ruptures and an ulcer results. The early ulcers have discrete slightly raised yellowish margins.[5] The ulcer bed is clean and is occasionally covered with fibrinous exudate. In severe cases, the ulcers become confluent over a segment of esophagus, with almost complete loss of mucosa. A typical pattern in severe herpes esophagitis is that of multiple punched out ulcers in the upper and mid-portions of esophagus and confluent lesions in the distal third. The disease stops abruptly at the gastroesophageal junction.

As seen on microscopic examination, the lesions generally begin in the squamous epithelium. Vesicle fluid accumulation in the mucosa is rarely detected. The espithelial cells undergo necrosis and slough, creating an ulcer bed. At the margins of the ulcer evidence of herpes simplex infection can be detected. The most characteristic change is formation of the eosinophilic intranuclear inclusion surrounded by a clear halo and by a thin layer of chromatin at the nuclear margin (Cowdry Type A inclusion, (Figure 13-1). Infected cells may show ballooning degeneration; nuclei may have a ground-glass appearance and may be clustered together to form

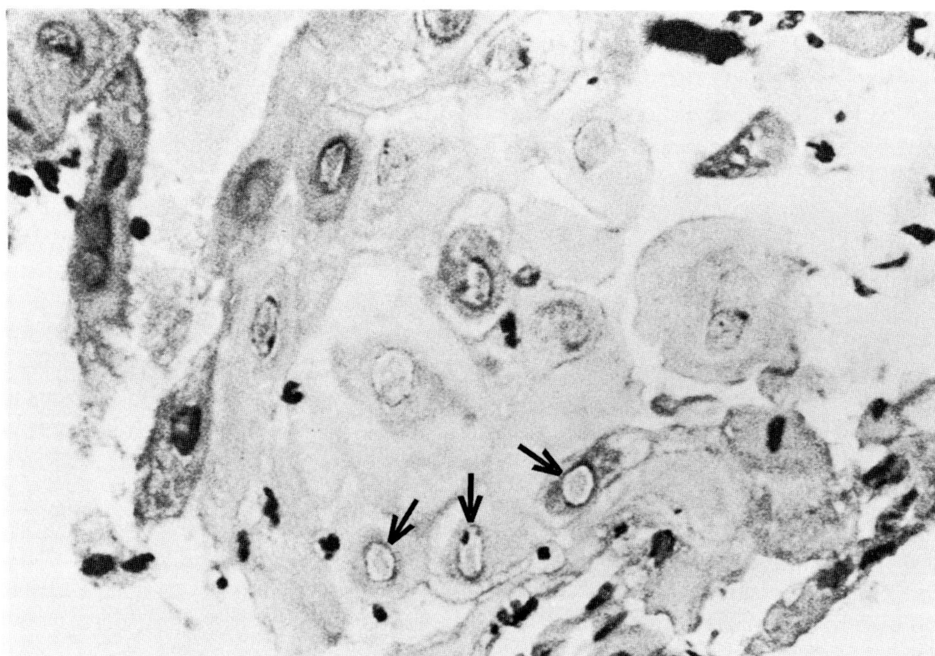

Fig. 13-1. Esophageal mucosa biopsy from patient with herpes esophagitis. Typical intranuclear inclusions (arrows) within esophageal epithelial cells are present (× 1280).

a giant cell. The bed of the ulcer shows acute and chronic inflammation, fibrin deposition, and necrotic debris. The ulcers are shallow and do not extend through the muscularis mucosa. Occasionally superinfection with Candida, with other fungi, or with bacteria is noted within the herpetic ulcers.

Many of the patients reported as having herpes esophagitis at autopsy were asymptomatic during life. When symptoms develop, the predominant features are dysphagia, odynophagia, and, occasionally, retrosternal burning. In several patients hematemesis has been the presenting feature.[9,11] Symptomatic infection has been documented in otherwise healthy patients,[12] but the illness develops mostly in cancer patients or in those immunocompromised by steroid, cytotoxic, or antineoplastic chemotherapy.[7-11]

The paucity of cases detected during life makes comment on the natural history of this infection difficult. However, progression from localized esophageal disease to disseminated skin or visceral involvement is rare, and most patients do not have active herpetic infections elsewhere, including in the oropharynx. In the few reports that document the duration of illness, symptoms often improve gradually over several weeks. Improvement may be spontaneous, occur when chemotherapy achieves tumor remission, or follow cessation of immunosuppressive drug therapy.

Levine et al.[10] described six cases of herpes esophagitis studied by double-contrast esophagrams. Examples of the lesions are shown in Chapter 3 in this volume, "Radiology of the Esophagus." Three patients had discrete widely separated ulcers on a background of relatively normal mucosa. Several ulcers had a stellate appearance with a surrounding zone of edema. Two patients had plaque-like defects without ulcerations, similar to findings in Candida esophagitis; and one patient had both discrete ulcers and plaque-like defects. The authors comment that discrete, widely separated ulcers on an otherwise normal mucosa are perhaps unique for herpetic esophagitis. Although Candida infections of the esophagus often produce ulcerations, these are usually multiple, causing the esophagus to assume a shaggy contour. These ulcerations can often be distinguished from the discrete ulcers that appear on otherwise normal mucosa in some patients with herpetic infection. Reflux esophagitis, Crohn's disease, Behcet's syndrome, and corrosive lye ingestion can also produce discrete esophageal erosions and should be considered in the differential diagnosis.

The appearance of herpetic esophagitis at esophagoscopy is similar to that from other causes of erosive esophagitis unless characteristic vesicles are detected. During esophagoscopy, specimens can be collected for cytology, histology, and viral culture. Although neither cytologic nor histologic findings can distinguish herpes simplex from varicella zoster virus, the absence of recognized varicella or zoster infection elsewhere makes infection with this latter virus unlikely. Cytologic examination is rapid (results usually available within 24 hours) and is a useful procedure to complement the yield obtained by biopsy. For the latter, best results occur if the margins of the ulcer are sampled.

Biopsy tissue or epithelial brushings should be sent for viral isolation. Herpes simplex is a rapid-growing virus, often isolated after 1 or 2 days' growth on a variety of tissue-culture cells.[11] Asymptomatic shedding of HSV occurs in the oropharynx of some patients; therefore, the esophagoscope can be contaminated by virus present in the mouth. This point must be kept in mind before assigning significance to isolation of the virus from esophageal specimens. Antibody testing on paired serum samples is an additional method used to establish a diagnosis of active herpes simplex infection.

Some patients with herpes simplex esophagitis do not require any specific therapy because the infection may improve spontaneously. However, those patients on immunosuppressive therapy who develop increasingly severe symptoms or whose symptoms fail to improve over several days can be treated by reducing the drug dosages. If patients are on large doses of steroids, one approach is to reduce the dose to the equivalent of 20 mg prednisone. A slower tapering over several days can then follow. If patients are on cytotoxic drugs, such as azothioprin, and are leukopenic (WBC count 4000/mm^3) these drugs should also be reduced or stopped. Patients on cancer chemotherapy should have treatment delayed until the esophagitis heals.

Vidarabine therapy for HSV is effective for disseminated neonatal herpes infections,[18] keratitis,[19] and encephalitis.[20] Several patients with esophagitis have been treated with this drug.[10] Proof of its efficacy for esophagitis, however, requires further study. Acyclovir, a potent new antiviral drug, is also effective against HSV.[21] Until more information becomes available, it seems reasonable to reserve antiviral chemotherapy for use in severely ill patients who do not respond to reduced chemo-

or immunosuppressive therapy or for those patients who cannot tolerate a reduction in immunosuppressive therapy.

Candida Esophagitis

Candida esophagitis was first described in 1860 by Virchow. The disease was well recognized by 1900; however, the causative organism remained unnamed until 1939. In recent years, fungal infections of the esophagus have been noted with increased frequency. The vast majority of these infections are caused by *Candida albicans* although a number of other Candida species and, occasionally, of other fungae have been associated with esophagitis.[22] Candida causes significant inflammatory lesions in any portion of the gastrointestinal tract. The esophagus is the most frequent gastrointestinal organ involved; in several autopsy series approximately 50% of the intestinal disease was found in that region.[23,24]

Candida is a ubiquitous yeast that rarely causes severe invasive disease in normal persons despite its frequent presence in the intestinal tract of healthy individuals. Gorbach et al. found Candida in 50% of mouth and 90% of stool cultures from healthy adults.[25,26] Predisposition to disease can involve a number of factors.[27-29] Prior antibiotic therapy allows for a selective increase in titers of Candida organisms. Esophageal irritation due to peptic esophagitis and poor esophageal drainage caused by achalasia, strictures, or tumors allow organisms to initiate infection more readily. Granulocytopenia, however, is the most common predisposing event for serious invasive disease.

The incidence of Candida esophagitis among 22,000 consecutive hospital admissions was found to be 0.1% (27 cases).[30] Over a 1-year period, 27 of 370 patients (7%) referred for endoscopy had evidence of Candida esophagitis.[30] Jensen found that 35 of 694 (5%) of cancer patients had Candida esophagitis during their illness,[22] whereas at autopsy, Eras noted that 44 of 251 (18%) cancer patients had this disease.[24]

The earliest histologic changes are white plaques several millimeters in dimension on an erythematous mucosa. As the infection progresses, edema increases and "cobblestoning" is seen. With further disease, patches of mucosa become necrotic and ulcerate. Gray-green pseudomembranes made up of mycelia and necrotic debris overlie the ulcers and erosions (Figs. 13-2 and 13-3). Less commonly, one may see mushroom-like excrescenses made up of large numbers of Candida. Advanced sequellae include diverticulae, stenosis, pseudotumors of heaped up granulation tissue, and areas of hemmorhage or perforation.

In a review of 13 patients with Candida esophagitis, Holt noted that odynophagia or dysphagia had been present in all of them and retrosternal pain in nine.[27] In the leukopenic patient, the combination of odynophagia, dysphagia, and retrosternal pain is the classical presentation. However, a number of authors have found that these symptoms are seen less frequently than they were in the patients in Holt's series. Jensen et al. noted odynophagia and dysphagia in 54% of 35 patients and retrosternal pain in only 9%.[22] In the largest review, by Eras et al., 30% presented with GI bleeding whereas 13% noted retrosternal pain or dysphagia

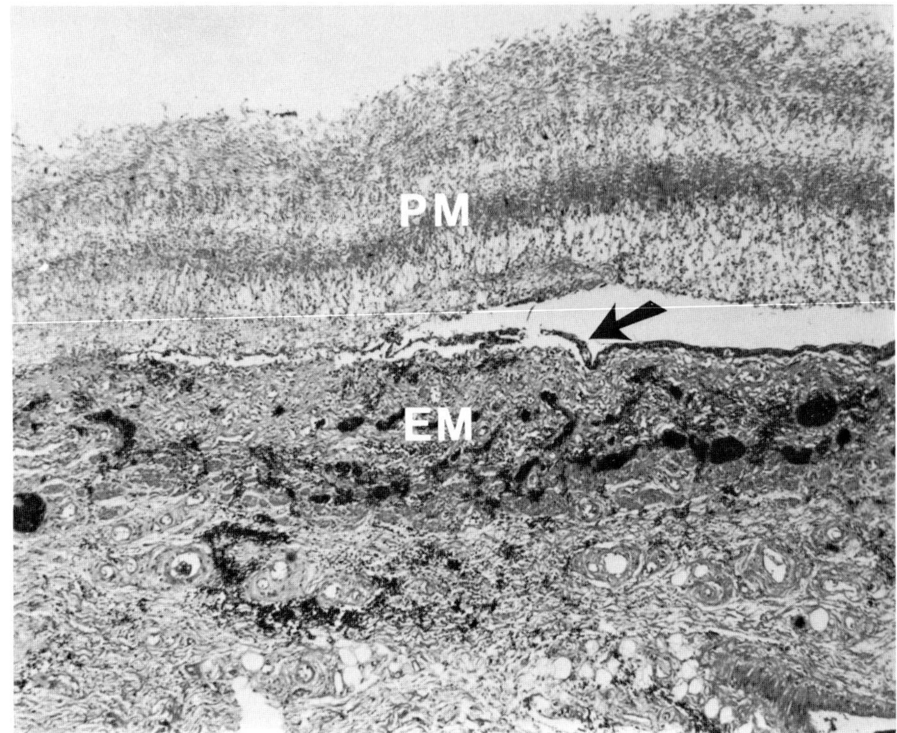

Fig. 13-2. Pseudomembrane consisting of mycelia and necrotic debris overlying sloughing squamous epithelium of the esophagus PM, pseudomembrane; EM, esophageal mucosa; arrow, sloughing epitheleal mucosa ($\times$ 40).

and 6% had odynophagia.[24] Nausea and vomiting are occasionally noted. Poor motility with resultant aspiration pneumonia can also occur. In general, approximately 25% of patients have no symptoms referrable to the esophagus. Oral thrush is a frequent occurrence in patients without esophagitis, and Candida esophagitis can occur without clinically apparent oral infection. Because advancing infection can destroy nerve endings and lead to anesthesia, occasionally patients note paradoxical improvement in pain as the disease progresses.

Serious complications include hemorrhage, dissemination of the yeast, and—though rare—perforation. Because esophageal symptoms may interfere with oral intake, the infection may also contribute to inanition in these patients.

The differential diagnosis that must be considered in patients presenting with the symptoms described above includes esophageal tumor, peptic esophagitis, herpes esophagitis, and esophagitis due to chemo- or radiation therapy.

The first description of the barium esophagram in esophageal candidiasis was by Andren and Theander in 1956.[31] The appearance can be quite variable, with up to 25% of esophagrams seeming normal. This occurs very early in the disease or occasionally very late if the entire esophageal mucosa has sloughed.[29] Progressive changes include granular, slightly irregular mucosa, nodularity (cobblestoning),

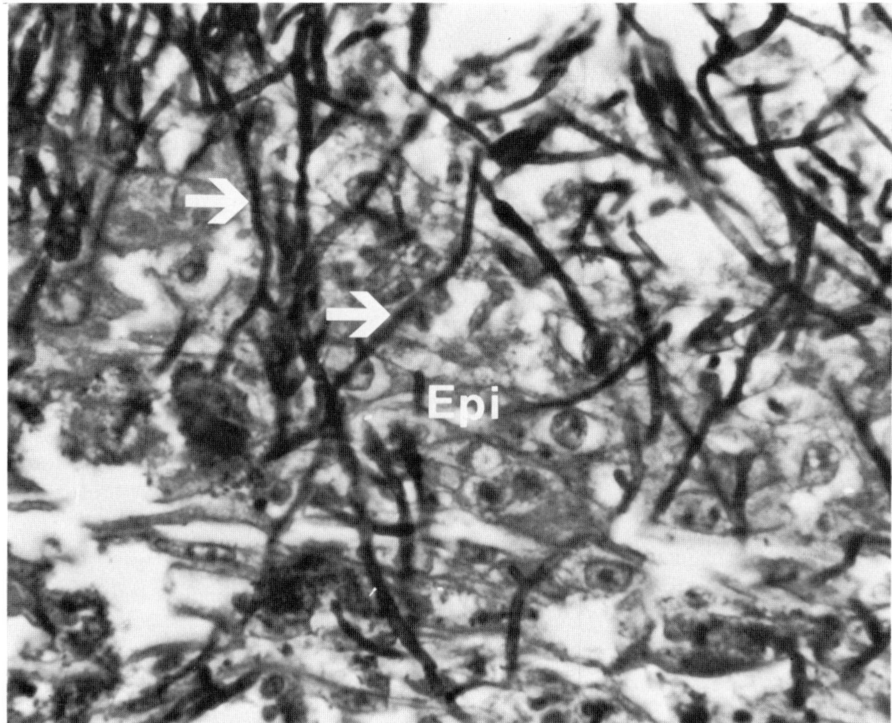

Fig. 13-3. Higher magnification of Candida pseudohyphae overlying squamous epithelial cells of the esophagus. Epi, esophageal epithelial cells; arrows, Candida pseudohyphae (× 650).

grossly shaggy mucosa secondary to ulcerations, and "tram-track" undermining of large patches of necrotic mucosa (see Ch 3). In addition, abnormal motility due to destruction of esophageal innervation has been noted.

Endoscopy is the most sensitive technique for establishing the diagnosis; however the mucosal appearance is variable and not necessarily specific for the etiology of the esophagitis. The findings include hyperemic and friable mucosa, erosions, ulcerations, pseudomembranes, and occasionally Candida masses or granulomatous masses. Esophagoscopy makes it possible to obtain material from which a specific diagnosis can be made. Cultures obtained at endoscopy are useful in identifying the specific organism and determining drug sensitivities but cannot distinguish colonization from true infection. Definitive diagnosis of fungal esophagitis can be made only by mucosal biopsy or by smears of the exudate.

Serologic diagnosis using Candida agglutinins has been found helpful by Kodsi et al.;[30] however, a positive test is not specific for recent disease, nor does it localize the infection to the esophagus. In additions, severely compromised patients may not be able to make sufficient antibodies to give a positive response.

A number of antimicrobial therapies are available for Candida esphagitis. There are no comparative studies, and the recommendations vary.

Nystatin can be an effective drug for cutaneous and vaginal Candida and has been used to treat Candida esophagitis with some success. There is potential difficulty with this drug; patients must be able to swallow, the time of contact between the drug and the organism is very short. In general, for the drug to be successful, it must be given very frequently; the minimal dosage is 500,000 units by mouthwash or oral tablet every 4 hours.

Amphotericin B is the standard therapy for those patients who do not respond to nystatin and for those sufficiently ill to require a more predictably effective drug. Medoff et al. reported remarkable success with very low dosages, in the range of 5–15 mg/day for 4–14 days.[32] This dosage avoids renal toxicity. Many authors recommend the full dosage (0.5 mg/kg/day) for severely immunosuppressed patients or for those with particularly severe disease.

Another drug to be considered for therapy is 5-fluorocytosine. A large number of Candida species, however, are not sensitive to this drug. Because sensitivities are unpredictable and because resistance to the drug may develop during therapy, it is probably best only to use this drug in combination with Amphotericin B in severely ill patients.

Intravenous miconazole has been used to treat Candida esophagitis with some success, although experience with purely esophageal candidiasis is limited. Jordan et al. noted response rates of only 41% for cancer patients with Candida infections of various types.[33] Since low-dose amphotericin B is effective and relatively safe, generally it is the preferred parenteral drug.

Finally, ketoconazole, an oral antifungal agent, appears to have some role in treating Candida infections. Best therapeutic results have been obtained in combatting mucocutaneous Candida infection. The efficacy of this drug in treating other forms of candidiasis is not yet well established. Because it is given orally, this drug may be difficult to use in patients with severe swallowing problems.

APPROACH TO DIAGNOSIS

Both Candida and herpes simplex infections occur predominantly in immunocompromised patients. Dysphagia, odynophagia, and retrosternal burning are common to both causes of esophagitis. If discrete ulcers are demonstrated on an esophagram, endoscopy should be performed to obtain cytology and biopsy samples for viral and fungal cultures. If the esophagram demonstrates multiple ulcers and plaques, empiric therapy for Candida esophagitis may be initiated. However, if no improvement occurs over several days, endoscopy should be performed with attempts at tissue and culture diagnosis.

SUMMARY

When considering the diagnosis of esphagitis one must remember several relevant facts. Candida and herpes virus are often found in the mouths of persons without esophageal infection, and esophageal infection frequently occurs without

signs of oral involvement. Patients with esophagitis may not have symptoms refera-
ble to the esophagus. The symptoms, esophagraphic findings, and endoscopic appearance are often not specific for a particular pathogen. The specific diagnosis
can be established only by smears of the esophageal exudate, cytology studies,
histologic examination of esophageal mucosa, and culture. Finally a number of
approaches to therapy exist. Choice of a specific drug is based on the severity of
the illness. Intravenous amphotericin B is currently the drug of choice for severe
Candida disease, whereas reduction in immunosuppressive therapy is often indicated
for herpetic esophagitis. The use of antiviral therapies can be considered in severe
infection, but proof of efficacy awaits results of controlled clinical trials.

ACKNOWLEDGMENT

We thank Dr. Francis X. McBrearty for providing Figures 2 and 3.

REFERENCES

1. Pearce J, Dagradi A: Acute ulceration of the esophagus with associated intranuclear
   inclusion bodies; report of four cases. Arch Pathol, 35:889–897, 1943.
2. Fingerland A, Vortel V, Endrys J: Oesophagitis herpetica. Cas Lek Cesk, 91:473–475,
   1952. (Abstract in English)
3. Berg JW: Esophageal herpes: a complication of cancer therapy. Cancer, 8:731–740,
   1955.
4. Rosen P, Hajdu SI: Visceral herpes virus infections in patients with Cancer. Am J
   Clin Pathol 56:459–465, 1971.
5. Nash G, Ross JS: Herpetic esophagitis: a common cause of esophageal ulceration. Hum
   Pathol, 5:339–345, 1974.
6. Buss DH, Scharyj M: Herpes virus infection of the esophagus and other visceral organs
   in adults: incidence and clinical significance. Am J Med, 66:457–462, 1979.
7. Lightdale CJ, Wolf DJ, Marcucci RA, Salyer WR: Herpetic esophagitis in patients
   with cancer: ante mortem diagnosis by brush cytotology. Cancer, 39:223–226, 1977.
8. Lasser A: Herpes simplex virus esophagitis. Acta Cytol, 21:301–302, 1977.
9. Shah SM, Schaefer RF, Araoz E: Cytologic diagnosis of herpetic esophagitis: a case
   report. Acta Cytol, 21:109–111, 1977.
10. Levine MS, Laufer I, Kressel HY, Friedman HM: Herpes esophagitis. AJR, 136:863–
    866, 1981.
11. Fishbein PG, Tuthill R, Kressel HY, et al.: Herpes simplex esophagitis: a cause of
    upper-gastrointestinal bleeding. Dig Dis Sci, 24:540–544, 1979.
12. Springer DJ, DaCosta LA, Beck IT: A syndrome of acute self-limiting ulcerative esopha-
    gitis in young adults probably due to herpes simplex virus. Dig Dis Sci 24:535–539,
    1979.
13. Skucas J, Schrank WW, Meyers PC, Lee CS: Herpes esophagitis: a case studied by
    air-contrast esophagography. Am J Roentgenol 128:497–499, 1977.
14. Pazin GJ: Herpes simplex esophagitis after trigeminal nerve surgery. Gastroenterology
    74:741–743, 1978.

15. Baringer JR, Swoveland P: Recovery of herpes simplex virus from human trigeminal ganglions. N Engl J Med 288:648–650, 1973.
16. Baringer JR: Recovery of herpes simplex virus from human sacral ganglions. N Engl J Med, 291:828–830, 1974.
17. Warren KG, Brown SM, Wroblewska Z, et al.: Isolation of latent herpes simplex virus from the superior cervical and vagus ganglions of human beings. N Engl J Med 298:1068–1070, 1978.
18. Whitley RJ, Nahmias AJ, Soong S-J, et al.: Vidarabine therapy of neonatal herpes simplex virus infection. Pediatrics 66:495–501, 1980.
19. Pavan-Langston D, Dohlman C: A double-blind clinical study of adenine arabinoside therapy of viral keratoconjunctivitis. Am J Opthalmol 74:81–88, 1972.
20. Whitley RJ, Soong S-J, Hirsch MSW, et al.: Herpes simplex encephalitis: vidarabine therapy and diagnostic problems. N Engl J Med, 304:313–318, 1981.
21. Mitchell CD, Gentry SR, Boen JR, et al.: Acyclovir therapy for mucocutaneous herpes simplex infections in immunocompromised patients. Lancet 1:1389–1392, 1981.
22. Jensen KB, Stenderup A, Thomsen JB, Bichel J: Oesophageal moniliasis in malignant neoplastic disease. Acta Med Scand 175:455–459, 1964.
23. Prolla JC, Kirsner JB: The gastrointestinal lesions and complications of leukemias. Ann Intern Med 61:1084–1103, 1964.
24. Eras P, Goldstein MJ, Sherlortz P: Candida infection of the gastrointestinal tract. Medicine 51:367–379, 1972.
25. Gorbach SL, Nahas L, Lerner PI: Studies of intestinal microflora I. Gastroenterology 53:845–855, 1967.
26. Gorbach SL, Plant AG, Nahas L, et al.: Studies of intestinal microflora II. Gastroenterology 53:856–864, 1967.
27. Holt JM: Candida infection of the esophagus. Gut 9:227–231, 1968.
28. Jones JM: Necrotizing candida esophagitis. JAMA 244:2190–2191, 1980.
29. Jones JM: The recognition and management of candida esophagitis. Hosp Pract. 64a–64v, 1981.
30. Kodsi BE, Wickremesinghe PC, Kozinn PJ, et al.: Candida esophagitis. Gastroenterology 71:715–719, 1976.
31. Andren L, Theander G: Roentgenographic appearances of esophageal moniliasis. Acta Radiol 46:571–574, 1956.
32. Medoff G, Dismukas WE, Meade, RH III, Moses JM: A new therapeutic approach to candida infections. Arch Intern Med 130:241–245, 1972.
33. Jordan WM, Bodey GP, Rodriquez V, et al.: Miconazole therapy for treatment of fungal infections in cancer patients. Antimicrob Agents Chemother 16:792–797, 1979.

14 | New Concepts in Esophageal Surgery

David B. Skinner
Alex G. Little

INTRODUCTION

Like all thoracic surgery, operations on the esophagus are relatively new. Advances in anesthesiology allowing control of ventilation with an open thorax, developments and refinements in surgical techniques and materials, blood banks, and the availability of antibiotics all combine to make esophageal surgery practical. As normal esophageal function and the pathophysiology of esophageal disorders become understood, surgery of the esophagus evolves. In this chapter, we discuss new ideas in esophageal surgery with special attention to the rationales and timing for surgery, patient selection for operation, surgical techniques, and the results that can be expected following surgery. No attempt at a comprehensive review is intended, but subjects are selected for which new concepts in diagnosis, pathophysiology, or treatment are changing the surgical approach or generating controversy.

BENIGN CONDITIONS

In this section we discuss three categories of disease: (1) gastroesophageal reflux, including the related problem of Barrett's esophagus, (2) motor disorders of the esophagus, and (3) portal hypertension with esophageal varices.

Gastroesophageal Reflux

It is now almost a cliché to state that attention has shifted from an anatomic fixation on hiatal hernia to a concern for the physiologic function of the cardia as an effective barrier to gastroesophageal reflux.[1] Whereas Type II or paraesophageal hernias require surgery because of the risk of incarceration and strangulation, Type I or sliding hiatal hernias are of no concern unless associated with abnormal gastroesophageal reflux. At present, the most frequent candidates for surgery to control reflux are those with ulcerative esophagitis documented by esophagoscopy. Without operation, such patients may have progression to stricture formation.[2] A smaller group of patients present with more severe complications of esophagitis such as bleeding, perforation, or stricture formation. Finally, patients with reflux but no ulcerative esophagitis may require surgical intervention if symptoms cannot be controlled by an adequate medical regimen or if they have recurrent pulmonary aspiration documented to be caused by reflux.

It is crucial to establish an accurate and objective diagnosis of gastroesophageal reflux in all these patients. Patients with the classical reflux symptoms of heartburn and regurgitation and findings of esophagitis on endoscopy are a straightforward group. More difficult are patients with typical symptoms but no esophagitis or those with atypical symptoms such as dyspepsia, gas, chest pain, cough, or hoarseness. In these patients, a careful search must be carried out for other causes of the symptoms such as cholelithiasis or coronary artery disease. Esophageal function tests may be essential to provide some objective measure of gastroesophageal reflux in the patients with atypical symptoms or without esophagitis.

Manometry defines the pressure and length characteristics of the distal esophageal segment (DES) and excludes the presence of a motor disorder in the body of the esophagus. The Bernstein acid-perfusion test is useful in demonstrating that the esophageal mucosa is acid sensitive, but does not diagnose endogenous gastroesophageal reflux.[3] Direct pH measurements to detect acid reflux in the distal esophagus, such as the Standard Acid Reflux Test (SART)[4] or 24-hour pH monitoring,[5] may be necessary. The SART is a useful test that measures reflux under stressful laboratory conditions. An acid load is introduced into the stomach, and a pH probe is positioned 5 cm proximal to the DES. The patient is asked to perform 4 respiratory maneuvers in each of 4 positions, thereby providing 16 opportunities for reflux. A patient with three or more reflux episodes is considered to have an incompetent cardia and abnormal reflux. At the University of Chicago we employ 24-hour pH monitoring in the distal esophagus in patients with suspected reflux using the methods originally developed by our colleagues Drs. DeMeester and Johnson.[6] While the pH probe is recording 5 cm proximal to the DES, the patient is permitted to eat and move about. Naturally occurring reflux can be quantitated and bouts of reflux can be correlated with the patient's symptoms. Results obtained in patients are compared to standards from normal controls. This is the most accurate and objective test for gastroesophageal reflux presently available.

The principles of successful antireflux surgery include reestablishment of an adequate infradiaphragmatic or intra-abdominal segment of esophagus to restore the normal sphincteric function. Clinical and experimental data show that creation of a 3–4-cm length of abdominal esophagus provides a competent cardia.[7] This permits intra-abdominal pressure to be applied equally both to the esophagus and to the stomach and prevents resting intragastric pressure from rising higher than distal esophageal pressure, thereby creating an opportunity for reflux to occur. In addition, the mechanical effect of a partial or complete wrap of stomach around the esophagus appears to play some role in the surgical creation of competency. The wrap serves to restrict the diameter of the esophageal swallowing tube as it enters the dilated gastric pouch, so that pressure and tension relationships, as described by the Law of LaPlace, act to discourage reflux.[8]

There are three operations that adhere to these principles. These are the Nissen fundoplication, the Belsey Mark IV procedures, and the posterior gastropexy of Hill. There are technical differences among these procedures such that the Nissen procedure creates a 360-degree wrap of fundus about the distal esophagus, the Belsey procedure a 270-degree wrap, and the Hill procedure a 180-degree wrap. The Hill procedure is done only through the abdomen and the Belsey procedure only through the chest, while the Nissen procedure may be done via either approach. We prefer the abdominal approach for nonobese patients without severe esophagitis who are undergoing their first operation for gastroesophageal reflux. This approach is used for patients with other concomitant intra-abdominal pathology that requires surgical treatment. The thoracic approach is preferred for obese patients, those with marked esophagitis, those who have undergone previous antireflux surgery, and for patients with other thoracic disorders requiring surgical treatment.

Good results are reported for each of these procedures. The most extensive long-term follow-up is reported for the Belsey Mark IV procedure, in which there is approximately a 15% recurrence rate after 10 years.[9] The single prospective randomized study reported to date shows that all three procedures significantly increase the distal esophageal pressures compared to preoperative levels with the Nissen procedure increasing pressure somewhat more than the other two.[10] In this study, the Nissen procedure more consistently curtails reflux in the early postoperative period. More comparative and long-term studies need to be carried out before a definitive recommendation can be made as to the most effective antireflux technique. The surgeon's choice of operation today is usually based on previous experience, level of expertise with the various procedures, and type of approach utilized, thoracic or abdominal.

Barrett's Esophagus. Barrett's original description of this disorder is of a patient having an ulcer in the midesophagus with columnar epithelium in the esophagus below this level.[11] As it is presently used, the term Barrett's esophagus is simply an esophagus lined in some part with columnar epithelium. Although there is still controversy, it appears that this epithelium develops as a result of destruction of esophageal squamous epithelium by refluxed gastric contents with subsequent upward migration of columnar epithelium from the cardia.[12] An important observation is that a Barrett's esophagus may be a premalignant condition.[13] Specifically, there is an increased incidence of atypia, dysplasia, and adenocarcinoma in this epithelium. In our series these adenocarcinomas are more aggressive than the typical squamous-cell cancers of the body of the esophagus, and show a tendency toward early extension and metastasis and, therefore, a poor prognosis. Physicians caring for patients with a Barrett's esophagus must be alert for neoplasia development. Multiple biopsies from the entire length of the columnar epithelium should be obtained, either through the esophagoscope or using a suction cup device. For long-term monitoring, either before or after surgery, the most practical form may be cytologic examination of brush specimens. Brushings performed on an outpatient basis are well tolerated by the patient, and are quite safe. This procedure is discussed in more detail in the section on malignant conditions.

The type of surgery performed in these patients varies. Patients with *in-situ* or invasive carcinoma require esophageal resection for palliation or possible cure. These adenocarcinomas are quite radio-resistant and an effective chemotherapeutic regimen is not yet validated. Patients presenting with esophagitis at the squamo–columnar junction or with symptoms of gastroesophageal reflux, in whom malignant changes can be excluded, should be treated by antireflux procedure. Reversion of the columnar epithelium to a normal squamous epithelium rarely, if ever, occurs after successful antireflux surgery. All patients with persisting columnar epithelium should undergo long-term follow-up as their propensity to develop esophageal cancer probably continues.

Motor Disorders of the Esophagus

Achalasia.   Patients with achalasia have dysphagia, which can be due to three factors: absence of peristalsis in the body of the esophagus, esophageal spasm (vigorous achalasia), or failure of the distal esophageal segment to relax with swallowing. It is said that these patients have a hypertensive distal esophageal sphincter contributing to the dysphagia, but this is not our experience. The distal segment simply does not relax with swallowing. The initial treatment for these patients is aimed at the distal esophagus and consists of either hydrostatic or pneumatic balloon dilatation or surgical myotomy. Up to a third of patients will be effectively palliated with a single pneumatic dilatation and another third can be handled with subsequent dilatations.[14] Patients who fail to respond adequately to dilatation require operation. Since the rate of esophageal rupture from balloon dilatation is approximately 5 percent and the permanent success rate is low, many physicians and patients opt for surgery as the initial treatment.[14,15]

The goal of surgery is to relieve dysphagia without creating new problems for the patient. Surgery cannot restore normal physiologic function to the esophagus or its distal sphincter. The present concepts evolve from the classic operation devised by Heller. The aim is both to relieve the obstruction from the nonrelaxing distal sphincter and to reduce obstruction from spasm of the esophageal body. To these ends, the patient is best served by a long myotomy that includes the entirety of the distal esophageal segment and extends as far proximally as is necessary. The proximal extension should include all the abnormal spastic esophagus demonstrated by manometry. In vigorous achalasia this frequently means extending the myotomy beneath the aortic arch. Controversy exists regarding the extent of the distal myotomy. Our practice is to include the entire distal sphincter with certainty in order to ensure complete relief of obstruction. To this end, we fully dissect the hiatus and carry the myotomy for a centimeter onto the stomach. It is then necessary to perform an antireflux procedure to avoid iatrogenically induced incompetency of the cardia. This is achieved by a modified Belsey Mark IV procedure. This technique prevents development of pathologic reflux, but does not create a significant barrier to swallowing or cause dysphagia.

Ellis takes a different approach to the extent of the distal esophagomyotomy. He advocates a longitudinal myotomy approximately 6–7 cm in length extending to the stomach performed without dissection of the hiatus. An antireflux procedure is not carried out. In his most recent follow-up report, Ellis finds a postoperative occurrence of gastroesophageal reflux in 3 percent of patients based on clinical criteria. In 8 percent of patients there is either no improvement or actual worsening of the patient's symptoms and in another 8 percent there is some improvement but continued difficulty with either dysphagia or regurgitation or both.[16]

In an earlier follow-up study, Belsey reports the necessity of reoperation for reflux esophagitis, stricture, or persistent obstruction in 17 percent of patients treated by Heller myotomy alone without dissection of the hiatus and extension of the myotomy onto the stomach. In conjunction with performance of an antireflux repair, he reports that none of 80 patients required reoperation.[17] Using this approach in our own series of 35 consecutive patients undergoing a first operation for achalasia, only one has required further dilatation and none have needed further operation for dysphagia or reflux esophagitis, confirming Belsey's experience. On the other hand, we have reoperated on 11 patients initially treated elsewhere by the less extensive myotomy without antireflux repair and who subsequently had unrelieved muscle obstruction (five patients) or developed a reflux stricture (six patients).

Cricopharyngeal Dysfunction.   It is becoming apparent that a Zenker's diverticulum is produced by dysfunction or discoordination of the pharyngeal and cricopharyngeal muscular mechanisms.[18] Careful manometric evaluation documents failure of the cricopharyngeus to relax in synchrony with pharyngeal contraction in many of these patients with the resultant production of a outpouching of mucosa between these two muscle groups. Follow-up studies show that the traditional surgical approach of simple diverticulectomy is associated with two complications. First, there is an incidence of suture-line leakage following this procedure, undoubtedly due to the presence of a functional distal obstruction, i.e., a nonrelaxing cricopharyngeus muscle. Second, there is a high postoperative recurrence rate in the ensuing months and years following simple excision of the diverticulum. With better understanding of the pathophysiology, the surgical approach is now different.

The cricopharyngeal muscle must be incised for its complete length so that pharyngeal contractions do not meet with resistance, and the swallowed bolus may proceed without obstruction. Cricopharyngeal myotomy is generally done through a left neck incision as the diverticulum itself tends to present somewhat to the left of the midline. Under direct vision, a myotomy is performed extending from the lower border of the inferior constrictor muscle down to the level of the clavicles, a length of approximately 5 cm. The muscle is dissected circumferentially for a short distance to allow the mucosa to pout out. Rather than resect the diverticulum with the attendant risk of suture-line leakage and development of infection, the diverticulum is suspended upside-down from the prevertebral fascia with a few stitches. This allows the sac to drain by gravity into the esophagus so that stasis does not occur.

With cricopharyngeal myotomy plus diverticulopexy, the postoperative course is routinely quite smooth with a low chance of sepsis. The patient is able to take liquids by mouth on the first postoperative day. When a careful myotomy is performed with complete division of all fibers of the cricopharyngeus and the mucosa is freed from the muscle for a short distance circumferentially to ensure that healing cannot occur between the two cut ends of muscle, our follow-up of 20 patients from 1 to 12 years shows no recurrence of the Zenker's diverticulum. Another advantage of this approach is that it can be performed utilizing a local anesthetic when necessary. Without need for a resection and closure of a suture line, the operation may be performed expeditiously and with minimal patient discomfort. This is a distinct advantage in the occasional patient who is thought to be a high risk for general anesthesia, and also obviates the risk of aspiration of pouch contents during induction of anesthesia.

Esophageal Varices

Patients with bleeding esophageal varices resulting from cirrhosis and portal hypertension are a desperate group. Except for the occasional patient with good liver function, both medical and surgical treatments yield poor results. Results from the standard end-to-side and side-to-side portacaval shunts, "H-graft" type mesocaval shunts, and standard splenorenal shunts do not show conclusively that life is prolonged in these patients. The shunts have a high operative mortality rate, and the survivors continue to have a high incidence of postoperative encephalopathy. Although the distal (Warren) splenorenal shunt is proposed to minimize the late development of encephalopathy this is not a particularly easy operation to perform, and long-term results remain equivocal. At the present time, we at the University of Chicago are evaluating alternative surgical methods to treat this problem: devascularization of the cardia and stomach for long-term control of bleeding and use of sclerotherapy for acute treatment of hemorrhage.

Sclerotherapy is a relatively old concept, dating back at least to the 1930's. Recent experiences in Europe and South Africa are encouraging, and call for reevaluation of this method. The technique we employ is advocated by Bengmark, Joelsson, and colleagues: injecting submucosally about the varices with sodium morrhuate, a known sclerosant.[19] The submucosal injection serves to compress and tamponade the varices acutely and to generate acute inflammation with subsequent development of fibrosis in the submucosa, hopefully leading to long-term protection against variceal bleeding. We use sclerotherapy in two groups of patients: (1) actively bleeding patients who fail to respond to standard medical interventions such as vasopressin infusion and are not considered candidates for urgent shunting, and (2) patients no longer actively bleeding who are considered a prohibitive risk for major surgery for a variety of medical reasons. In these latter patients the repeated sclerotherapy is proposed as definitive treatment. Initial control of acute bleeding by sclerotherapy is gratifying, but long-term observation is necessary to decide whether it provides useful results in permanent control of bleeding.[20]

The concept of devascularization of the cardia for treatment of variceal bleeding is not new. Various procedures are described which have the goal of preventing portal venous flow from reaching the cardia and distal esophagus. This objective is attractive as it permits continued portal perfusion of the liver to minimize the risk of future development of hepatic insufficiency and encephalopathy. However, most of these procedures have limited success because of recurrent bleeding due to incomplete devascularization or complications related to leakage from an esophageal suture line. Direct observations of the bleeding site show that variceal rupture almost always occurs in the distal esophagus within a centimeter or two of the gastroesophageal junction. Three factors explain this. The insertion of the phrenoesophageal membrane into the distal esophageal submucosa at the cardia places the venous channels immediately under the mucosa at this level. The abrupt step-off in luminal pressure due to the abodmino–thoracic differential favors variceal distention at this point; finally, this is the location where reflux esophagitis is most apt to erode the mucosa.

Based upon these pathophysiological observations and prior experiences with various attempts to interrupt varices, a full devascularization operation first developed in 1965 is used in selected patients who are not candidates for a shunt.[21] The operation is performed through a left thoracotomy and the diaphragm is detached peripherally to provide exposure to the upper abdomen. The distal esophagus and the entire gastric blood supply (including right and left gastric, right and left gastroepiploic and splenic arteries) is divided and a splenectomy is performed. The gastroesophageal junction is completely separated from the hiatus but the vagus nerves are saved. A short transverse incision is made in the gastric fundus and varices at the cardia and distal esophagus are oversewn with full thickness permanent sutures to create a submucosal barrier to intramural blood flow through the cardia. The final step of the operation involves construction of a fundoplication about the distal esophagus and narrowing of the hiatus. This operation obliterates the varices in the critical distal esophageal zone, raises intra-abdominal pressure in the distal esophagus, and prevents reflux. As complete a devascularization as possible is accomplished consistent with gastric and esophageal survival. The gastric suture line heals more reliably than does an esophageal suture line. Based upon effective long-term control of bleeding without encephalopathy in the first six patients followed through 5 years, and comparable results being reported by other surgeons, use of this operation is being extended. A similar extensive devascularization developed independently by Sugiuro, but including an esophageal anastomosis, is being evaluated by others as well.[22] At present, patients considered to be acceptable surgical candidates for either devascularization or porta–caval shunt operations are being treated alternatively by these procedures. Results of this study should help to clarify the value of these procedures both in the control of bleeding, avoidance of encephalopathy, and long-term survival.

MALIGNANT CONDITIONS

Surgery for carcinoma of the esophagus is traditionally considered a palliative rather than curative form of therapy. Surgical palliation can be achieved by limited resection with esophagogastrostomy or by colon or stomach bypass, without resection of the primary tumor. The goal of palliative surgery is to restore the ability to swallow so that the patient does not drown in his own secretions and is able to eat and drink relatively normally until the cancer causes death. Although reasonable paliation is achieved by these measures, the patient is doomed with an average survival measured in months. At the University of Chicago a more aggressive approach to esophageal neoplasms is taken with hopes of both improving patient survival and extending the duration of palliation.

The factor limiting curability of esophageal carcinoma is the extent of spread at the time symptoms develop. At initial presentation, many patients are found to have direct invasion of other mediastinal structures as well as lymphatic extension and distant metastases. The reason for this is probably related to the distensibility of the esophagus, which allows the patient to continue swallowing and remain asymptomatic until the tumor becomes nearly circumferential. As shown in China and Japan, early detection of esophageal carcinomas, before widespread extension and distant metastases occur, significantly improves chances for cure.[23] An early detection program in high-risk patients, using esophageal brushing with cytologic examination of obtained material, as developed by Dowlatshahi et al; shows promise that esophageal cancer can be diagnosed in a presymptomatic stage with an increase in both the resectability rate and long-term survival.[24] We utilize this technique in selected patients considered to be at high risk including those with documented Barrett's esophagus, long-standing reflux, achalasia, and patients with a history of lye ingestion. The technique is simple and easily performed in an office setting. The esophagus is intubated transnasally with a small tube containing a brush that is passed up and down the esophagus several times and then removed. A slide is prepared and examined in the cytology laboratory for atypia, dysplasia, or definite neoplasia. Although mass screening using this technique may not be cost effective in this country, its use in high-risk patients may play an important role in their long-term follow-up.

Most patients with esophageal carcinoma have some degree of malnourishment, and many are frankly cachetic. This state of protein–calorie deprivation is detrimental in two fashions: poor wound healing and increased risk of anastomotic failure, and suppression of the cellular immune system. The latter can be documented to be impaired by cutaneous anergy, as shown by a negative DNCB skin test, depressed absolute lymphocyte counts and T-lymphocyte numbers and depressed mitogenic responsee to phytohemagglutinin. A compromised cellular immune response is correlated with poor clinical outcome in many groups of cancer patients. Nutritional repletion and reversal of negative nitrogen balances both reverses the *in vitro* evidence of immunoparesis and restores the protein reserve and wound healing capacity of the patient.[25] Correction of these two factors improves patient prognosis. For that reason, many groups emphasize nutritional support during preoperative preparation of patients with esophageal cancer. Patients with protein–calorie malnutrition are immediately begun on total parenteral nutrition at time of admission. This is continued through the time of operation and into the postoperative period until the patient is consuming an adequate diet. Alternatively, at operation a small catheter jejunostomy is placed and utilized postoperatively for nutritional support until the patient is able to sustain himself with adequate oral intake.

The usual surgical approach to carcinoma of the esophagus in this country, as mentioned, is oriented toward palliation. In patients without evidence of distant metastasis or medical contraindications, we use a more aggressive approach in hopes of achieving cure in some patients. This is based on the well-established surgical principles for radical cancer operations: wide resection of the tumor-bearing organ with sufficient margins to ensure complete removal of the primary tumor and resection in continuity of the primary lymphatic drainage basins. For carcinoma of the esophagus, this means 10-cm margins on both sides of the lesion must be obtained because of the extensive submucosal spread which frequently occurs. The entire posterior mediastinum is dissected and removed to insure complete extirpation of adjacent lymphatic networks. For tumors of the cardia or distal third of the esophagus, splenectomy, omentectomy, and removal of all left gastric and celiac nodes is practiced. Results of this radical esophagectomy or posterior mediastinectomy procedure are being assessed in 80 patients treated to date. Among the first 45 operated more than 3 years ago, 30-day hospital mortality is 7 percent and absolute 3-year survival is 22 percent. The operation is used in approximately 45 percent of all patients referred with esophageal cancer. For those not suitable for radical resection because of extent of tumor or medical contraindications, a palliative resection is done when possible (9 percent of cases). In others, radiation therapy or palliative bypass is employed to reduce dysphagia.

Patients with carcinoma of the mid-third of the esophagus are at risk for development of tracheo- or broncho-esophageal fistulae. Some patients have this complication at the time of initial presentation, but a fistula more commonly follows a course of radiotherapy. The tumor bridging the distal trachea or either mainstem bronchus and the esophagus undergoes necrosis leaving a fistulous communication. The patient immediately begins to soil the tracheo–bronchial tree with salvia, swallowed materials, and retained esophageal contents. Each swallow leads to paroxysmal coughing so that sleep is only possible for moments at a time. Inevitably, the patient develops a necrotizing broncho-pneumonia and succumbs to this complication. Not uncommonly, these patients have no evidence of widespread or distant disease at autopsy and might be able to survive for a year or more with radiation therapy if the fistula is controlled. For this reason, we attempt to achieve surgical palliation of the fistula in patients without extensive or distant disease. This requires an urgent operation to isolate the fistula by dividing the cardia and the cervical esophagus. If pneumonia is not severe, a substernal bypass of the involved area utilizing either the left colon or stomach is done at the same time. An anastomosis is performed in the neck between the upper esophagus and either stomach or colon. The excluded body of the esophagus is initially drained through a catheter passed out through a neck stab wound. When this catheter is removed, the esophagus decompresses itself through the fistula. If the pneumonia is severe, only a cervical esophagostomy and gastrostomy are done after the esophagus is divided above and below the fistula. A later bypass can be done or oral alimentation restored by an extracorporeal esophageal replacement tube. In the 14 patients treated for fistula to date, this approach is well tolerated as documented by an operative mortality rate of 14 percent. The ability to eat and drink is restored and patients are able to resume home life during and after radiation therapy for periods up to 20 months before succumbing to the inevitable spread of their disease.

REFERENCES

1. Skinner DB, DeMeester TR: Gastroesophageal reflux. In Current Problems in Surgery, Vol. XIII, No. 1, January, 1976.
2. Little AG, DeMeester TR, Kirchner PT, O'Sullivan GC, and Skinner DB: Pathogenesis of esophagitis in patients with gastroesophageal reflux. Surgery 88:101–107, 1980.
3. Bernstein LM, Baker LA: A clinical test for esophagitis. Gastroenterology 34:760–766, 1958.
4. Skinner DB, Booth DJ: Assessment of distal esophageal function in patients with hiatal hernia and/or gastroesophageal reflux. Ann Surg 172:627–637, 1970.
5. Johnson LF and DeMeester TR: Twenty-four-hour distal esophageal pH monitoring and gastroesophageal reflux. Gastroenterology 66:717–725, 1974.
6. DeMeester TR, Wang CI, Wernly JA, Pellegrini CA, Little AG Klementschitsch P, Bermudez G, Johnson LF and Skinner DB: Technique, indications, and clinical use of 24 hour esophageal pH monitoring. J Thorac Cardiovasc Surg 79:656–670, 1980.
7. DeMeester TR, Wernly JA, Bryant GH, Little AG, and Skinner DB: Clinical and in vitro analysis of determinants of gastroesophageal competence. a study of the principles of anti-reflux surgery. Am J Surg 137:39–46, 1979.
8. Pettersson GB, Bombeck CT, Nyhus LM: The lower esophageal sphincter: mechanisms of opening and closure. Surgery 88:307–14, 1980.
9. Orringer MB, Skinner DB, and Belsey RH: Long-term results of the Mark IV operation for hiatal hernia any analysis of recurrences and their treatment. J Thorac Cardiovasc Surg 63:25–33, 1972.
10. DeMeester TR, Johnson LF, Kent AH: Evaluation of current operations for the prevention of gastroesophaageal reflux. Ann Surg 180:511–525, 1974.
11. Barrett NR: Chronic peptic ulcer of the esophagus and "oesophagitis." Brit J. Surg 38:175–182, 1950.
12. Mossberg SM: The columnar-lined esophagus (Barrett Syndrome)—an acquired condition. Gastroenterology 50:671–676, 1966.
13. Naef AP, Savary M, Ozzello L: Columnar-lined lower esophagus: an acquired lesion with malignant predisposition. J Thorac Cardiovasc Surg 70:826–835, 1975.
14. Sanderson DR, Ellis FH, Olsen AM: Achalasia of the esophagus: results of therapy by dilatation. Chest 58:116–121, 1970.
15. Okike N, Payne WS, Neufeld DM, Bernatz PE, Pairolero PC, Sanderson DR: Esophagomyotomy versus forceful dilatation for achalasia of the esophagus: results in 899 patients. Ann Thorac Surg 28:119–125, 1978.
16. Ellis FH, Gibb SP, Lazier RE: Esophagomyotomy for achalasia of the esophagus. Ann Surg 192:157–161, 1980.
17. Belsey R.: Functional disease of the esophagus. J Thorac Cardiovasc Surg 52:164–175, 1966.
18. Palmer ED: Disorders of the cricopharyngeus muscle: a review. Prog Gastroenterol 71:510–519, 1976.
19. Bengmark S, Borjesson B, Hoerek J, Joelsson B, Lunderquist A., Owman, T.: Obliteration of esophageal varices by PTP. Ann Surg 190:549–554, 1979.
20. Palani CK, Abuabara S, Kraft AR, Jonasson O.: Endoscopic sclerotherapy in acute variceal hemorrhage. Am J Surg 141:164–168, 1980.
21. Skinner DB: Transthoracic, transgastric interruption of bleeding esophageal varices. Arch Surg 99:447, 453, 1969.
22. Suguira M, Futagawa S: A new technique for treating esophageal varices J Thorac Cardiovasc Surg 66:677–685, 1973.

23. Co-ordinating group for research on esophageal cancer. Clin Med J 2:113–120, 1976.
24. Dowlatshahi K, Daneshibod A, Mobarhan S: Early detection of cancer of oesophagus along Caspian littoral. Lancet 125–126, January, 1978.
25. Haffejee AA, Angorn IB: Nutritional status and the nonspecific cellular and humoral immune response in esophageal carcinoma. Ann Surg 189:475–479, 1979.

Index

Note that page numbers followed by (f) represent figures and those followed by (t) represent tables.